Gunshot Wounds
Practical Aspects of Firearms, Ballistics, and Forensic Techniques

ELSEVIER SERIES IN
**PRACTICAL ASPECTS OF CRIMINAL
AND FORENSIC INVESTIGATIONS**

VERNON J. GEBERTH, BBA, MPS, FBINA, *Series Editor*

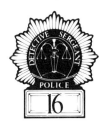

**Practical Homicide Investigation: Tactics, Procedures,
  and Forensic Techniques**
Vernon J. Geberth

**Friction Ridge Skin: Comparison and Identification
  of Fingerprints**
James F. Cowger

**Gunshot Wounds: Practical Aspects of Firearms,
  Ballistics, and Forensic Techniques**
Vincent J.M. Di Maio, M.D.

Gunshot Wounds

Practical Aspects of Firearms, Ballistics, and Forensic Techniques

VINCENT J.M. DI MAIO, M.D.

Chief Medical Examiner
Director, Regional Crime Laboratory, County of Bexar
San Antonio, Texas

Elsevier
New York • Amsterdam • Oxford

Elsevier Science Publishing Co., Inc.
52 Vanderbilt Avenue, New York, New York, 10017

Distributors outside the United States and Canada:
Elsevier Science Publishers B.V.
P.O. Box 211, 1000 AE, Amsterdam, The Netherlands

Library of Congress Cataloging in Publication Data

Di Maio, Vincent J. M.
    Gunshot wounds.

    (Elsevier series in practical aspects of criminal and forensic investigations)

    Includes bibliographies and index.
    1. Gunshot wounds. 2. Forensic ballistics.
    3. Forensic pathology. 4. Firearms. 5. Ballistics.
    I. Title. II. Series.
RA1121.D56 1985   614'.1   84-21128
ISBN 0-444-00928-0

Current printing (last digit)
10 9 8 7 6 5 4 3

Manufactured in the United States of America

To My Parents

Contents

Foreword xi

Acknowledgments xiii

1 An Introduction to Firearms and Ammunition 1

  Small Arms 1

    Handguns 1

    Rifles 9

    Shotguns 9

    Submachine Guns 9

    Machine Guns 10

  Caliber Nomenclature for Rifled Weapons 10

  Ammunition 11

    Cartridge Cases 12

    Head Stamps 13

    Primers 14

    Propellants 17

    Bullets 19

  Flintlock and Percussion Weapons 22

  References 24

2 The Forensic Aspects of Ballistics 25

  Class and Individual Characteristics of Bullets 30

  Comparison of Bullets 31

  Cartridge Cases 33

  Base Markings 34

  Fingerprints 35

  Black Powder Firearms 36

  Discharge of a Weapon 37

  References 40

3 Wound Ballistics   41
Loss of Kinetic Energy   45
References   49

4 An Introduction to the Classification of Gunshot Wounds   51
Contact Wounds   51
Near-Contact Wounds   53
Intermediate-Range Gunshot Wounds   57
  Powder Soot   60
Distant Gunshot Wounds   66
  Entrance Versus Exit Wounds   67
Atypical Entrances   77
Intermediate Targets   80
Pseudo-Powder Tattooing   84
Pseudo-Soot   88
Ricochet Bullets   88
Bone   92
Bullet Wounds of the Skull   94
Caliber Determination from Entrance Wounds   97
Bullet Wipe   97
References   97

5 Wounds from Handguns   99
Contact Wounds   100
  Contact Wounds over Bone   103
Near-Contact Wounds   109
  Hair   110
  Gas Injuries   110
Intermediate-Range Wounds   111
Cylinder Gap   120
Distant Wounds   120
Addendum: Centerfire Handgun Cartridges   121
  .25 Auto   121
  .32 Auto   123
  .32 Smith & Wesson and .32 Smith & Wesson Long   123
  .38 Smith & Wesson   123
  .38 Special   123
  .357 Magnum   124
  .380 Automatic   124
  .38 Colt Super Auto   124
  9-mm Luger   124
  .45 ACP   125
  .44 Smith & Wesson Magnum   125
References   125

6 Wounds from .22 Caliber Rimfire Weapons   127

.22 Short, Long, and Long Rifle Cartridges   129
   .22 Short Cartridge   131
   .22 Long Ammunition   131
   .22 Long Rifle Ammunition   131
CB and BB Caps   134
Frangible Ammunition   134
Wounds due to Rimfire Ammunition   135
   Contact Wounds   135
   Intermediate-Range Wounds   136
   Distant Wounds   137
References   137

7 Wounds from Centerfire Rifles   139

Centerfire Rifle Bullets   143
High-Velocity Rifle Wounds   146
Powder Tattooing   152
X-Rays   155
Perforating Tendency of Centerfire Rifle Bullets   157
Intermediary Targets   157
Addendum: Rifle Calibers   158
   .222 Remington   159
   .223 Remington   159
   .30-30 Winchester   161
   .30-06 Springfield   161
   .270 Winchester   161
   .308 Winchester   161
   .243 Winchester   161
   .30 M-1 Carbine   162
References   162

8 Wounds from Shotguns   163

Shotgun Ammunition   166
Shot   175
Birdshot   175
Buckshot Ammunition   176
Shotgun Slugs   179
Wound Ballistics of the Shotgun   182
Shotgun Wounds   183
   Window Screens as Intermediate Targets   200
Wounds from Buckshot   201
Sawed-Off Shotguns   203
   Shotgun Diverters   203
   Automatic Ejection of Fired Hulls   204
Shotgun Shells Exclusive of Buckshot   204

Remington-Peters   204
Winchester-Western   204
Federal Ammunition   206
Miscellaneous Shotgun Ammunition   207
Brass Shotgun Shells   207
Winchester Tracer Rounds   207
Remington Modi-Pac   207
References   208

9 Gunshot Wounds: Miscellaneous   **209**

Bloody Bodies and Bloody Scenes   209
Physical Activity Following Gunshot Wounds   210
Concealed Wounds   211
Minimal Velocities Necessary to Perforate Skin   213
Bullet Emboli   216
Gunshot Wounds of the Brain   217
Bone Chips   217
Secondary Fractures of the Skull   217
Shape of the Bullet Tracks   218
Point of Lodgment of the Bullet   218
Intrauterine Gunshot Wounds   220
Lead Poisoning from Retained Bullets   221
Location of Fatal Gunshot Wounds   222
Behavior of Ammunition and Gunpowder in Fires   223
Blunt Force Injuries from Firearms   224
References   226

10 Weapons and Ammunition: Miscellaneous   **227**

Air Weapons   227
Zip Guns   231
Stud Guns   233
Sympathetic Discharge of Rimfire Firearms   233
Bullets without Rifling Marks   234
Elongated Bullets   237
Cast Bullets   237
Sabot Ammunition   237
Tandem Bullets   239
New Forms of Handgun Ammunition   240
Hollow-Point Ammunition   240
Glazer Round   241
Exploding Ammunition   241
Multiple Bullet Loadings   242
KTW Ammunition   244
NYCLAD® Revolver Cartridges   244

Handgun Shot Cartridges   245
Plastic Training Ammunition   246
Flechettes   247
Blank Cartridge Injuries   248
Electrical Guns   251
Interchangeability of Ammunition in Weapons   251
Markings and Foreign Material on Bullets   254
Effect of Environmental Temperature on Bullet Velocity   255
References   255

11 **X-Rays**   **257**
References   265

12 **Detection of Gunshot Residues**   **267**
Gunshot Wounds Through Clothing   275
Analytical Examination of Clothing for Range
    Determination   280
Range Determination in Decomposed Bodies   281
References   283

13 **Correct Handling of Deaths from Firearms**   **285**
The Autopsy Report   288

14 **Suicide by Firearms**   **293**
Accidental Deaths from Firearms   302
References   307

Appendix A   Hollow-Point Ammunition:
                   Myths and Facts   **309**
Appendix B   The Forensic Autopsy   **313**
Appendix C   Gunshot Residue Procedures   **319**
Index   **321**

Foreword

Today, in the United States, there are approximately 20,000 persons murdered each year. Clearly, murder is no stranger to society. Guns are the most frequently used weapons and firearms account for almost 50% of the slayings.

Gunshot Wounds: Practical Aspects of Firearms, Ballistics, and Forensic Techniques, written by Vincent J. Di Maio, M.D., is a practical hands-on guide to the subject of gunshot injuries. The experience of the author has given him insight and understanding to create a text for the working practitioner involved in the investigation of gunshot injuries.

I have known Dr. Vincent Di Maio for over ten years and consider him to be one of the nation's foremost authorities in the sphere of gunshot wounds and forensic techniques as they relate to firearm injuries. *Gunshot Wounds: Practical Aspects of Firearms, Ballistics, and Forensic Techniques* is based upon Dr. Di Maio's personal observations, experience, and research of gunshot wounds and firearms. Dr. Di Maio, who is presently the Chief Medical Examiner of San Antonio, was previously associated with Southwestern Institute of Forensic Sciences at Dallas. Both facilities combine the Medical Examiner's Office and the Crime Laboratory under one administrative entity in which the Chief Medical Examiner acts as Director of the Crime Lab.

Dr. Di Maio has been able to view gunshot wounds at the same time as the weapons and ammunition used to inflict them. He has also been able to discuss the weapons and ammunition with firearms examiners at the time of autopsy. This text combines over twelve years of medicolegal investigation with practical experience.

The book begins with an excellent presentation regarding firearms and ammunition and acquaints the reader with some basic knowledge of firearms and the terminology used by ballistics and firearms examiners. The text then describes the practical aspects of ballistics, wound ballistics, and the classification of various wounds pertaining to handguns, rifles, and shotguns. The final chapters deal with autopsy technique and procedure, as well as the very pertinent laboratory analysis relating to weapons and gunshot evidence.

The book is written clearly and concisely; the text is accented by numerous photographs that depict exactly what to look for and how to interpret gunshot evidence.

Collectively, the chapters are a source and definitive guide for professional law enforcement officers, Medical Examiners, forensic pathologists, lawyers, and forensic crime laboratories.

Gunshot Wounds: Practical Aspects of Firearms, Ballistics, and Forensic Techniques is, without a doubt, the most comprehensive text on gunshot wounds available today.

Vernon J. Geberth
Homicide Commander
New York City Police Department

Acknowledgments

I wish to thank the following individuals who aided me in preparation of this book:

Don Calhoun (photographer, Southwestern Institute of Forensic Sciences at Dallas) for taking many of the photographs used in this book;

Patrick Besant-Matthews, M.D., for supplying additional photographs;

Doro Olivan Martinez for typing the final manuscript and Annelotte Weber for typing portions of the original manuscript;

Lars Haga, for the original artwork.

An Introduction to Firearms and Ammunition

1

In order to interpret gunshot wounds, a certain basic knowledge of firearms and ammunition is necessary. This chapter will attempt to convey such information.

Small Arms

There are five general categories of small arms: handguns, rifles, shotguns, submachine guns, and machine guns.

Handguns

There are four basic types of handguns:

Single-shot pistols

Derringers

Revolvers

Auto-loading pistols (automatics)

A single-shot pistol has one firing chamber integral with the barrel, which must be loaded manually each time the weapon is to be fired (Figure 1–1). Derringers are a variant of single-shot pistols. Derringers are small pocket firearms having multiple barrels, each of which is loaded and fired separately. The traditional derringer has two barrels (Figure 1–1).

The revolver is the most common type of handgun in the United States. Revolvers have a revolving cylinder that contains several chambers, each of which holds one cartridge. The cylinder is rotated mechan-

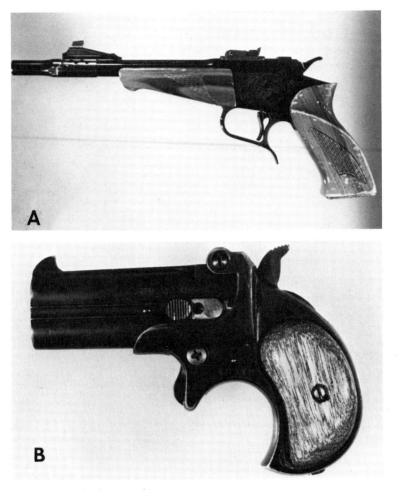

Figure 1–1 A. Single-shot pistol. **B.** Derringer.

ically so as to align each chamber successively with the barrel and firing pin. The first revolver was produced by Samuel Colt in 1835–1836.

There are three types of revolvers, the most common of which is the "swingout" form (Figure 1–2A). On pressing the cylinder latch, which is normally found on the left side of the frame, and pushing the cylinder to the left, the cylinder swings out, exposing the chambers. Each individual chamber is then loaded with a cartridge. The cylinder is swung back into the frame, engaging the cylinder latch. The weapon is now ready to be fired. After discharge of all the cartridges, the release catch is pressed and the cylinder is swung out. An ejector rod, affixed to the front of the cylinder, is pressed to the rear, ejecting the fired cases. The cylinder is ready to be reloaded.

In break-top revolvers, the frame is hinged at the rear such that, on release of a top catch, the barrel and cylinder swing down, exposing the back of the cylinder for loading (Figure 1–2B). The opening action will

Figure 1–2 A. 9-mm revolver, swing-out type, with cylinder swung open exposing chambers. **B.** Break-top revolver with action open.

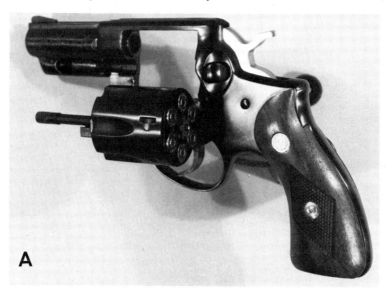

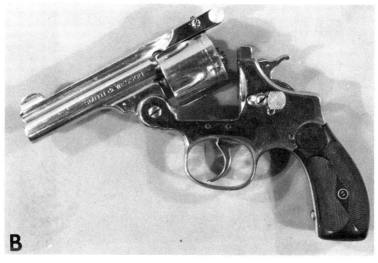

also eject empty cases from the cylinder. This form of weapon is relatively uncommon in the United States, but it has been the traditional form of revolver in Great Britain. In the United States only one firm, Harrington and Richardson, currently manufacture break-top revolvers.

The solid-frame revolver is the oldest form of revolver, dating back to Colt's original weapons (Figure 1–3). In this weapon the cylinder is held in the frame by a central pin, around which it rotates. The back of this cylinder is never exposed completely by either "swinging out" or "breaking open." Each chamber in the cylinder is loaded individually through a loading gate on the right side of the frame. The hammer of the weapon is placed on half cock, and the cylinder is then manually rotated so that a chamber is aligned with the loading gate. A cartridge is inserted. The cylinder is then manually rotated to the next chamber and a second cartridge is inserted. This procedure is continued until the cylinder is completely filled. After the weapon is discharged, the cylinder has to be manually rotated again and aligned with the loading gate, and each cartridge case must be ejected through the gate. This type of construction is most commonly encountered in single-action revolvers and the early model Saturday Night Specials. The latter term, dating back to the turn of the century, refers to a cheap weapon usually of poor construction and does not refer to concealability.

Revolvers may be either single-action or double-action types. In single-action revolvers the hammer must be cocked manually each time the weapon is to be fired. Cocking the hammer revolves the cylinder, aligning the chamber with the barrel and the firing pin. Pressure applied to the trigger then releases the hammer, discharging the weapon. In

Figure 1–3 Solid-frame revolver with loading gate swung open. Arrow points to loading port where individual cartridges are inserted.

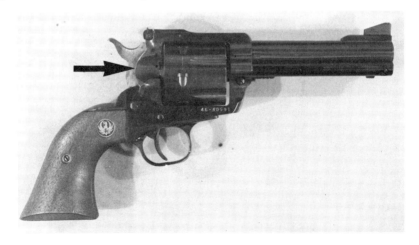

double-action revolvers a continuous pressure on the trigger revolves the cylinder, aligns the chamber with the barrel, and cocks and then releases the hammer, firing the weapon. With rare exceptions, all double-action revolvers may be fired in a single-action mode. The amount of pressure on a trigger necessary to fire a well-made double-action revolver varies from 12 to 15 lb. If these weapons are cocked and fired in single-action mode, less pressure is necessary to fire them. The double-action trigger pull for cheap, poorly made revolvers is usually much greater, while single-action trigger pull may vary from less than a pound to as much as the double-action pull in a well-made revolver.

Most single-action revolvers have a "half-cock" notch in the cocking hammer that lies between the position of "full cock" and "fired." The purpose of the half-cock notch is to catch the hammer if it accidentally slips from the thumb as it is being manually cocked. Many individuals incorrectly consider the half-cock notch a safety position and will carry weapons on "half cock". Dropping a weapon when on half cock may cause the hammer to disengage, fly forward, and discharge the weapon. Some single-action revolvers will fire from the half-cock position if the trigger is pulled. Ruger single-action revolvers equipped with a safety bar do not have a half-cock notch.

The cylinder of a revolver may rotate either clockwise (Colt revolvers) or counterclockwise (Smith & Wesson revolvers). This difference has resulted in a number of deaths among individuals playing Russian roulette. Such an individual loads one chamber of a revolver and spins the cylinder. He or she then "peeks" to locate the cartridge. If it is in any cylinder except the one that will be rotated into firing position on pulling the trigger, the gun is then put to the head and the trigger pulled. If the cartridge is in the lethal chamber, the player makes some excuse to spin the cylinder again. This system of playing Russian roulette is perfectly safe if one knows which way the cylinder rotates. A person used to playing the game with a Colt revolver may try it with a Smith & Wesson revolver in which the cylinder rotates in the other direction and may experience a fatal conclusion to the game.

Auto-loading or automatic pistols make up the fourth category of handguns. The term "automatic pistol" is a misnomer, as this form of pistol is an auto-loader in which the trigger must be pulled for every shot fired. This pistol uses the forces generated by the fired cartridge to operate the mechanism that extracts and ejects the empty cases, loads the fresh cartridge, and returns the mechanism into position to fire the next round (Figure 1–4). The cartridges are stored in a removable magazine in the grip of the pistol. Some earlier automatic pistols—for example, the Mauser Model 1896—had the magazine in front of the trigger guard. The term "clip" is often used synonomously with the term "magazine." In fact, a clip is a device designed to facilitate the loading of

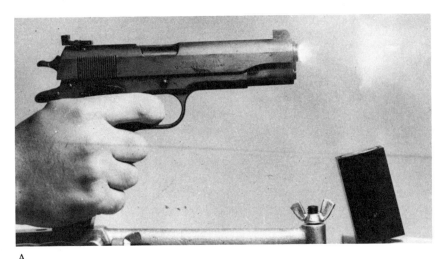

A

B

Figure 1−4 A. The weapon has just been fired. The slide has begun to recoil with the bullet a few inches in front of the muzzle. **B.** The slide has recoiled all the way back and the fired cartridge case is being ejected. The slide will now come forward, chambering a new round and cocking the weapon.

a number of cartridges into a magazine, but most people use the terms interchangeably. The first commerical automatic pistol was produced in 1893 by Borchardt; this weapon was the predecessor of the Luger.

There are five methods of operation of automatic pistols: blow-back, delayed or retarded blow-back, blow forward, recoil, and gas. Only two of these methods are in widespread use now: blow-back and recoil. In blow-back action, the pressure of the gas produced by combustion of the powder forces an unlocked slide to the rear, thus starting the cycle of extraction, ejection, and reloading.

In a recoil-operated automatic pistol, the barrel and the slide are locked together at the moment of firing. As the bullet leaves the barrel, the rearward thrust of the propellant gas on the cartridge case starts the barrel and slide moving to the rear. After a short distance, the barrel is halted, and the locking device is withdrawn from the slide (Figure 1–5). The slide then continues to the rear, ejecting the fired case and starting the reloading cycle.

Virtually all automatic pistols have at least one manually operated safety device (Figure 1–6). Manual safeties are thumb pieces or buttons that are mounted in either the slide or receiver. Putting on the safety locks the firing mechanism (hammer, striker, and sometimes sear) and prevents the weapon from discharging. Less commonly, automatic pistols are equipped with grip safeties (Figure 1–6), movable pieces mounted in the grip which prevent connection between the trigger and the sear except when the pistol is held firmly in the hand, ready for shooting. The grip safety is held out by springs when at rest. Grasping the grip pushes the piece in and permits connection between the trigger and sear and thus firing of the weapon. Many automatic pistols have magazine safeties. This device prevents discharge of the weapon when the magazine has been removed from it.

Walther and Smith & Wesson automatic pistols as well as a number of

Figure 1–5 Locking action of recoil operated locked breech automatic pistol. On firing, the slide (**A**) and barrel (**B**), which are locked together by the ribs (**C**), recoil. After a short distance, the barrel is haltered by a bar (**D**) engaging the barrel lug (**E**). The ribs disengage and the slide continues backward to extract and eject the fired cartridge case. The slide then comes forward to chamber a new round and cock the weapon.

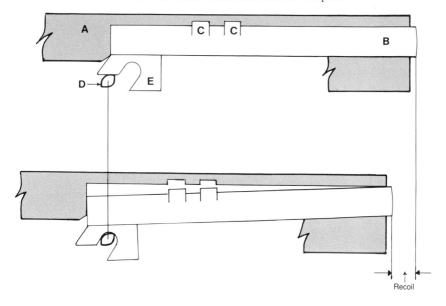

Recoil

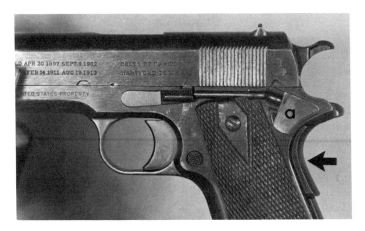

Figure 1-6 Left side of Colt .45 automatic pistol with manual safety (**a**) and grip safety (**arrow**).

other pistols have a thumb piece on the left side of the frame which externally resembles the usual safety lever. When this thumb piece is pushed down, the hammer falls. The weapon will not discharge, however, as the thumb piece locks the firing pin and/or rotates a steel surface between the hammer and the firing pin to prevent contact between the two.

With rare exceptions, currently manufactured revolvers do not have manually operated safety devices. There is an imported single-action revolver with a manually operated metal bar that can be rotated between the firing pin and the cocked hammer. Although thumb safeties are not present on modern revolvers, some revolvers manufactured in the recent past are equipped with grip safeties.

Preparing an automatic pistol to fire involves two steps. First, the loaded magazine is inserted into the grip. The slide is grasped, pulled rearward, and released. A spring drives the slide forward, stripping the cartridge from the magazine and loading it into the firing chamber. The weapon is now cocked and ready to be fired. Most automatic pistols must be fired in a single-action mode for the first shot. Thus, the hammer must be in a cocked position before pressure on the trigger will fire the gun. After the first shot, the operating mechanism of the automatic pistol automatically cocks the hammer. Some auto-loading pistols—for example, the Walther P-38—are equipped with a double-action trigger that will cock and fire the first shot as a result of continuous pressure on the trigger. After this, the weapon automatically cocks itself for each succeeding shot fired. Even in double-action automatic pistols, however, the slide must be pulled back initially to chamber a cartridge.

Rifles

A rifle is a firearm with a rifled barrel which is designed to be fired from the shoulder. Barrel length is immaterial in classifying a firearm as a rifle. However, U.S. federal law requires rifles to have a minimum barrel length of 16 in. The types of rifles commonly encountered are single-shot, lever-action, bolt-action, pump-action, and auto-loading. A single-shot rifle has one firing chamber integral with the barrel which has to be manually loaded each time the weapon is fired. A lever-action rifle has a lever beneath the grip which is used to open the rifle action, to extract the cartridge case, and, in closing the action, to insert a fresh cartridge in the firing chamber and to cock the gun.

In a bolt-action rifle, a handle projects from a bolt. Pulling back and pushing forward on this projection causes the bolt to extract and eject a cartridge case and then to insert a new cartridge while cocking the gun. The slide-action rifle uses the manual movement of a slide under and parallel to the barrel to open the action, extract and eject a cartridge, load a fresh cartridge, and cock the weapon.

In auto-loading or semiautomatic rifles, the weapon fires, extracts, ejects, reloads, and cocks with each pull of the trigger using the force of gas pressure or recoil to operate the action. After each shot the trigger must be released and then pulled again to repeat the cycle. Auto-loading rifles are commonly but incorrectly called "automatic rifles." A true or fully automatic rifle is one that utilizes the force of gas pressure or recoil to eject the fired case, load the next round, fire it, and then eject it. This cycle is repeated until all the ammunition is used or the trigger is released. Automatic weapons are generally used only by military and police organizations.

Shotguns

A shotgun is a weapon that is intended to be fired from the shoulder; it has a smooth bore and is designed to fire multiple pellets from the barrel. Again, barrel length is immaterial in classifying a firearm as a shotgun, although U.S. federal law requires a minimal barrel length of 18 in. A shotgun may be classified as single-shot, over-and-under, double-barrel, bolt-action, lever-action, pump-action, or auto-loading. The over-and-under shotgun has two barrels one above the other, and the double-barrel version has its barrels side by side. The two barrels in these weapons are often of different choke.

Submachine Guns

A submachine gun or machine pistol is a weapon that is designed to be fired from either the shoulder or the hip. It is capable of fully automatic fire, has a rifled barrel, and fires pistol ammunition. It is often incorrectly called a "machine gun."

Machine Guns

A machine gun is a weapon that is capable of fully automatic firing and that fires rifle ammunition. It is generally crew-operated, but some forms may be fired by single individuals. Most machine guns have the ammunition fed by belts, although some use clips.

Caliber Nomenclature for Rifled Weapons

Rifles and handguns have rifled barrels; that is, spiral grooves have been cut the length of the interior or bore of the barrel (Figure 1–7). Rifling consists of these grooves and the metal left between the grooves—the lands.

In the United States the caliber of a rifle or handgun is supposed to be the diameter of the bore, measured from land to land. This measurement represents the diameter of the barrel before the rifling grooves were cut. However, caliber may be given in terms of bullet, land, or groove diameter. Caliber specification using the U.S. system is neither accurate nor consistent. Thus, the .303 Savage fires a 0.308-in.-diameter bullet, while the .303 British cartridge has a 0.312-in.-diameter bullet. Both the .30-06 and the .308 Winchester cartridges are loaded with bullets having a diameter of 0.308 in. The "06" in .30-06 refers to the year of adoption of this cartridge. American cartridges that originally used black powder are designated by caliber, the original black powder charge, and, in some cases, bullet weight. Thus, the .45-70-405 cartridge has a 405-gr bullet, 0.45 in. in diameter and propelled by 70 grains of black powder. The term "grains" refers to the weight of powder, not

Figure 1–7 Cross-section of barrel showing lands and grooves.

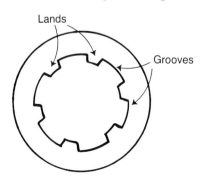

the number of grains or granules of powder. A few of the smokeless powder cartridges that came out in the late nineteenth century also use this method of designation. Thus, the .30-30 cartridge has a 0.308-in.-diameter bullet originally propelled by 30 gr of smokeless powder. However, with the development of newer types of powder, this powder charged is no longer used.

The best example of difficult and confusing caliber designation and the one most significant to the forensic pathologist involves .38 Special and .357 Magnum cartridges. Weapons chambered for these calibers have barrels with the same bore and groove diameters. Bullets loaded in each of these cartridges have identical dimensions. The .357 Magnum chambers and fires all .38 Special ammunition, although a weapon chambered for a .38 Special cartridge cannot ordinarily chamber and should never use the .357 Magnum cartridge.

The .357 Magnum cartridge case is, in fact, the .38 Special cartridge case lengthened and loaded with additional propellant. Except for the difference in the length of the cartridge cases, all other physical dimensions are the same for both calibers.

The European system of cartridge designation, which uses the metric system, is more thorough and logical than the U.S. system. It clearly and specifically identifies a cartridge by giving the bullet diameter and the case length in millimeters, as well as by designating the type of cartridge case. Thus, the Russian rimmed service round becomes the 7.62 × 54 mm R. The 7.62 refers to the diameter of the bullet; 54 mm indicates the length of the cartridge case, and R indicates that the round is rimmed. The letters SR are used for semirimmed cases, RB for rebated cartridge cases, and B for belted cases. No letter is used to describe rimless cartridge cases. Thus, the .30-06 in the metric designation is the 7.62 × 63 mm.

The term "Magnum," when used in connection with rifle or pistol cartridge cases, refers to an extra-powerful load in a given cartridge obtained by using more powder or a different type of powder.

A Wildcat cartridge is a nonstandard cartridge produced by a small company, independent gunsmith or other individual; it is not available from major ammunition manufacturers.

Ammunition

A small arms cartridge consists of a cartridge case, a primer, propellant (gunpowder), and a bullet or projectile (Figure 1−8). Blank cartridges are sealed with paper disks instead of bullets or have a crimped neck. Dummy cartridges have neither a primer nor powder. Some dummy cartridges contain inert granular material that simulates powder.

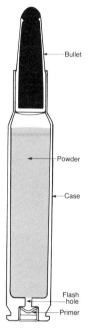

Figure 1–8 Small arms cartridge with bullet, powder, cartridge, case and primer.

Cartridge Cases

Cartridge cases are usually made of brass, a composition of 70% copper and 30% zinc. Less commonly, they are made of steel. Aluminum, zinc, and plastic materials have been used experimentally. Brass, plastic, and paper are used for shotshell tubes.

The main function of the cartridge case is to expand and seal the chamber against rearward escape of gases when the cartridge is fired. When a brass cartridge is fired in a weapon, the gas pressure produced by burning of the propellant expands the case tightly against the walls of the chamber. If the brass is tempered to the correct hardness, it will spring back to approximately its original dimensions and make the case easy to extract. If the brass is too soft, it will not spring back and will make extraction difficult. If the brass is too hard—that is, brittle—it will crack.

There are three general shapes for cartridge cases: straight, bottleneck, and tapered. Almost all pistol cartridges are straight, whereas almost all rifle cartridges are bottlenecked. The bottleneck design permits more powder to be packed in a shorter, fatter cartridge than would be possible in a straight cartridge, where the lumen is approximately the diameter of the bullet. Cartridges with tapered cases are virtually obsolete.

Cartridge cases are classified into five types according to the configuration of their bases (Figure 1−9):

Rimmed

Semirimmed

Rimless

Belted

Rebated

Rimmed cartridge cases have an extractor flange that is larger than the diameter of the cartridge case body. The letter R is added after case length numbers in the metric system of caliber designation.

Semirimmed cartridge cases have an extractor flange that is larger in diameter than the cartridge case body, but they also have a groove around the case body just in front of the flange. The metric designation for these cartridges is SR.

Rimless cartridge cases have an extractor flange whose diameter is the same as that of the cartridge case body and also have a groove around the body of the case in front of the flange. In the metric system of caliber designation, no letter is used for this type of cartridge case.

A rebated cartridge case has an extractor flange that is smaller than the diameter of the case. A groove around the body of the case is present in front of the flange. The metric designation is RB.

A belted cartridge case has a pronounced, raised belt encircling the cartridge case body in front of the groove in the body. The diameter of the extractor flange is immaterial. The metric designation is B.

Head Stamps

Virtually all cartridge cases have head stamps on their bases (Figure 1−10). The head stamp is a series of letters, numbers, symbols, and/or tradenames. They are either imprinted or embossed on a cartridge case head for identification purposes. Civilian cartridges are usually marked

Figure 1−9 Cartridge case head designs. **a.** Belted. **b.** Rebated. **c.** Rimless. **d.** Semirimmed. **e.** Rimmed.

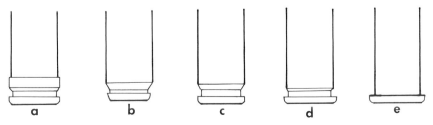

a   b   c   d   e

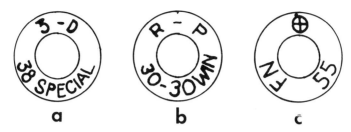

Figure 1-10 Headstamps on centerfire cartridges. **a.** A .38 Special cartridge manufactured by 3D. **b.** A rifle cartridge manufactured by Remington-Peters of caliber .30-30 Winchester. **c.** A rifle cartridge manufactured by Fabrique Nationale in 1955 with a NATO symbol.

with the initials or code of the manufacturer, as well as the caliber. Military cartridges are usually marked with the manufacturer's initials or code plus the last two numerals of the year of manufacture. The caliber may be designated as well. American military Match ammunition has the word "Match" or the letters "NM" (National Match) imprinted on it. 7.62 NATO ammunition carries the NATO symbol which is a cross within a circle (Figure 1-10).

Head stamps are not necessarily reliable indicators of the caliber of the particular cartridge case or the manufacturer because a cartridge case may have been reformed to another caliber. Thus a .308 cartridge case may have been necked down to a .243 cartridge. Commercial concerns that buy large quantities of ammunition, such as Sears, may have the tradename stamped on the cartridge cases rather than the designation of the actual manufacturer.

Ammunition manufactured by Russia and Japan during World War II and some 7.62 × 39 mm ammunition manufactured by the U.S. government during the Vietnam war do not have head stamps. Occasionally, a cartridge case may be seen with a surcharge. These are markings added to the base of the cartridge after the original head stamp has been formed. They are not necessarily applied in the plant that performs the original head stamp operation on the cartridge case, and they may indicate that the cartridge has been reloaded.

Primers

Small-arms cartridges are classified as centerfire or rimfire, depending on the location of the primer. In centerfire cartridges, the primer is located in the center of the base of the cartridge case. There are two types of primers: Boxer and Berdan. American centerfire cartridges have Boxer primers. A Boxer primer consists of a brass or gilding-metal cup, a pellet containing a sensitive explosive, a paper disk and a brass anvil (Figure

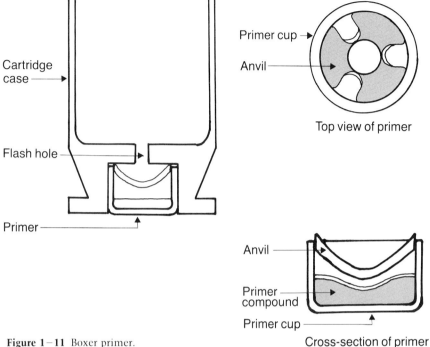

Figure 1–13 Cross-section of base of .22 rimfire cartridge with primer composition in rim of case (**arrow**).

Cartridge case

Primer cup →

Anvil

Top view of primer

Flash hole

Primer

Anvil

Primer compound

Primer cup

Cross-section of primer

Figure 1–11 Boxer primer.

detonation. The primer mixture
factured by Winchester and C
barium. Federal ammunition u
antimony. Remington rimfire am
lead.

Propellants

Until the end of the nineteenth c
black powder. Black powder is a
sium nitrate. These materials w
mechanically mixed, ground tog
moisture and pressed into hard ca
the desired granulation. In such a
the potassium nitrate is the oxyge
the mixture more density and w
ignitable. When black powder bu
its original weight in gases and
residues appear principally as a c

In 1884, Vieille, a French che
practical form of what is now k
alcohol and ether, he reduced n
which was rolled into sheets and
developed a slightly different form
cellulose that was not as highly

1–11). These component parts are assembled to form a complete
primer. The Boxer primer has a single large flash hole in the bottom of
the case.

European cartridges traditionally are loaded with Berdan primers. The
Berdan primer differs from the American Boxer primer in that it has no
integral anvil. Instead, the anvil is built into the cartridge case and forms
a projection in the primer pocket (Figure 1–12). Berdan primers have
two flash holes in the primer pocket.

Primers made for rifles and pistols differ in construction in that the
cups of pistol primers are made with thinner metal. The rifle primer also
has a mixture that burns with a more intense and sustained flame.

Primers come in four sizes—large rifle, small rifle, large pistol and
small pistol. The large primers measure .210 in. diameter, whereas
the small measure 0.175 in. in diameter. Magnum primers (either rifle or
pistol) produce a more intense and sustained flame, which is necessary
for better ignition in Magnum cartridges.

When a weapon is fired, the firing pin strikes the center of the primer
cup, compressing the primer composition between the cup and anvil

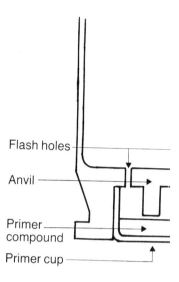

Flash holes

Anvil

Primer
compound

Primer cup

and causing the composition
flame to pass through the fl.
to ignite the propellant.

Primer compounds origina
firing, however, free mercur
brass of the cartridge case, m
In addition, storage of ammu
periods of time led to deterio
Mercury compounds were
Unfortunately, on firing the
severe rusting of the barrels.

All U.S.-made primers curi
ents that are nonmercuric ai
used vary: Lead styphnate,
commonly used; U.S. center
tain all three compounds. T
tutes the basis for tests to de
firearm. A German concern i
ther lead nor barium in thei

Rimfire ammunition—for
primer assembly. Instead, the
of the cartridge case with the
composition (Figure 1–13). O
cartridge case, compressing t

colloided it with nitroglycerine and then dried, rolled, and cut it into
flakes. These two types of smokeless powder are known as single-base
and double-base, respectively. The physical configuration of individual
powder grains can be disk, flake, or cylinder, whether the powder is
single- or double-base.

The next major step in the development of smokeless powder was the
introduction of ball powder by Winchester in 1933.[2] In ball powder, the
nitrocellulose instead of being colloided is dissolved completely and the
resultant lacquer is agitated under conditions to make it form into small
balls that constitute the powder grains. By manipulation of the process,
the diameter of the balls of powder can be controlled, whereas in an
extra operation the balls of powder may be flattened between rollers,
thus altering the surface area and thus the burning rate of the powder.
True or classical ball powder consists of small, uniform silver-black
spheres or ovals having a shiny, reflective surface. Grains of flattened
ball powder appear as irregular, flattened chips with a silver-black shiny
surface. In most flattened ball powder one can find nonflattened spheres
and ovoid grains. Between the extremes of classical ball and flattened
ball powders is a wide spectrum of variations.

Smokeless powder theoretically is converted completely into gaseous
products. Unlike black powder, it does not leave a significant residue in
the bore. Smokeless powders burn at the surface only. Thus, the burning
surface decreases continuously as the grains are consumed. This degres-
sive burning, an unfavorable characteristic, can be overcome to a degree
by putting a hole in the individual powder grain, with a resultant
increase in the surface area as the grain burns. More commonly, chemical coating deterrents are applied to powder grains to slow the burning
initially in order to make progressive burning powder. These grains of
powder burn slowly at first and then burn rapidly. The grains of powder
may also be coated with graphite to eliminate static electricity and
facilitate the flow of powder while the cartridges are loaded. Rather than
having a shiny silver-black appearance, uncoated grains of ball powder
are a pale green color. Ball powder grains recovered from the skin may be
green secondary to having their coats burned away.

The weight of the propellant charge in a cartridge is adjusted for each
lot of propellant to give the required muzzle velocity for the weight of
the bullet with a chamber pressure within the limits prescribed for the
weapon.

Pyrodex®, a "synthetic" black powder, was developed to replace black
powder in weapons in which only black powder can be used. It was
developed for two reasons: First, there is a shortage of black powder;
second, in the United States there are a number of restrictions put on the
sale and storage of black powder because of its explosive properties.
As Pyrodex® is a nitrocellulose-based powder, it is considerably safer than

black powder and avoids these restrictions. The problem with developing a replacement for black powder is that black powder burns at substantially the same rate whether unconfined or fired in a weapon. Smokeless powder, however, burns slowly when unconfined, requiring about 1000 lb/in.^{2} of pressure to burn consistently. As pressure increases, it burns at an increasing rate, producing pressures that exceed those that can be tolerated by black powder firearms.

Pyrodex® has more bulk than black powder, with an equal volume of Pyrodex® having about 88% of the weight of black powder. In weapons chambered for black powder, Pyrodex® is loaded bulk for bulk with black powder, not by weight. The pressures and velocities generated are compatible with those achieved with black powder.

Bullets

The bullet is the part of the cartridge that leaves the muzzle of the firearm when it is discharged. Bullets were originally lead spheres. These worked satisfactorily with smooth-bore weapons, in which accuracy and long range were not expected. By the early nineteenth century, however, the superiority of the muzzle-loading rifle over the smoothbore musket was accepted. These rifled weapons had a greater range and considerably more accuracy. The main difficulty, however, was in reloading. To make such a rifle shoot accurately, the bullet had to fit the bore, but this qualification made the gun difficult to load and decreased the rate of fire. The bullet had to be forced down the barrel with a mallet. American riflemen developed a more rapid way of loading their rifles. They used a bullet that was slightly under bore diameter. This bullet was wrapped in a greased patch of fabric, and the patch and the spherical bullet were rammed down the barrel together. This step speeded up the rate of loading to some degree, but it did not solve the problem of long-range accuracy. The sphere has a very poor aerodynamic shape and loses velocity rapidly. The solution to these problems with muzzle-loading rifled weapons was to develop a bullet with a diameter less than the bore which would expand to fit the rifling grooves on firing and also would have a better aerodynamic shape than the ball. The solution was the Minie bullet, developed by Captain Charles Minie of the French Army.[3] It originally consisted of a conical-shaped, hollow-based lead bullet into whose base an iron wedge was inserted. The bullet was smaller in diameter than the bore. On firing, the gases of combustion would drive the wedge into the base of the bullet, expanding the base of the Minie bullet to fit the rifling grooves and to seal the propellant gases behind the bullet. Subsequent research found that the wedge could be eliminated and that the propellant gases working on the hollow base alone were sufficient to flare out the base of the bullet and seal the bore.

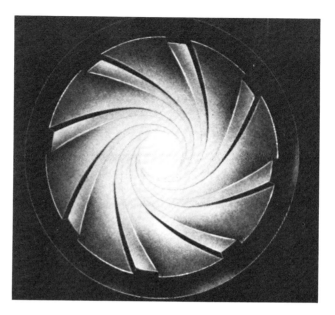

Figure 2–1 Cross-section of barrel with traditional rifling. Right-hand twist.

clockwise twist. The Mark III, manufactured by Colt, was a temporary exception to the manufacturer's policy in that for a number of years this weapon was produced with a right-hand twist. A minority of foreign handgun manufacturers also use a left-hand twist. The majority of domestic and foreign handgun manufacturers use a right-hand twist. Polygonal rifling has a right-hand twist.

Figure 2–2 A. Cross-section of barrel showing polygonal rifling. **B.** Cross-section of barrel with micro-groove* rifling. (From DiMaio, V.J.M. Wounds caused by centerfire rifles. Clin. Lab. Med. 3:257–271, 1983. (Used with permission.)

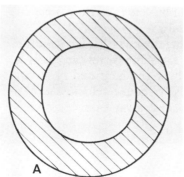

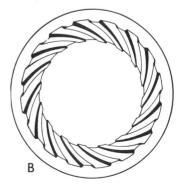

Table 2–1 *(continued)*

	Ruger Winches Mossber Marlin

Caliber	Man
Handguns	
.22 S, L, LR	Colt CDM, Ber Hi-stanc Smith & Rohm
.22 Magnum	Colt Wincheste Smith & Rohm
.25 ACP	Colt, Astr Titan, Ber
.32 ACP–.380 ACP	Colt Browning, Walther
.32 S & W, S & W Long	Colt, Cler Smith & Rohm, Ch Arminius
9-mm Parabellum	Colt Browning Walther
.38 S & W	Colt Smith & Enfield
.38 Special	Colt, Mir Smith & Ruger D. Colt MK Arminius Charter A Rohm, A
.357 Magnum	Colt Smith & Ruger I

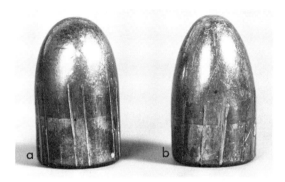

Figure 2–3 Two 9-mm bullets fired from weapons with (**a**) left twist and (**b**) right twist to their rifling.

Figure 2–3 shows two bullets, one fired in a weapon with left twist and the other in a weapon with a right twist. Figure 2–4 shows two .45 ACP bullets, one with traditional rifling marks and the other with markings from polygonal rifling.

The number of lands and grooves in a weapon can range from 2 to 22. Most modern weapons have four, five, or six grooves (Table 2–1). Colt handguns traditionally have had six lands and grooves with a left-hand twist, while Smith & Wesson has had five lands and grooves with a right-hand twist. Most centerfire rifles have four or six grooves with a right-hand twist. Rifle barrels with two grooves were manufactured during World War II for the M-1 carbine, the .30-06 Springfield rifle, and the British .303 Enfield.

Rifles manufactured by Marlin and sold under their own and other names have Micro-Groove® rifling (Figure 2–2). Micro-Groove® rifling was developed by Marlin in the early 1950s. Instead of 4 to 6 deep rifling grooves, their barrels have 12 to 22 shallow grooves (Table 2–2). Marlin manufactures rifles in the following calibers: .22 rimfire, .22 rimfire Magnum, .357 Magnum, .30-30, .35 Remington, .44 Magnum, .444 Marlin, and .45/70. They formerly produced a rifle chambered for the .30

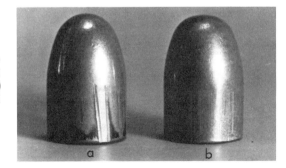

Figure 2–4 Two .45 ACP bullets: one (**a**) with traditional rifling marks, the other (**b**) with markings from polygonal rifling.

Table 2–1 Rifling Characteris[

Caliber	
Centerfire Rifles	
.223	AR-15 (
	Ruger N
	Heckler
	Reming
.243	All Rem
	Winc
	rifles
	Mossbe
.270	Winche
	Reming
.30 Carbine	Numerc
.30–06	M 1917
	Springfi
	Winche
	Reming
.30-30	Winche
	Marlin
.32 Winchester Special	Marlin
	Winche
.303 British	Lee Enf
	No. 1
	No. 4
.308	Winche
	M 14
	Reming
7.62 × 39	AK-47

	M
.22 Rimfire Rifles	
	Wincl
	Remi
	Remi

Table 2–1 Rifling Characteristics of Rifles and Handguns (*continued*)

Caliber	Manufacturer	Direction of twist	Number of lands and grooves
	Colt Mk III, Dan Wesson,	R	06
	Ruger SA/DA	R	06
	Ruger SA	R	08
.41 Magnum	Smith & Wesson	R	05
	Ruger	R	06
.44 Magnum	Smith & Wesson	R	05
	Ruger SA	R	06
	Ruger Carbine R	R	12
.45 ACP	Colt	L	06
	Star, Llama	R	06

[a] This is the most common rifling for this weapon.
[b] This is the most common rifling for this manufacturer.
[c] This is the most common rifling for these guns.

Table 2–2 Micro-Groove® Rifling

Caliber	Number of lands and grooves[a]
.22 S, L, LR	16
.22 Magnum	20
.30 Carbine	12
.30-30	12
.35 Remington	12
.357 Magnum	12
.44 Magnum	12
.444 Marlin	12
.45/70	12

[a] All right-twist.

Carbine cartridge. Recovery of a bullet with Micro-Groove® rifling indicates that the individual was shot with a rifle, as such rifling is not found in handguns.

Class and Individual Characteristics of Bullets

When a bullet is fired down a rifled barrel, the rifling imparts a number of markings to the bullet that are called "class characteristics." These markings may indicate the make and model of the gun from which the bullet had been fired. They result from the specifications of the rifling, as laid down by the individual manufacturer. These characteristics are:

1. Number of lands and grooves
2. Diameter of lands and grooves
3. Width of lands and grooves
4. Depth of grooves
5. Direction of rifling twist
6. Degree of twist

In addition to these class characteristics, imperfections on the surfaces of the lands and grooves score the bullets, producing individual characteristics. For lead bullets these individual characteristics are more pronounced where the grooves score the bullet. In contrast, for jacketed bullets, the land markings are the most pronounced.[1] These individual characteristics are peculiar to the particular firearm that fired the bullet and not to any others. They are as individual as fingerprints. No two barrels, even those made consecutively by the same tools, will produce the same markings on a bullet. Thus, while the class characteristics may be identical on bullets fired by two different weapons, the individual characteristics will be different. In addition to markings on the bullets, the magazine, firing pin, extractor, ejector, and breech face of a weapon may all impart class and individual markings to a cartridge case or primer.

Comparison of Bullets

When a gun is discharged, the bullet is forced down the barrel by the gases of combustion. Both class and individual characteristics are imparted to the bullet, whether it is lead or jacketed. Because lead is softer, one might postulate that bullet markings on lead bullets are more distinctive than those found on jacketed bullets. In fact, markings on jacketed bullets are usually superior, because the jacket of harder metal is less likely to have the rifling marks wiped off by the target.

In order to recover bullets for ballistic comparison, bullets have traditionally been fired into cotton waste. The tumbling of the bullet through this material may cause a wipe-off of some of the finer individual characteristics if the bullet is made of soft lead. This trait is especially true for the .22 rimfire bullets. Therefore, many ballistic laboratories now use water, in which loss of fine markings does not occur.

The individual characteristics that a barrel imparts to a bullet may be destroyed by rust, corrosion, or the firing of thousands of rounds of jacketed ammunition down a barrel. Accumulation of large quantities of dirt and grease from multiple firings may also alter to some degree the markings imparted to a bullet.

If a bullet with a diameter smaller than that intended for the specific weapon is fired, the bullet will be unable to follow the rifling suffi-

In rimfire cartridge cases, the firing pin impression is the most important identifying mark. Extractor, ejector, and breech block marks are less useful.[1]

Occasionally one will encounter a fired rifle cartridge case having a series of parallel longitudinal markings impressed on the case (Figure 2–6). Such markings are a consequence of a fluted chamber in the rifle. During manufacture, small parallel grooves have been cut into the chamber to allow the neck of the cartridge case to "float" on gas, thus aiding extraction. Heckler-Koch rifles have fluted chambers.

Base Markings

On discharge of a weapon, powder grains may be propelled against the base of the bullet with sufficient force to mark the base. Such markings are most evident in bullets with a lead base, that is, lead bullets or full

Figure 2–7 a. Base of unfired full metal jacketed bullet with exposed lead core. **b.** Pitting of base of similar bullet due to ball powder. **c.** Circular and linear marks on base of lead bullet due to disk powder. **d.** Peppered appearing base of lead bullet due to black powder.

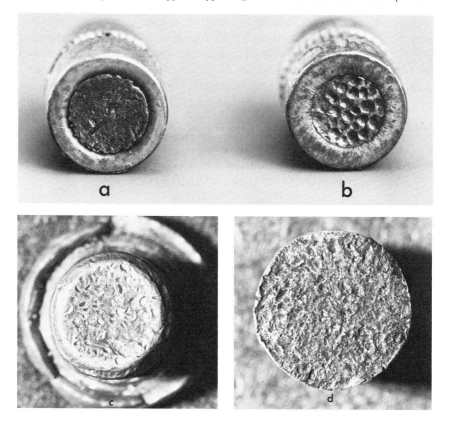

metal jacketed bullets whose lead core is exposed at the base. The shorter the barrel, the more numerous and the deeper the powder marks.[2] Different forms of powder produce different marks. Spherical ball powder produces numerous deep circular pits, disk powder shallow, circular imprints as well as linear markings (powder flakes striking on edge), and black powder a characteristic peppered appearance (Figure 2–7).

Powder marks are more prominent on the exposed lead base of full metal-jacketed bullets than on the base of all lead bullets. Bullets with a jacketed base (partial metal-jacketed bullets) can but usually do not show very faint powder markings on the base.

Powder grains may become adherent to the base of a bullet and be carried into and even through a body. This usually involves bullets with a lead base though on very rare occasions this has been seen in a bullet with a jacketed base (Figure 2–8).

Fingerprints

In contrast to what is seen on television and read in mystery books, it is rare for an identifiable fingerprint to be left on a firearm, especially a handgun. Only a small surface area is suitable for leaving prints, and the recoil of the weapon causes the fingers to slide and produce smudges.

Figure 2–8 Powder adherent to base of full metal-jacketed .357 Magnum bullet.

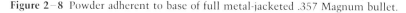

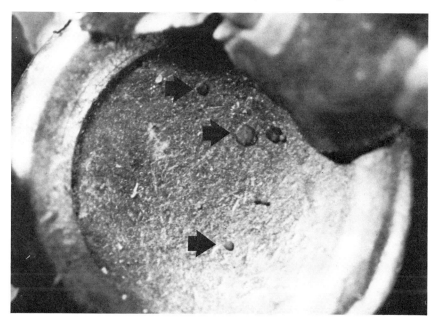

Both public and many police agencies do not realize, however, that identifiable fingerprints may be obtained from fired cartridge cases.[3] Thus, ejected cartridge cases at a crime scene should be collected in such a manner as to preserve prints that might be found on such casings.

Black Powder Firearms

Black powder weapons are rarely involved in fatal shootings. Most of such cases involve percussion revolvers. As these weapons have rifled barrels, rifling marks will appear on the spherical or conical bullets fired from them. In addition, the loading rammer used to ram the bullet into the chamber may leave markings on the bullet of sufficient clarity and with individual characteristics that make ballistic comparison possible.

Figure 2–9 shows a .44 caliber ball removed from the arm of a woman accidentally shot with a percussion revolver. Examination of the bullet

Figure 2–9 0.44-caliber ball showing **(a)** shearing of one surface, and **(b)** marking from loading rammer. Opposite surface has a peppered appearance due to black powder **(c)**.

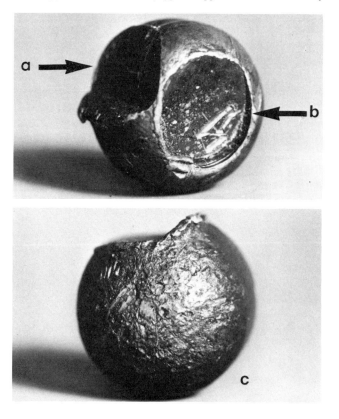

reveals absence of rifling, shearing of one surface, and markings from a loading rammer. The first two findings indicate that this bullet was not fired down the barrel but came out the side of the gun from a chamber that was not in line with the barrel.

When a black powder revolver is fired, a large amount of flame and sparks is produced that can ignite the powder in an adjacent chamber. In such a case, as the ball emerges from the chamber no rifling will be imparted to it and lead will be sheared off the side of the ball. Figure 2–9 illustrates this pattern. Ballistic comparison might still be possible, however, from an examination of the marks left on the bullet by the rammer.

Discharge of a Weapon

Now that we have attained a basic knowledge of firearms and ammunition, let us consider the sequence of events that occurs when one brings the two elements together. Pulling the trigger causes release of the firing pin. This strikes the primer, crushing it, igniting the primer composition, and producing an intense flame. The flame enters the main chamber of the cartridge case through one or more vents, igniting the powder and producing a large quantity of gas and heat. This gas, which may be heated to 5200° F, exerts pressure on the base of the bullet and sides of the cartridge case that may vary anywhere from a few tons to 25 tons per square inch.[4] The pressure of the gases on the base of the bullet propels it down the barrel. As the bullet travels down the barrel, some of the gas leaks past the bullet, emerging from the muzzle ahead of it. The bulk of the gas and any unburnt powder, however, emerge after the bullet (Figure 2–10).

When the bullet emerges from the barrel of the gun, it is accompanied by flame, gas, powder, soot, primer residue, metallic particles stripped from the bullet and vaporized metal from the bullet and cartridge case. The powder results from incomplete combustion of the propellant, as burning of smokeless powder is never really complete. Thus, partially burnt, burning, and unburned grains of powder invariably emerge with the bullet from the barrel. The amount of unburned or partially burned powder exiting depends largely on the burning properties of the powder and the length of the barrel. Contrary to popular misconception, smokeless powder does not explode; rather, it burns. The rate of burning can be controlled by the manufacturer by means of varying the size and shape of the powder grains, as well as by coating them with substances that retard combustion. The size and shape affect the burning rate by controlling the amount of surface area exposed to the flame. The greater the surface area, the faster the combustion.

38

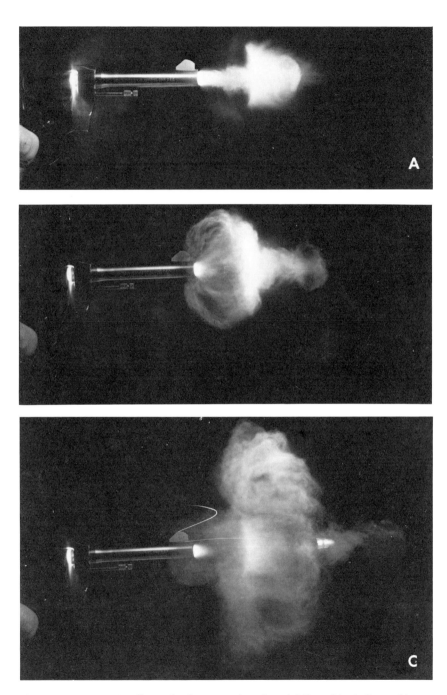

Figure 2–10 A–C. Small gas cloud emerges from barrel followed by bullet and larger cloud of gas (.38 Special Colt revolver).

The object of controlling the burning rate of powder is to achieve "progressive burning." Ideally, the propellant should start burning slowly, gradually increasing its rate of combustion until it is completely consumed just as the bullet leaves the muzzle. Such ideal burning powder is never achieved because the same powder is used to propel bullets of various calibers and weighs down barrels of different lengths.

Bullet weight affects variations in burning by altering the pressure of the gases in the firing chamber. When powder is ignited and gas forms, the bullet does not begin to move immediately. There is a small interval of time necessary for the gas to overcome the inertia of the bullet and the resistance of its passing down the barrel. This interval increases with the weight of the bullet if everything else remains constant. As the interval increases, the pressure increases, causing the powder to burn faster and give off more heat. The heat in turn raises the gas pressure. If there is an ideally progressive burning powder for a specified bullet weight and that weight is increased, the interval will increase and the powder will burn faster. Therefore, the powder will be burned before the bullet leaves the barrel. Lightening the weight of the bullet would cause the opposite effect; in this case, not all the powder will be burned before the bullet emerges from the muzzle.

Varying the length of the barrel also affects how much powder exits the muzzle. Shortening the barrel causes more unburned powder to emerge. Lengthening the barrel results in the consumption of more powder before the bullet emerges.

When a bullet exits the barrel, it is accompanied by a "flame" consisting of incandescent superheated gases. This flame is usually no more than 1 to 2 in. in length in handguns. The flame is of little significance except in contact and near-contact wounds, where it may sear the skin around the entrance wound. It cannot ignite clothing. Accounts of close-range firing igniting clothing date back to the use of black powder in cartridge cases.

The gases produced by ignition of gunpowder are oxygen-deprived. When they emerge from the barrel at extremely high temperatures, they react with the oxygen in the atmosphere, producing what is commonly known as the "muzzle flash." This should not be confused with the flame.

In revolvers, in addition to the gas, soot, vaporized metals, and powder particles emerging from the muzzle of the weapon, similar material emerges from the gun at the cylinder-barrel gap (Figure 2–11). If the cylinder of the weapon is not in perfect alignment with the barrel, fragments of lead will be avulsed from the bullet as it enters the barrel and will also emerge from this gap. In revolvers made to close tolerances, the amount of gas, soot, and powder escaping is relatively small and fragments of lead will be absent. In less well-made guns, however,

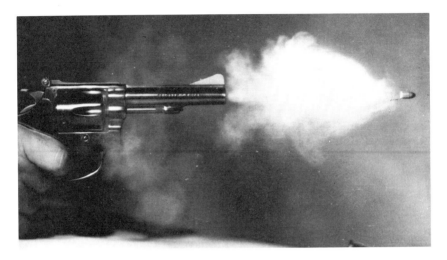

Figure 2-11 A cloud of gas can be seen emerging from the cylinder-barrel gap.

considerable debris may emerge from the cylinder-barrel gap. In either case, the soot and powder emerging from the gap may cause powder blackening and powder tattooing of the skin, if the weapon is held in close proximity to the body. The fragments of lead shaved from the bullet as a result of the misaligned cylinder may impact and become embedded in the skin.

References

1. Mathews, J.H. *Firearms Identification* (3 vol). Springfield, IL: Charles C. Thomas 1972.
2. Experiments by author.
3. Given, B.W. *Latent Fingerprints on Cartridges and Expended Cartridge Casings.* J. Forensic Sci. 21(3):587–594, 1976.
4. Lowry, E.D. *Interior Ballistics: How a Gun Converts Chemical Energy into Projectile Motion.* Garden City, NY: Doubleday and Co., 1968.

Wound Ballistics

3

Ballistics is the science of the motion of projectiles. It is divided into interior ballistics, external ballistics, and terminal ballistics. Interior ballistics is the study of the projectile in the gun; exterior ballistics, the study of the projectile through air; and terminal ballistics, the study of penetration of solids by the missile. Wound ballistics can be considered a subdivision of terminal ballistics concerned with the motions and effects of the projectile in tissue. In this chapter we shall review wound ballistics.

A moving projectile, by virtue of its movement, possesses kinetic energy. For a bullet, this energy is determined by its weight and velocity: K.E. = $WV^2/2\ g$, where g is gravitational acceleration, W is the weight of the bullet, and V is the velocity.[1] From this formula, it can be seen that velocity plays a greater role in determining the amount of kinetic energy possessed by a bullet than does weight. Doubling the weight doubles the kinetic energy, but doubling the velocity quadruples the kinetic energy.

In the concept of a gunshot wound held by most individuals, the bullet goes through a person like a drill bit through wood, "drilling" a neat hole through structures that it passes through. However, this concept is erroneous. As a bullet moves through the body, it imparts kinetic energy to the surrounding tissue, flinging it away from the bullet's path in a radial manner (direction) and producing a temporary cavity considerably larger than the diameter of the bullet.[1,2] This temporary cavity, which has a lifetime of 5 to 10 msec from initial rapid growth until collapse, undergoes a series of gradually smaller pulsations and contractions before it finally disappears, leaving the permanent would track. (Figure 3–1).

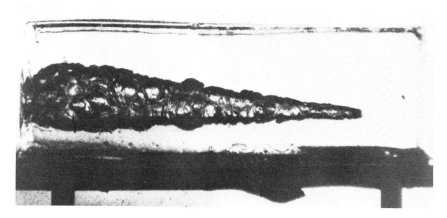

Figure 3–1 Temporary cavity produced in gelatin block by 110-gr semijacketed hollow-point .38 Special bullet.

The size and the shape of the temporary cavity depend on the amount of kinetic energy lost by the bullet in its path through the tissue, how rapidly the energy is lost, and the elasticity and cohesiveness of the tissue. The maximum volume and diameter of this cavity are many times the volume and diameter of the bullet. Maximum expansion of the cavity does not occur until some time after the bullet has passed through the target. The temporary cavity phenomenon is significant because it has been found to be the most important factor in determining the extent of wounding in an individual in regard to the interaction of a bullet with the body. In the case of low-velocity missiles, e.g., pistol bullets, the bullet produces a direct path of destruction with very little lateral extension within the surrounding tissues. Only a small temporary cavity is produced. To cause significant injuries to a structure, a pistol bullet must strike that structure directly. The amount of kinetic energy lost in the tissue by a pistol bullet is insufficient to cause the remote injuries produced by a high-velocity rifle bullet.

The picture is radically different in the case of a high-velocity missile. As the bullet enters the body, there is a "tail splash," or the backward hurling of injured tissue. The bullet passes through the target, creating a large temporary cavity whose maximum diameter may be up to 30 times the diameter of the original bullet.[3] The maximum diameter of the cavity occurs at the point at which the maximum rate of loss of kinetic energy occurs. This cavity will undulate for 5 to 10 msec before coming to rest as a permanent track. In high-velocity centerfire rifles, the expanding walls of the temporary cavity are capable of doing severe damage. Local pressures in the order 100 to 200 atm may develop.[4] This pressure may produce injuries to blood vessels, nerves, or organs that are a considerable distance from the path of the bullet. Fractures can occur even without direct contact between the bone and a rifle bullet. Positive and negative pressures alternate in the wound, with resultant sucking of foreign material and bacteria into the wound track from both entrance and exit.

The size of both the temporary and the permanent cavities is determined not only by the amount of kinetic energy deposited in the tissue but also by the density and elastic cohesiveness of the tissue. Because liver and muscle have similar densities (1.01 to 1.02 and 1.02 to 1.04), both tissues absorb the same amount of kinetic energy per centimeter of tissue traversed by a bullet.[4] Muscle, however, has an elastic, cohesive structure; the liver has a weak, less cohesive structure. Thus, both the temporary and the permanent cavities produced in the liver are larger than those in the muscle. In muscle, except for the bullet path, the tissue displaced by the temporary cavity returns to its original position. Only a small rim of cellular destruction surrounds the permanent track. In liver struck by high-velocity bullets, however, the undulation of the temporary cavity loosens the hepatocytes from the cellular supporting tissue and produces a permanent cavity approximately the size of the temporary cavity. Lung, with a very low density (specific gravity of 0.4 to 0.5) and high degree of elasticity, has only a very small temporary cavity formed with very little tissue destruction.[4]

Energy loss along a wound track is not uniform. Variations may be due either to behavior of the bullet or changes in the density of the tissue as the bullet goes from one organ to another. An increase in kinetic energy loss is reflected by an increase in the diameter of the temporary cavity. A full metal-jacketed rifle bullet will produce a cylindrical cavity until it begins to tumble. At this time, the bullet's cross-sectional area will become larger, and the drag force will be increased. The result is an increase in kinetic energy loss and thus an increase in the diameter of the temporary cavity (Figure 3−2). With hunting ammunition, the picture is radically different. The bullet will begin to expand shortly after entering the body, with a resultant rapid loss of kinetic energy. A large temporary cavity is formed immediately as the bullet enters the body (Figure 3−2).

A lead shotgun pellet produces a cone-shaped temporary cavity with the base of the cone at the entrance (Figure 3−2). The diameter of the cavity gradually lessens as the velocity of the pellet decreases. The loss of velocity is much more rapid for shotgun pellets because of their unfavorable ballistic properties (large cross-sectional area in relation to mass).

It has been found that above a certain critical velocity (800 to 900 m/sec or 2625 to 2953 ft/sec), the character of a wound changes radically with tissue destruction becoming much more severe.[2] Trans- or super-

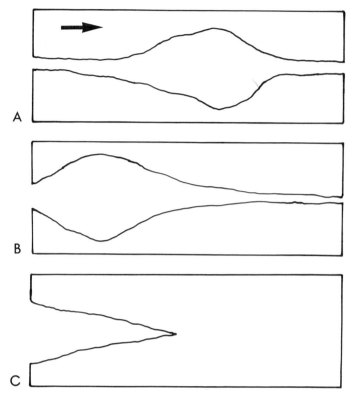

Figure 3–2 Appearance of temporary cavities in gelatin blocks due to (**A**) full metal jacketed rifle bullet, (**B**) hunting rifle bullet, and (**C**) shotgun pellet.

sonic flow within the tissue causing strong shockwaves has been assumed to be responsible for this effect.[3] In experiments by Rybeck and Janzon, 6-mm steel balls weighing 0.86 gm were fired at the hind legs of dogs.[5] They found that at a velocity of 510 m/sec, the volume of macroscopically injured muscle was only slightly larger than the diameter of the bullet. At 978 and 1313 m/sec, the volume of devitalized muscle was seen to be 20 to 30 times the volume of the permanent cavity.

These experiments as well as observations by other authorities have involved either steel balls or full metal jacketed military bullets, that is, essentially nondeforming missiles. In civilian practice, however, the critical velocity appears to be lower because of the different construction of the ammunition encountered. The only full metal-jacket ammunition routinely seen in civilian practice is low-velocity automatic pistol ammunition. The centerfire rifle bullets encountered are not full metal-jacketed but semijacketed expanding hunting bullets. Centerfire rifle wounds due to hunting bullets do not generally appear any different in severity regardless of the caliber and muzzle velocity.

It is the author's belief that rather than there being a critical velocity above which the severity of wounds increases dramatically, there is instead a critical level of kinetic energy loss. This level is different for each organ or tissue. When a bullet exceeds this kinetic energy threshold, it produces a temporary cavity that the organ or tissue can no longer contain, i.e., one that exceeds the elastic limit of the organ. When the elastic limit is exceeded, the organ "bursts." For full metal-jacketed bullets or steel balls to reach that level of kinetic energy and thus a particular size of temporary cavity, these missiles must be traveling at very high velocities (greater than 800 to 900 m/sec). For soft-point or hollow-point rifle bullets, however, the same loss of kinetic energy will occur at lower velocity as a result of the deformation of the bullets. Thus, for hunting ammunition, the critical velocity, in the author's experience, appears to be between 1500 and 2000 ft/sec (457.2 to 609.6 m/sec).

High-velocity missile wounds of the head are especially destructive because of formation of a temporary cavity within the cranial cavity. The brain is enclosed by the skull, a closed, rigid structure that can relieve pressure only by "bursting." Thus, high-velocity missile wounds of the head tend to produce bursting injuries. That these bursting injuries are the result of temporary cavity formation can be demonstrated by shooting through empty skulls. A high-velocity bullet fired through an empty skull produces small entrance and exit holes with no fractures. The same missile fired through a skull containing brain causes extensive fracturing and bursting injuries.[6]

With a high-velocity rifle bullet, the permanent cavity in tissue is usually larger in diameter than the bullet. With a low-energy projectile such as a pistol bullet, the permanent track is often distinctly smaller in diameter. Tissue elasticity with contraction of the surrounding tissue accounts for this latter phenomenon. If, however, the elastic limit of the tissue has been exceeded by the pistol bullet, the tissue tears, and a large irregular wound track is produced. This latter phenomenon is seen most often in the liver.

Loss of Kinetic Energy

The severity of a wound is directly related to the amount of kinetic energy lost in the tissue, not the total energy possessed by the bullet. If a bullet penetrates a body—i.e., does not exit—all the kinetic energy will be utilized in wound formation. On the other hand, if the bullet perforates the body—i.e., goes through it—only part of the kinetic energy is used in wound formation. Thus, bullet A with twice the kinetic energy of B may produce a wound less severe than B, because A perforates the body whereas B does not.

The amount of kinetic energy lost by a bullet depends on four main factors.[1] The first is the amount of kinetic energy possessed by the bullet at the time of impact. This, as has been discussed, is dependent on the velocity and mass of the bullet.

The second factor is the angle of yaw of a bullet at the time of impact.[1] The yaw of a bullet is defined as the deviation of the long axis of the bullet from its line of flight. When a bullet is fired down a rifled barrel, the rifling imparts a gyroscopic spin to the bullet. The purpose of the spin is to stabilize the bullet's flight through the air. Thus, as the bullet leaves the barrel, it is spinning on its long axis, which in turn corresponds to the line of flight. As soon as the bullet leaves the barrel, however, it begins to wobble or yaw. The amount or degree of yaw of a bullet depends on the physical characteristics of the bullet—that is, its length, diameter, cross-sectional density, and so forth—and the rate of twist of the barrel and the density of the air.

Angles of yaw have been determined with certainty only in military weapons. The maximum angle of yaw at the muzzle may vary from 1.5 degrees for a .30-caliber, 150-gr Spitzer bullet, to 6 degrees for a 55-gr .223 bullet.[7] Extremes in temperature can increase yaw and thus the stability of the bullet. Altering the rate of twist in the barrel can also alter the angle of yaw. The AR-15 as originally designed had a barrel twist of 1/14 in. This twist was too slow, however, so that bullets fired from the weapon were so unstable as to cause significant problems in accuracy. In order to correct this flaw and to stablize the bullet, the twist rate was changed to 1/12 in.

The greater the angle of yaw, when a bullet strikes the body, the greater the loss of kinetic energy.[1] Because retardation of a bullet varies as the square of the angle of yaw, the more the bullet is retarded, the greater is the loss of kinetic energy.

As the bullet moves farther and farther from the muzzle, the maximum amplitude of the yaw—the degrees of yaw—gradually decreases. At 70 yd, the degree of yaw for the .223-caliber bullet decreases to approximately 2 degrees.[7] This stabilization of the bullet as the range increases explains the observation that close-up wounds are often more destructive than distant wounds. It also explains the observation that a rifle bullet penetrates deeper at 100 yd than at 10 ft.

Although the gyroscopic spin of the bullet along its axis is sufficient to stabilize the bullet in air, this spin is insufficient to stabilize the bullet when it enters the denser medium of tissue. Thus, as soon as the bullet enters the body, it will begin to wobble.[1] As the bullet begins to wobble, its cross-sectional area becomes larger, the drag force increases, and more kinetic energy is lost. If the path through the tissue is long enough, the wobbling will increase to such a degree that the bullet will be completely unstable and will tumble end-over-end through the tissue.

Tumbling of a bullet causes a much larger cross-sectional area of the bullet to be presented to the target. This in turn results in greater loss of kinetic energy and a larger temporary cavity. The sudden increase of the drag force or tumbling puts a great strain on the bullet which may eventually break up. A short projectile will usually tumble sooner than a longer one.[8]

The third factor that influences the amount of kinetic energy lost in the body is the bullet itself: its caliber, construction, and configuration. Blunt nose bullets, being less streamlined than spitzer (pointed) bullets are retarded more by the tissue and therefore lose greater amounts of kinetic energy. Expanding bullets, which "open up" in the tissue, are retarded more than streamlined full metal-jacketed bullets, which resist expansion and lose only a minimum amount of kinetic energy as they pass through the body.

The caliber of a bullet and its shape—i.e., the bluntness of the nose—are important in that they determine the initial value of the area of interphase between the bullet and the tissue and thus the "drag" of the bullet. Shape and caliber decrease in importance when deformity of the bullet occurs. The amount of deformation in turn depends on both the construction of the bullet (the presence or absence of the jacketing; the length, thickness, and hardness of the jacket material; the hardness of the lead used in the bullet; and the presence of a hollow point) and the bullet velocity. A lead round-nose bullet will deform at a velocity above 340 m/sec (1115 ft/sec) in tissue. For hollow-points, it is above 215 m/sec (705 ft/sec).[9]

Soft-point and hollow-point centerfire rifle bullets not only tend to expand as they go through the body, but also shed lead fragments. This shedding occurs whether or not they strike bone. The pieces of lead fly off the main bullet mass, acting as secondary missiles, contacting more and more tissue, and increase the size of the wound cavity and thus the severity of the wound. Such a phenomenon—i.e., shedding lead fragments—does not appear to happen with pistol bullets, even if they are soft-point or hollow-point, unless they strike bone. Breaking up of missiles appears to be related to the velocity. The velocity of pistol bullets, even of the new high-velocity loadings, is insufficient to cause the shedding of lead fragments seen with rifle bullets.

A fact not often appreciated is that even full metal-jacketed bullets may break up in the body without hitting bone. This phenomenon has not been seen in the .30-06 M-1 round but has gained some medical attention in the 5.56-mm M-16 round. Thus, there have been a number of press and medical reports stating that this bullet "blows up" in the body. This claim is nonsense! The M-16 bullet does tend to break up, but it does not blow up. Although the 5.56-mm round has a reputation for causing extremely severe wounds, the amount of kinetic energy lost by this round is less than that seen with the relatively low velocity .30-30 hunting ammunition.

The tendency of a 5.56-mm bullet to break up in the body is due to its greater tendency to tumble.[10] When the bullet tumbles, its projected cross-sectional area becomes much larger, with a resultant increase in the drag force acting on the bullet. The sudden increase in this drag force puts a great strain on the structure of the bullet, producing a greater tendency to break up. All this causes a greater loss of kinetic energy with an increase in the severity of the wound. Callender and French, commenting on the tendency of high-velocity, full metal-jacketed bullets to break up, observed that blunt-nosed bullets break up from the tip, whereas pointed bullets break up from the base.[2] In both types of full metal-jacketed bullets, the lead core can be squeezed out the base if the bullet is exposed to severe stress, due to tumbling.

Breakup of the military 5.56-mm bullet begins with the bullet losing its core through the open base.[10] The bullet then tends to flatten on its longitudinal axis and bend at the cannula. Breakup of the 7.62-mm NATO bullet starts at the cannula. This bullet does not ordinarily lose any of its core from the bottom.[10]

To investigate the breakup of military ammunition in targets, the author conducted a number of tests using gelatin blocks and comparing the M-14, M-16, SKS-46 and M-1 rifles and the M-1 carbine. For experimental purposes, 20 percent gelatin can be substituted for human tissue if it is kept at 10° C. Tests were conducted at a range of 10 yd. Twenty-four rounds of .30-06, 20 rounds of .30 carbine, and 10 rounds of 7.62 × 39 military ball ammunition were fired through gelatin blocks. Not one of these bullets tumbled or broke up in the block. Twenty 7.62 NATO ball rounds were then fired through gelatin blocks. Eighteen of these bullets tumbled, with three fragmenting. Twenty rounds of 5.56 ball ammunition were then fired from an M-16. Eighteen of these bullets tumbled, with five fragmenting.

The fourth characteristic that determines the amount of kinetic energy lost by a bullet is the density, strength, and elasticity of the tissue struck by a bullet as well as the length of the wound track. The denser the tissue the bullet passes through, the greater the retardation and the greater the loss of kinetic energy. Increased density acts to increase the yaw as well as shortening the period of gyration. This increased angle of yaw and the shortened period of gyration lead to greater retardation and increased loss of kinetic energy.

References

1. French, R.W., Callender, G.R. Ballistic characteristics of wounding agents. In Beyer, J.C. (ed.), *Wound Ballistics*. Washington, D.C.: Superintendent of Documents, U.S. Government Printing Office, 1962.
2. Callender, G.R., French, R.W. Wound ballistics: studies in the mechanism of wound production by rifle bullets. Mil. Surg. 77:177−201, 1935.
3. Rybeck, B. Missile wounding and hemodynamic effects of energy absorption. Acta Chir. Scand. [Suppl] 450:1−32, 1974.
4. Amato, J.J., Billy, L.J., Lawson, N.S., Rich, N.M. High velocity missile energy: an experimental study of the retentive forces of tissue. Am. J. Surg. 127:454−459, 1974.
5. Rybeck, B., Janzon, B. Absorption of missile energy in soft tissue. Acta Chir. Scand. 142:201−207, 1976.
6. Harvey, E.N., McMillen, H., Butler, E.G., Puckett, W.O. Mechanism of wounding. In Beyer, J.C. (ed.) *Wound Ballistics*. Washington D.C.: Superintendent of Documents, U.S. Government Printing Office, 1962.
7. Personal Communication. Edgewood Arsenal.
8. Berlin, R., Gelin, L.E., Janzon, B., Lewis, D.H., Rybeck, B., Sandegrad, J., Seeman, T.: Local effects of assault rifle bullets in liver tissues. Acta Chir. Scand. [Suppl.] 459: 1976.
9. Bruchey, W.J., Frank, D.E. Police Handgun Ammunition: Incapacitation Effects. Volume I. Evaluation. Washington, D.C.: Superintendent of Documents, U.S. Government Printing Office, 1984.
10. Nordstrand, I., Janzon, B., Rybeck, B. Break-up behavior of some small calibre projectiles when penetrating a dense medium. Acta Chir. Scand [Suppl.] 489:81−90, 1979.

General References

La Garde, L.A. *Gunshot Injuries*, 2nd ed. New York: William Wood & Co, 1916.

Evaluation of Wound Data and Munitions Effectiveness in Vietnam (Vol. 1). Joint Tech. Coord. Group for Munitions Effectiveness, December 1970.

Scott, R. *Projectile Trauma. An Enquiry Into Bullet Wounds*. Crown Copyright.

Scott, R. Pathology of injuries caused by high-velocity missiles. In DiMaio, V.J.M. (ed.), *Forensic Pathology. Clinics in Laboratory Medicine*. 3(2):273−274, 1983.

An Introduction to the Classification of Gunshot Wounds

4

Gunshot wounds are either penetrating or perforating. Penetrating wounds occur when a bullet enters an object and does not exit; in perforating wounds, the bullet passes completely through the object. A wound, however, can be both penetrating and perforating. A bullet striking the head may pass through the skull and brain before coming to rest under the scalp, thus producing a penetrating wound of the head but a perforating wound of the skull and brain.

Gunshot wounds can be divided into four broad categories, depending on the range from muzzle to target: contact, near contact, intermediate, and distant.

Contact Wounds

In contact wounds, the muzzle of the weapon is held against the surface of the body at the time of discharge. Contact wounds may be hard, loose, angled, or incomplete (a variation of angled). In hard contact wounds, the muzzle of the weapon is jammed "hard" against the skin, indenting it so that the skin envelops the muzzle. In hard contact wounds, the immediate edges of the entrance are seared by the hot gases of combustion and blackened by the soot (Figure 4–1). This soot is embedded in the seared skin and cannot be completely removed either by washing or by vigorous scrubbing of the wound.

In loose contact wounds, the muzzle, while in complete contact with the skin, is held lightly against it. Gas preceding the bullet, as well as the bullet itself, indents the skin, creating a temporary gap between the skin and the muzzle through which gas can escape. Soot carried by the gas is deposited in a band around the entrance (Figure 4–2). This soot can be wiped away easily.

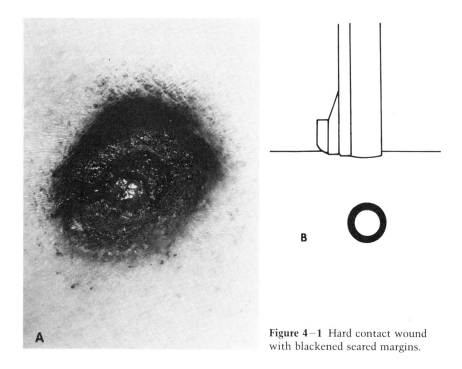

Figure 4−1 Hard contact wound with blackened seared margins.

Figure 4−2 Loose contact wound with soot deposited in band around entrance.

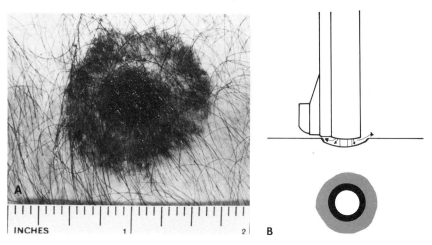

In angled contact wounds, the barrel is held at an acute angle to the skin so that the complete circumference of the muzzle is not in contact with it. Gas and soot escaping from the gap where contact is not complete radiate outward from the muzzle, producing an eccentrically arranged pattern of soot. The soot is arranged in two different zones. The most striking zone and often the only one seen is a blackened seared area of skin or cloth having a pear, circular, or oval configuration (Figure 4–3). Less prominent is a larger fan-shaped zone of light gray soot that radiates outward from the muzzle. On the skin this light zone is usually

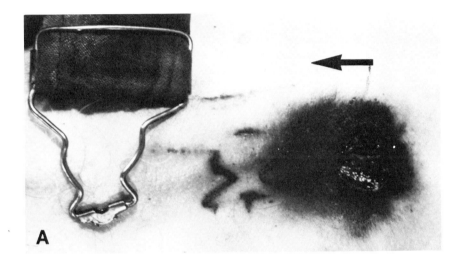

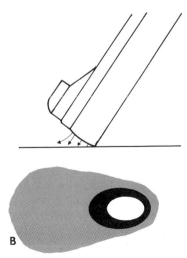

Figure 4–3 Angled contact wound with seared blackened zone of skin on opposite side of wound from muzzle pointing the way the gun was directed.

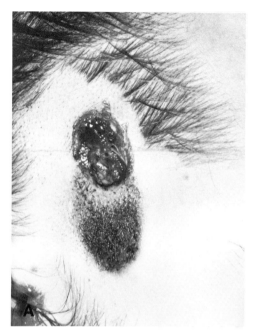

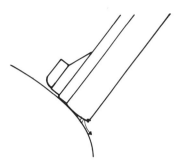

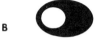

Figure 4–4 Incomplete contact wound.

washed away or obscured by bleeding or removed in cleaning the wound for examination.

The entrance wound is usually present at the base of the seared blackened zone. As the angle with the skin increases, the entrance hole will be found more toward the center of the zone. All or at least the majority of the seared blackened zone will be on the opposite site of the wound from the muzzle, and thus it "points" the way the gun was directed.

Incomplete contact wounds are a variation of angled contact wounds. In these, the muzzle of the weapon is held against the skin, but, because the body surface is not completely flat, there is a gap between the muzzle and the skin. A jet of soot-laden gas escapes from this gap producing an area of seared, blackened skin. The location of this seared, blackened zone can be anywhere in relationship to the muzzle circumference, depending on where the gap is. Incomplete contact wounds are often seen on the head with the seared, blackened zone directly opposite to the direction the bullet is traveling (Figure 4–4).

In all contact wounds, soot, powder, and vaporized metals from the bullet, primer, and cartridge case as well as carbon monoxide are deposited in and along the wound tract.

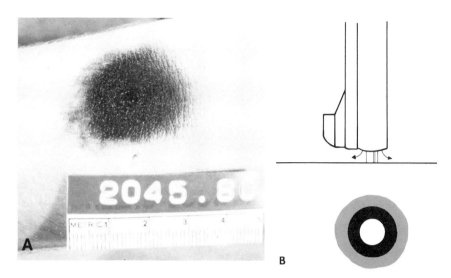

Figure 4–5 Near contact wound with wide zone of powder soot overlying seared blackened skin.

Near Contact Wounds

Near-contact wounds lie in a gray zone between contact and intermediate-range wounds. In these wounds, the muzzle of the weapon is not in contact with the skin, being held a short distance away. The distance, however, is so small that the powder grains emerging from the muzzle do not have a chance to disperse and mark the skin, producing the individual powder tattooing that is the sine qua non of intermediate-range wounds. In near contact wounds, there is an entrance wound, surrounded by a wide zone of powder soot overlying seared, blackened skin (Figure 4–5). The zone of searing is wider than that seen in a loose contact wound. The soot in the seared zone is baked into the skin and cannot be completely wiped away. However, as there is an overlap between the appearance of near and loose contact wounds, it is not always possible to differentiate the two, especially if the muzzle of the weapon is held perpendicular to the skin.

In near-contact angled wounds (Figure 4–6), just as in angled contact wounds, soot radiates outward from the muzzle creating two zones: the pear-shaped, circular, or oval blackened seared zone and the light gray fan-shaped one. The location of the blackened seared zone to the entrance hole is different from what is seen in angled contact wounds, however. In near-contact angled wounds, the bulk of the blackened, seared zone is on the same side as the muzzle, i.e., pointing toward the weapon. This is the opposite of what is found in angled contact wounds.

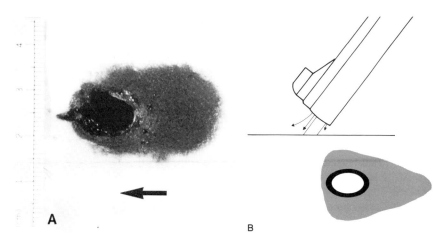

Figure 4-6 Angled near contact wound with blackened seared zone on same side as muzzle, i.e., pointing toward the weapon.

The importance of understanding the difference in the distribution of soot deposition for angled near-contact and contact wounds is that the direction in which the muzzle was pointing at the time of discharge cannot be deduced by looking at the soot pattern alone. In both contact and near-contact angled wounds, one gets an eccentric area of seared blackened skin. In contact wounds, however, this area lies on the side opposite to the muzzle, pointing the direction in which the bullet was fired. In near-contact wounds, the area lies on the same side as the muzzle of the weapon. By correlating the location of the blackened, seared zone with the path of the bullet through the body, one can differentiate an angled contact wound from a near-contact wound. Thus, if both the bullet and the zone point in the same direction, an angled contact wound has occurred. If, however, the zone is on one side of the wound with the bullet going the other way, an angled near-contact wound has taken place.

This interpretation assumes the ideal presentation of contact and near-contact angled wounds. Things are never as simple as one might wish, however. Thus, in angled contact wounds, the entrance wound should be present at the base of the seared, blackened zone. By increasing the angle to the skin, however, this entrance will move toward the center of the zone. This same picture can also be produced by a near-contact angled wound if the distance from muzzle to target is approximately 5 mm. In such an instance one cannot always differentiate between a contact and a near-contact angled wound. When the distance from muzzle to target increases to 10 mm in near-contact angled wounds, there is usually no difficulty differentiating it from an angled contact wound. The seared, blackened zone on the side of the muzzle is much wider than it is on the opposite side. Powder grains may be seen in the seared zone on the side opposite to the muzzle.

Intermediate-Range Gunshot Wounds

An intermediate-range gunshot wound is one in which the muzzle of the weapon is held away from the body at the time of discharge yet is sufficiently close so that powder grains expelled from the muzzle along with the bullet produce "powder tattooing" of the skin (Figure 4−7). These markings are the sine qua non of intermediate range gunshot wounds.

Just as there is a gradual transition from loose contact to near-contact wounds, there is also a gradual transition from near-contact to intermediate wounds. The powder grains emerging from the muzzle may be deposited in the seared zone around near-contact wounds so that individual tattoo marks are not seen. As soon as one sees individual tattoo marks, however, one is dealing with an intermediate-range wound. For handguns, powder tattooing begins at a muzzle-to-target distance of approximately 10 mm.

Figure 4−7 Powder tattooing of skin due to flake (disk) powder.

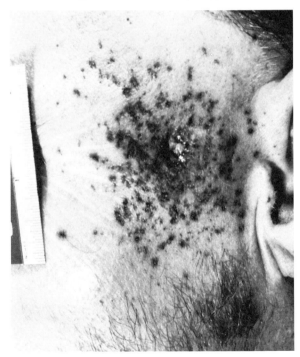

Tattooing consists of numerous reddish-brown to orange-red punctate lesions surrounding the wound of entrance. The distribution around the entrance site may be either symmetric or eccentric, depending on the angle of the gun to the target at the time of discharge, the nature of the target (flat or angled), and any covering of the skin by hair or clothing which may prevent powder grains from reaching the skin. When the muzzle of the weapon is at an angle to the skin, the skin under the muzzle—i.e., on the same side as the barrel—will show denser tattooing than the skin on the other side of the entrance hole (Figure 4–8).

Powder tattooing is an *antemortem* phenomenon and indicates that the individual was alive at the time he or she was shot. If the individual was dead before being shot, although the powder may produce marks on the skin, these marks have a moist grey or yellow appearance rather than the reddish-brown to orange-red coloration of an *antemortem* wound. There should be no difficulty with differentiating the two.

Powder tattoo marks are produced by the impact of powder grains on the skin. They are not powder burns, but rather are punctate abrasions. Similar markings can be produced by noncombustible particles such as polyethylene granules. The term "powder burns" should never be used, because one does not know to what phenomenon the term is being applied. Some individuals use the term "powder burns" to signify

Figure 4–8 Intermediate-range gunshot wound with muzzle of weapon at angle to skin. Powder tattooing of skin on same side as barrel. **Arrow** indicates direction of bullet.

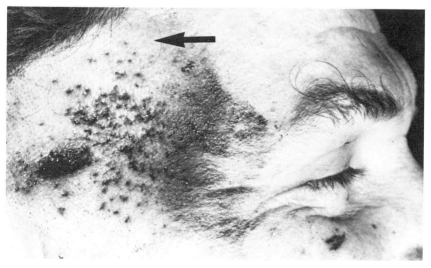

powder tattooing, whereas others use it to signify searing and black-ening of the skin due to the hot gases that occur from combustion of the propellant.

The term "powder burns" dates back to the black powder era, when burning grains of black powder emerged from the muzzle and were deposited on the skin and clothing, where they smoldered, apparently producing actual burns on the skin. Black powder grains could also penetrate into the dermis and produce literal tattooing. These burning grains of black powder are capable of setting clothing on fire, a character-istic not possessed by smokeless powder.

The punctate abrasions of smokeless powder tattooing cannot be wiped away. Powder tattoo marks usually heal completely if the individ-ual survives. This is logical, as the injuries are generally confined only to the superficial layers of the epidermis. Grains of ball powder, and less commonly flake powder, however, may penetrate into the upper dermis thus producing actual tattooing of the skin.

The author has never seen powder tattooing of the palms or soles caused by powder emerging from the muzzle of a gun though he has seen cases in which powder grains were embedded in the palms without any vital reaction, i.e., tattooing (Figure 4–9). It is probable that the thick-ness of the stratum corneum in this area protects the dermis from any trauma-direct or indirect; thus there is no vital reaction and therefore no tattooing.

Figure 4–9 Intermediate range gunshot wound of palm with entrance at base of thumb, soot on thenar eminence and powder grains embedded in skin of palm. No powder tattooing present.

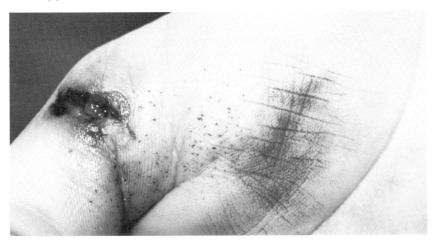

Powder Soot

When a weapon is discharged, in addition to powder, soot produced by combustion of the gunpowder emerges from the muzzle of the weapon. The soot, which is carbon, contains vaporized metals from the primer, bullet, and cartridge case. If the muzzle is held close to the victim, this soot may be deposited on the body. The size, intensity, and appearance of the soot pattern and the maximum range out to which it occurs depend on a number of factors:

1. Range
2. Propellant
3. Angle of the muzzle to the target
4. Barrel length
5. Caliber of the weapon
6. Type of weapon
7. Target material and the state of the target, i.e., bloody or nonbloody

As the range from the muzzle to the target increases, the size of the zone of powder soot blackening will increase, whereas the density will decrease. Beyond a certain point, however, the overall dimensions of the powder soot pattern will begin to decrease, and it will be impossible to delineate exactly the outer border of the soot, as it has become so faint.

The propellant is a determinant as to the amount of powder soot present in that some powders burn more cleanly than others. Thus, in a test using a .22-caliber revolver with a 6-in. barrel, two forms of .22 Long rifle ammunition were fired at white cotton cloth. One form of ammunition was loaded with flake powder, the other with ball powder. The flake powder produced powder soot deposition out to a maximum of 30 cm, whereas soot from the ball powder disappeared between 20 cm and 25 cm. Powder loaded in Federal centerfire cartridges seems to be "dirtier" than that of other manufacturers.

Differences in the barrel length of a weapon may affect the amount of soot reaching the target. Thus, Remington 158-grain .38 Special cartridges loaded with flake powder were fired at white cotton cloth. A 6-in. barrel weapon produced soot out to a maximum of 30 cm; a 4-in. barrel weapon to 25 cm, and a 2-in. barrel weapon, out to 20 cm. The longer barreled weapons produced a soot pattern that was denser and more concentrated. The tattoo pattern produced by the 6-in. weapon also appeared denser and smaller in size.

On the basis of the author's experience, the maximum distance out to which powder soot deposition occurs for handguns is 20 to 30 cm.

The orientation of the muzzle of the weapon to the target will determine whether the soot deposit around the wound of entrance in the skin or clothing is symmetric (concentric) or eccentric. If the muzzle is at a

90-degree angle to the target, the soot pattern should be circular in shape, with the entrance hole in the center. At ranges from loose contact up to 1 to 2 cm, there is usually a circular area of extremely dense dark black powder blackening surrounded by a zone of light gray powder blacking. Beyond this range (1 to 2 cm), one begins to get the blossom or petal pattern described by Barnes and Helson.[1] As the range increases farther, this pattern increases in diameter, reaches a maximum size, and then gradually begins to shrink and fade, disappearing by 15 to 25 cm of range. In some instances the classical petal or blossom pattern will not be present; rather, there will be a dense black center surrounded by a lighter gray outer zone, with this zone possibly having a scalloped appearance.

In addition to the soot pattern produced by soot emerging from the barrel, in revolvers a powder soot pattern can be produced by soot escaping from the cylinder-barrel gap. If the weapon is held parallel to the skin or clothing at the time of discharge, the jet of soot-laden gas escaping from the cylinder-barrel gap may produce linear, L-shaped or V-shaped gray sooty deposit (Figure 4–10). The skin or cloth on which the soot is deposited may be seared. If the clothing is 100% synthetic, the hot gas may burn completely through the material with formation of the soot pattern on the underlying skin. If the gun is held at an acute angle to the body, there will be the soot mark of the cylinder gap as well as searing and soot deposition at the entrance from the muzzle. Measurements from the cylinder mark to the hole of entrance will give an approximation of the barrel length (Figure 4–11).

Attachments to the muzzle of a weapon can alter the powder soot patterns. A silencer attached to a pistol may filter out most of the soot present; thus, soot deposits from a .22 Long rifle pistol may extend only out to a range of 2.5 to 8 cm.

Silencers are rarely encountered, however; more common is a muzzle-break. This device is present at the muzzle of target pistols. It works by directing some of the gas emerging from the barrel in an upward-forward direction, thus dampening the muzzle climb and permitting a shooter to stay on target more readily. Some individuals who fire Magnum revolvers cut slits on the top of the barrel at the muzzle to accomplish the same purpose. In contact wounds, the jets of gas escaping out the slits at the muzzle end of such weapons may produce characteristic soot patterns on the skin or clothing. Figure 4–12 shows a "rabbit ear" pattern produced by a .22-caliber target pistol with a muzzle break having two slits.

Modern military rifles and some civilian rifles have flash suppressors at the muzzle. These devices are intended to break up the "fireball" that emerges from the muzzle of the rifle when fired at night. Such a device is useful in combat to decrease the possibility of counterfire. Flash sup-

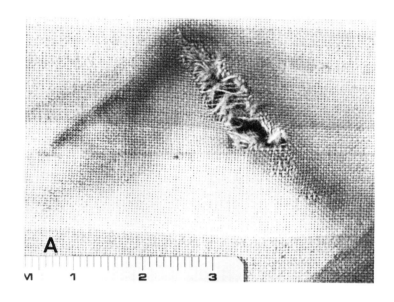

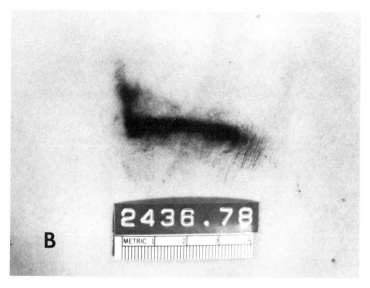

Figure 4–10 A. V-shaped deposit of soot from cylinder gap. **B.** L-shaped deposit of soot on skin from cylinder-barrel gap.

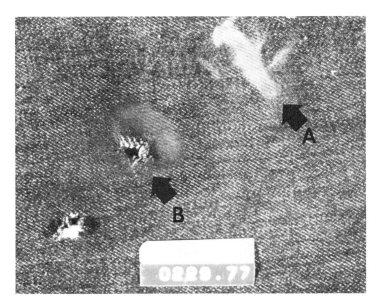

Figure 4 – 11 Angled near contact gunshot wound through blue jeans. The arrows indicate (**A**) a strip of seared material due to the hot gases from the cylinder-barrel gap and (**B**) the point of entrance of the bullet seared by the hot muzzle gases. The distance between these two points indicates the weapon was a short barrel revolver.

Figure 4 – 12 "Rabbit ear" pattern of soot on T-shirt produced by .22 caliber target pistol with muzzle break at end. Two slits on top of the muzzle break directed gas upward and forward, producing the soot pattern.

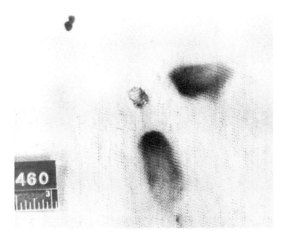

pressors generally consist of a cylinder having a number of longitudinal slits along its length that is attached to the muzzle of the weapon (Figure 4–13). On firing, the gas emerging from the muzzle is bled out the slits rather than emerging as one large cloud. Soot is present in this cloud of gas. If the muzzle of such a weapon is held in contact with the body, the flash suppressor will produce an unusual flower-like pattern of soot and seared skin (Figure 4–13B). The number of slits will determine the number of "petals" to the "flower," and may give one an idea of the type of weapon used. The M-16 rifle used to have a flash suppressor with three slits; thus, a three-petal "flower" was produced. The newer M-16 flash suppressor has six slits; the M-14 has five. The skin underlying these linear deposits of soot is seared, with the soot often being baked into the skin.

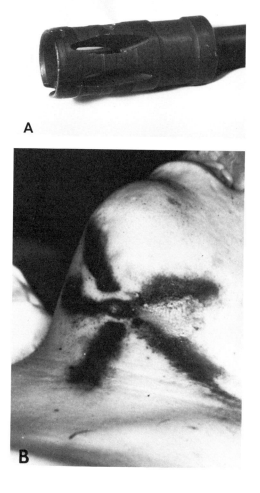

A

B

Figure 4–13 **A.** Flash suppressor. **B.** Flash suppressor burns on undersurface of chin due to self-inflicted wound with M-14 rifle.

Gas-operated centerfire semiautomatic rifles have gas ports where the gas, after operating the gun's mechanism, is vented. In Remington semiautomatic centerfire rifles, there are two slots on the top of the forearm—one on each side of the barrel—through which soot-laden gas is vented. The author has a case of suicide with such a weapon where the right forearm overlaid the vents as the deceased reached for and pushed the trigger. A linear deposit of soot from one of these vents was present on the forearm (Figure 4−14). This documented the position of the deceased's arm at the time the weapon was fired, adding additional evidence that the case was a suicide.

An unusual powder pattern may be due to specific peculiarities of a gun. Thus, in the case illustrated, a 20-year-old Puerto Rican male shot himself twice in the chest (Figure 4−15A). The two contact wounds showed extensive blackening of the skin. Approximately 3.2 cm above each entrance wound there was a small, irregular area of powder soot deposit. The weapon used to inflict the wounds was a .22-caliber starter pistol (Figure 4−15B) whose barrel had been reamed open. On the top of the barrel was a vent that was intended to channel off gases when blank cartridges were fired. When the two live rounds were fired, the vent in the weapon directed some of the gases in an upward and forward direction, causing the observed patterns. The two bullets recovered from the body were free of rifling.

Figure 4−14 Soot on arm from a gas port.

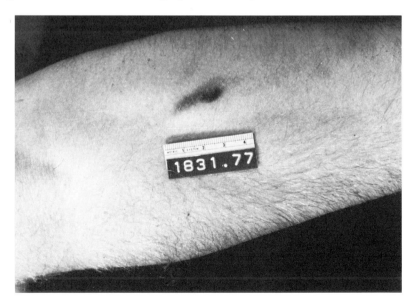

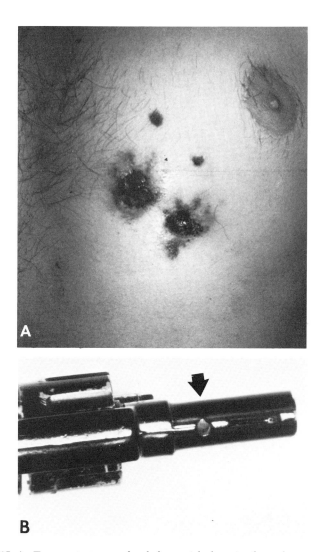

Figure 4–15 A. Two contact wounds of chest with deposit of powder soot above the wound entrances. **B.** Top view of .22 caliber starter pistol barrel with vent visible.

Thus, some weapons at contact range can cause unusual and characteristic soot patterns. Tentative identification of the general type of weapon sometimes can be made from these patterns.

Distant Gunshot Wounds

In distant wounds, the only marks on the target are those produced by the mechanical action of the bullet in perforating the skin.

Entrance Versus Exit Wounds

Entrance wounds. Most entrance wounds, no matter what the range, are surrounded by a reddish zone of abraded skin—the abrasion ring (Figure 4–16). This is a rim of flattened, abraded epidermis, surrounding the entrance hole.

The abrasion ring occurs when the bullet abrades, or "rubs raw," the edges of the hole as it indents and pierces the skin (Figure 4–16). It is not

Figure 4–16 A. The bullet indents the skin, punching a hole through it and abrading the margins of the entrance wound in the skin. **B.** Typical entrance wound with abrasion ring of margins.

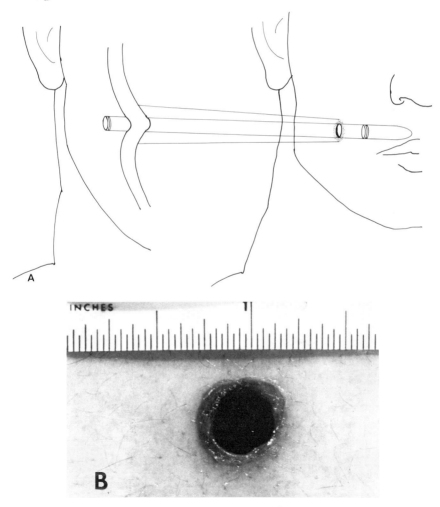

due to the bullet's rotational movement as it goes through the skin, as even the fastest rotating bullet makes only one complete rotation in 8 in. of horizontal travel.

Fresh entrance wounds have an abrasion ring with a moist, fleshy appearance. As the abrasion ring dries out, however, it assumes a more typical and familiar appearance.

The abrasion ring can vary in width, depending on the caliber of the weapon, the angle at which the bullet entered, and the anatomic site of entrance. Entrance wounds in the scalp generally have a wider abrasion ring than those in other parts of the body, possibly due to reinforcement of the scalp by the bone of the skull.

The abrasion ring around an entrance hole can be concentric or eccentric, depending on the angle between the bullet and the skin. A bullet striking perpendicular to the skin should produce a concentric abrasion ring (Figure 4–16). If the bullet penetrates at an oblique angle, the zone of abrasion in the skin will be eccentric, with the zone wider on the side from which the bullet comes (Figure 4–17). This however, assumes that the skin is flat. But people are three-dimensional, with curves, depressions, and projections. Thus, the bullet may be fired perpendicular to the body but strike a projecting surface—for example, the breast—so that an eccentric abrasion ring wound is produced even though the bullet is going straight into the body. Thus, it is never possible to say with certainty in which direction a bullet has traveled through the body from examination of the entrance wound alone.

Figure 4–17 Entrance wound with eccentric abrasion ring due to bullet striking skin at angle. **Arrow** indicates direction of bullet.

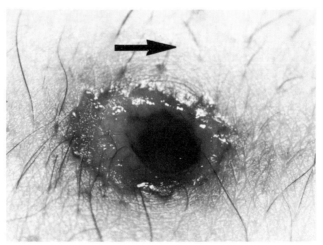

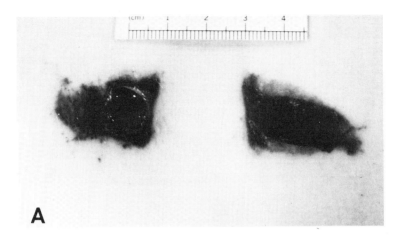

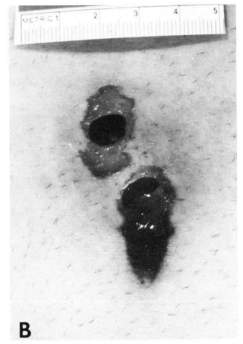

Figure 4−18 A. Two areas of abrasion (compound abrasion ring) due to single bullet as deceased was bent over at time bullet impacted. **B.** Two entrance wounds with markedly different abrasion rings, though trajectory of bullets through body was identical.

Abrasion rings may have very unusual configurations due to the position of the individual when he or she was shot. Thus, in Figure 4−18A, the abrasion ring, besides being markedly eccentric, is divided into two sections. The medial end of each is "squared" off. At the time the deceased was shot, he was bent over with a "depression" between two "rolls" of flesh. The bullet abraded the crest of the two adjacent rolls on entering. The individual shown in Figure 4−18B was crouching when shot. Both bullets followed the same path through the body. Their abrasion rings, however, are markedly different because of the irregular dips and peaks in the skin caused by bending over.

Occasionally an entrance wound will not have an abrasion ring observable either by naked eye or by dissecting microscope. This ring can occur with entrance wounds of the palm or sole, high-velocity centerfire rifle entry wounds, entrance wounds from jacketed or semijacketed handgun bullets (usually of high velocity, such as the .357 Magnum; see Figure 5–19) and re-entry wounds in the axilla and scrotum.

Distant gunshot wounds of the palm and sole differ from wounds of the skin in other areas in that the entrance is usually stellate, with tears 1 to 3 mm in length radiating from the entrance perforation. These wounds typically have no abrasion ring (Figure 4–19).

Wounds from high velocity centerfire rifle bullets often show small splits or tears radiating outward from the edges of the perforation (Figure 7–10). These "micro-tears" usually involve the complete circumference of the entrance wound, though like abrasion rings they may involve only a partial circumference. Although micro-tears are not very noticeable with the naked eye, they are very obvious with the dissecting microscope. Micro-tears are also seen, though rarely, in entrance wounds from partial metal-jacketed .357 Magnum bullets.

There is usually no difficulty determining that an entrance wound without an abrasion ring is truly an entrance. With the exception of palm and sole, these wounds are oval to circular with a punched-out clean appearance totally unlike that of exit wounds. The exception to this are reentry wounds of the axilla, which may be slit-shaped and

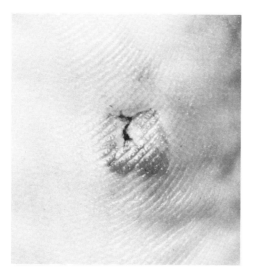

Figure 4–19 Entrance wound of palm without abrasion ring.

resemble exits. Fortunately, these reentry wounds are virtually all penetrating rather than perforating. Thus, one is not often presented with
two "exits," one of which is an entrance.

In rare instances, a circular punched-out entrance without an abrasion ring is associated with an exit that also has a circular punched-out
appearance, leading to confusion as to which wound is the entrance and
which the exit. In such an instance a determination as to which is the
entrance and which the exit from the appearance of the wounds in the
skin alone may not be possible.

In a case seen by the author, the victim had a through-and-through
gunshot wound of the left calf with wounds on the lateral and posterior-
medial surfaces of the calf. Both wounds appeared identical, having a
circular punched-out appearance and no abrasion ring. It was the
author's opinion on examining these wounds that the lateral wound was
the entrance and the posterior-medial wound the exit. An x-ray,
however, showed a fracture of the fibula with bone fragments following
a lateral path, thus indicating that the bullet entered the posterior-
medial aspect of the calf and exited from the lateral aspect (Figure 4–20).

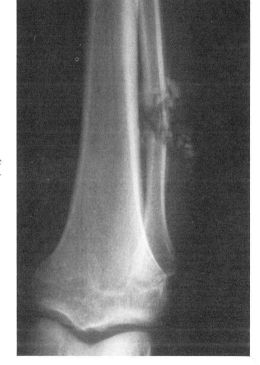

Figure 4–20 X-ray showing fracture
of fibula, with bone fragments following lateral path.

Because he still had doubts concerning this interpretation, the fibula and the bulk of the bone fragments were removed from the leg. When the bone was reassembled from the fragments, it was obvious that the x-ray was correct; the entrance in the leg was posterior-medial and the exit was lateral.

Microscopic sections through a gunshot wound of entrance show a progressive increase in alteration of the epithelium and dermis as one proceeds from the periphery of the abrasion ring to the margin of the perforation. The most peripheral margin of the abrasion ring shows a zone of compressed, deformed cells many of which show nuclear "streaming." As one proceeds centrally, there is loss of superficial cellular layers so that only the rete pegs remain adjacent to the perforation.[2] Such epithelial changes occur in contact, near contact, intermediate and distant wounds. In contact and near-contact wounds, black amorphous material probably representing soot is found in the abrasion zone and wound track. Positive identification of this material as soot cannot be made microscopically.

In intermediate-range wounds, the skin adjacent to the perforation will show embedded grains of powder. The grains of powder are for the most part embedded in the epidermis. Ball powder and occasionally flake may perforate the epidermis and come to rest in the upper dermis. Although ball powder quite commonly penetrates the dermis, flake powder for the most part bounces off the skin. Occasionally, fragments or whole flakes of powder become imbedded in the skin and are seen projecting from the surface. The type of flake powder that can penetrate into the dermis consists of small, thick disks unlike the more common larger thin disks.

There is no histologic method of proving that the black amorphous material seen embedded in skin or along a wound track is definitely powder. Nitrate and nitrite stains are not specific. Identification of a wound as contact or intermediate should be done not histologically, but with either the naked eye or a dissecting microscope. Positive identification of a material as powder can usually be made in accordance with the shape of the powder grains if they are intact. If they are partially burned and there is no definite shape, the material can be analyzed by thin-layer chromatography to identify the material positively as powder.[3] A cruder test involves touching what appears to be a powder grain with a red-hot probe. This will cause the powder to burn.

The dermis underneath the abrasion ring and adjacent to the wound track shows alterations in the collagen. These alterations have been ascribed to the thermal effects of hot gases in close range wounds and the thermal effects of a "hot bullet" in distant wounds.[2] The collagen fibers stain from deep red to gray-blue and appear swollen and homogeneous. Although the changes in collagen in contact and near-contact wounds may be due to heat, the changes in intermediate- and distant range wounds are not. Rather, the changes are due to the mechanical action of the bullet stretching the epidermis and dermis as it pushes its way through the skin. Bullets are never "red-hot." In fact, a bullet never gets hot enough to sterilize itself. This fact has been proved in experiments in which bullets were dipped in a bacterial culture, fired, and recovered; the bacteria was then plated from the fired bullet.[4,5]

In the late nineteenth century, Von Beck conducted experiments to determine the amount of heat imparted to both lead bullets of large caliber and jacketed .30-caliber rifle bullets.[5] He found that the temperature of a lead bullet of .45 caliber when recovered was 69° C, whereas that of a steel jacketed .30-caliber bullet was 78° C and that of a copper-jacketed .30-caliber rifle bullet was 110° C. The missiles were handled by the fingers and never possessed sufficient heat to burn skin.

Exit Wounds. Exit wounds, whether they are the result of contact, intermediate, or distant firing, all have the same general characteristics. They are typically larger and more irregular than entrance wounds and, with rare exceptions, do not possess an abrasion ring. Exit wounds can be stellate, slitlike, crescent, circular, or completely irregular (Figure 4–21). Stellate exit wounds can be seen in the scalp and may be confused with contact wounds.

The larger but more irregular nature of exit wounds is due to two factors. First, the spin that stabilized the bullet in the air is not effective in tissue because of the greater density of the tissue. Thus, as the missile travels through the body, its natural yaw is accentuated; if it travels through enough tissue it will eventually tumble end over end. Second, the bullet may be deformed in its passage through the body. Both factors result in the presentation of a larger area of bullet at the site of exit, with resultant larger and more irregular exit wounds. That deformation and tumbling of the bullet are the reasons why the exit wound is usually larger and more irregular than the entrance was proved by a number of experiments in which steel balls were fired through animals at high velocities.[6] These balls were not deformed by the tissue, and because of their configuration they could not tumble. The exit wounds produced were smaller than the entrance wounds because the missiles had less energy at the time of exit compared to when they entered the body.

In unusual circumstances, exit wounds will have abraded margins (Figure 4–22). These are called shored exit wounds. In such wounds the skin is reinforced, or "shored," by a firm surface at the instant the bullet exits. Thus, individuals shot while lying on the floor, leaning against a wall, or sitting back in a chair may have shored exit wounds. As it exits, the bullet everts the skin, with the everted margin impacting against the wall, floor, or back of a chair, thus being abraded or "rubbed

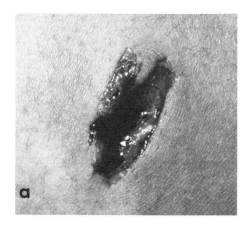

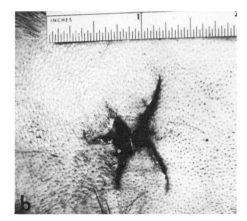

Figure 4–21 a–c. Exit wounds.

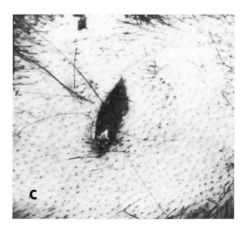

raw." Shored exit wounds can also occur from tight supportive garments, such as girdles, brassieres, and belts, as well as from tight clothing.

Occasionally, a bullet traveling through the body will lose most of its forward velocity such that, while it may have sufficient velocity to create an exit wound, any resistance to its exiting the body by either an overlying garment or an object such as a seat back or wall will prevent the bullet from exiting. The "exit," however, may show shoring of its edges due to impaction with the object that prevented the bullet from exiting.

Fresh shored wounds have a moist succulent appearance. The pattern of the material overlying the shored exit may be imprinted on the edges of the wound. Shored wounds may have very wide abrasion collars and when dry may simulate contact wounds.

The size and the shape of the exit wound are dependent to a certain degree on the location of the exit. In lax skin, the exit wounds tend to be small and slit-shaped. In contrast, where the skin is stretched tightly across a bony surface—e.g., the scalp—exit wounds tend to be larger and more irregular, often with a stellate configuration.

Although exit wounds are typically larger than entrance wounds, it is possible for an exit to be smaller than the entrance and in fact smaller in diameter than the bullet. The last phenomenon is due to the elastic nature of the skin. Another significant fact to be remembered concerning exit wounds is that the shape of an exit wound does not correlate with the type of bullet used, e.g., roundnose, hollow-point, and so forth.

Figure 4–22 Shored exit.

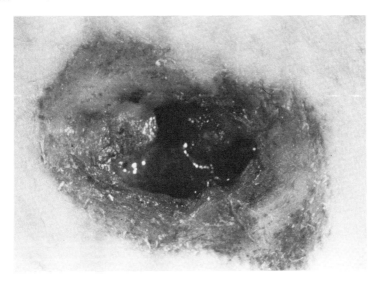

If one examines the whole spectrum of incomplete, partial, and complete exit wounds, one sees a progression in their development. First is the bullet lodged subcutaneously without disruption of the overlying skin. Next is the incomplete exit, consisting of one or two small slit-like lacerations in the skin with the bullet still in the underlying subcutaneous tissue. These lacerations do not communicate directly with the bullet or wound tract. They are apparently "tears" in the skin produced by eversion of the skin as the bullet attempts to exit. The elastic limit of the skin is exceeded, and the skin tears. The paired lacerations may represent the opposite ends of a bullet attempting to exit sideways. Next is the bullet that breaks the skin but cannot exit and rebounds back into the wound because of the elasticity of the skin. The exit may or may not be shored. The missile had sufficient velocity to cause the exit but insufficient velocity to leave the body. Then comes the bullet that exits, hits a hard surface and is deflected back into the exit wound (Figure 4–23). Such exits are virtually always shored exits. Last is the complete exit.

A common and seemingly logical assumption that is not always true is that a bullet on exiting the body will continue in a straight path that is a continuation of the path the bullet had in the body. As a bullet passes through the body, however, it becomes unstable and its yaw increases. If the path is sufficiently long, the bullet will eventually tumble end over end. Thus, an exiting bullet may be wildly yawing or even tumbling. In such an instance, as the bullet moves farther from the exit, the probability rises that the bullet will drift off at an angle from its projected trajectory. If in passing through the body the bullet undergoes deformation, this may also contribute to the tendency of the bullet to wobble or tumble after exiting. Knowledge of this phenomenon is important in

Figure 4–23 Incising the skin lateral to the shored exit reveals the bullet to be present.

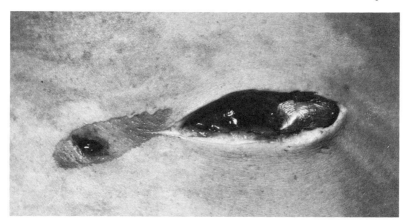

trying to reconstruct the shooting scene. Thus, with bullets embedded in a wall, one can accurately and confidently determine their point of origin—i.e., where they were fired from—by projecting backward along their trajectory only if these bullets have not passed through a body.

Atypical Entrances

A graze wound is one in which a bullet strikes the skin at a shallow angle, producing an elongated area of abrasion without actual perforation or tearing of the skin (Figure 4−24). In a tangential wound, the injury extends down through to the subcutaneous tissue (Figure 4−25). The skin is torn, or "lacerated," by the bullet.

In both graze and tangential wounds, it may be very difficult to tell the direction in which the bullet was traveling when it produced the wound. Examination of the two ends of a tangential wound will often but not always reveal the entrance end to have a partially abraded margin, i.e., a cap of abraded tissue, while the exit end will be split. Tears along the margin of a tangential wound point in the direction the bullet moved (Figure 4−25).

Superficial perforating wounds are shallow through-and-through wounds in which the entrance and exit are close together. They may be difficult to interpret. The entrance will usually have a complete but

Figure 4−24 Graze wound. **Arrow** indicates direction of bullet.

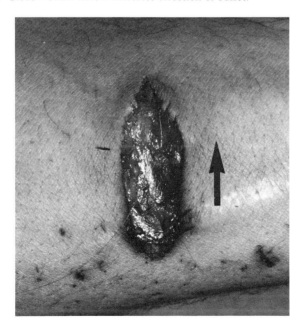

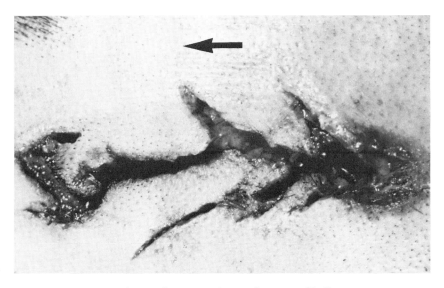

Figure 4−25 Tangential wound. **Arrow** indicates direction of bullet.

eccentric abrasion ring, whereas the exit will have abrasion of only a portion of the circumference. The abrasion at the exit points the way the bullet was moving; the eccentric abrasion of the entrance, the way the bullet was coming from.

Reentry wounds occur when a bullet has passed through one part of the body and then reentered another part. Most commonly, this occurs when a bullet perforates an arm and enters the thorax. The reentry wound is usually characterized by a wide, irregular abrasion ring and a large irregular entrance hole whose edges are ragged (Figure 4−26).

Reentry wounds of the axilla caused by missiles that have passed through the arm often have a very atypical appearance. Such wounds may be oval to slit-shaped with a very thin or even absent abrasion ring (Figure 4−27). They often so nearly resemble a wound of exit rather than entrance that they cannot be differentiated from an exit wound if considered alone.

Associated with a reentry wound of the thorax may be shoring of the exit site in the upper extremity. This occurs when the arm was against the chest at the time the bullet perforated the arm and entered the chest. The chest "shores up" the exit. Irregular abrasions may also be present on the chest around a reentry wound (Figure 4−28). These shored entrance wounds are apparently due to skin around the reentry site slapping against the arm that was against the chest.

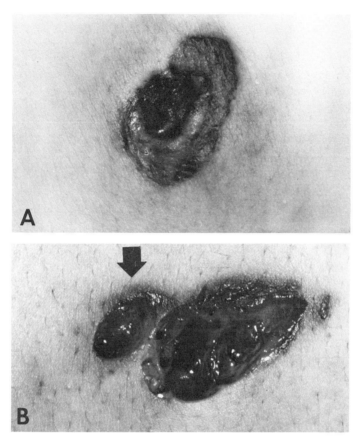

Figure 4–26 A. Reentry wound with wide irregular abrasion ring and large irregular entrance hole. **B.** Primary entrance wound (as indicated by **arrow**) adjacent to large irregular reentry wound.

Figure 4–27 Exit and reentry wound (indicated by **arrow**) of axilla.

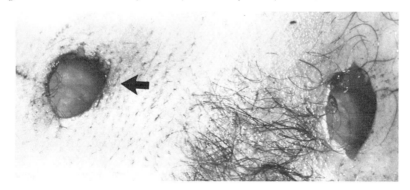

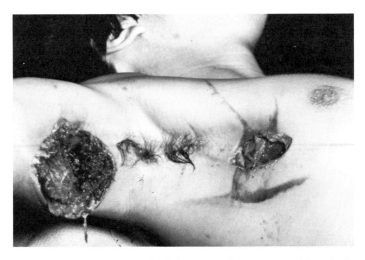

Figure 4–28 Irregular abrasions of side of chest around reentry wound from high-velocity bullet that exited arm.

Intermediate Targets

Passage of a bullet or pellets through an intermediate object before striking a victim can result in alteration in the appearance of the wound or the wounds incurred. In the case of shotgun pellets, the object will cause the pattern to "open up" sooner than it would have otherwise. The fact that the pellets passed through an intermediate target has to be taken into account when conducting range determinations based on the size of the pellet pattern on the body. Increased dispersion of pellets by an intermediate object can lead to the conclusion that the individual was shot at a greater range than he or she actually was if the intermediate target is not taken into account.

In passing through an object, a bullet may propel fragments of the object outward from the bullet path. If the victim is close to the object, these fragments may strike the individual, embedding themselves in the clothes and skin and producing pseudo-powder tattoo marks in the latter instance. The author has seen fragments of wood from doors and wire from screens embedded in the skin (Figure 4–29). With wire screens, the pattern of the wire may also be imprinted on the tip of the bullet. In lead or lead-tipped bullets that have passed through glass, glass fragments may be embedded in the tip of the bullet; these can be seen with a dissecting microscope.

The gyroscopic spin that stabilizes a bullet as it travels through the air is insufficient to stabilize the bullet as it passes through a solid object. Because of this, the bullet' yaw is accentuated and the bullet may

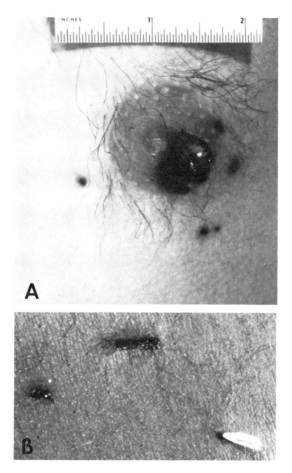

Figure 4–29 A, B. Wood fragment marks.

wobble violently. In addition, the bullet may be deformed in its passage through the object. As a result of these factors, when the bullet does strike the victim, the entry wound is usually atypical (Figure 4–30). The perforation will be larger and more irregular with ragged margins. The surrounding abrasion ring will be irregular and wider.

Passage of a semijacketed bullet through an intermediate target can result in separation of the jacket and the core. Thornton found that this occurred in half the instances when a .38 Special jacketed hollow-point bullet passed through a tempered-glass automobile window.[7]

In one of the author's cases, a .223 semijacketed soft-point bullet was fired through a wood door. On passing through the wood, the jacket and

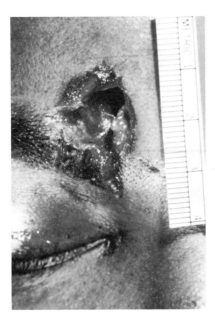

Figure 4−30 Irregular entrance wound from .38-caliber bullet that passed through windshield.

core separated with a 16-gr fragment of jacket penetrating into the brain of a woman, killing her.

The most common intermediate targets seen in forensic medicine are the upper extremities, doors, and car windows. As previously stated, in about half the instances when a semijacketed bullet passes through the tempered glass window of a car, there will be jacket and core separation. The core, because of its greater mass, tends to continue the original trajectory, retaining most of the impact velocity and thus can readily penetrate the victim. The jacket, because of its light weight, rapidly loses velocity and usually flies off at an angle from the path of the core. If the jacket does hit the victim, it can bounce off or penetrate. Occasionally both jacket and core will penetrate, and the victim will have two entry wounds from one bullet (Figure 4−31). The jacket usually does not penetrate the body to any significant degree with handgun bullets.

Rarely, the bullet on hitting glass may completely disintegrate, showering the individual with fragments of lead, jacket, and glass. This is shown in Figure 4−32, where the individual was shot through the side window of a car by a police officer using 110-gr semijacketed hollow-point ammunition.

In the past 2 years, the author has seen three individuals shot through car doors with centerfire rifles. The caliber of the weapon was .30-30 in two instances and .223 in the third. The .30-30 ammunition was hunting, whereas that of the .223 was full metal-jacketed. On passing through the metal door, all three bullets broke up, inflicting multiple

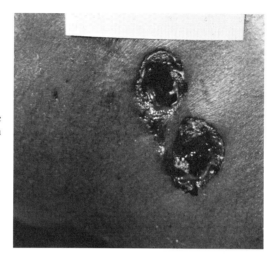

Figure 4–31 Separate entrance wounds of jacket and core from same bullet.

Figure 4–32 Fragment wounds of left side of chest due to disintegration of bullet and side window of car.

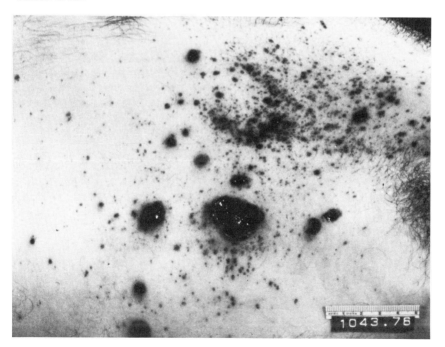

entry wounds on the victims. All the wounds were penetrating rather than perforating. In all three instances, a plug of steel from the car door was recovered from the body. This plug of metal was propelled ahead of the bullet as it passed through the door. (See Chapter 7.)

Semijacketed bullets passing through hands or arms before impacting the body usually do not undergo separation of the jacket and core. The reentry wound in the body, however, is almost invariably large and irregular with a widely abraded and irregular abrasion ring.

In his paper on the effects of tempered glass on bullet trajectory, Thornton has made some other observations.[7] Tempered-glass automobile windows are usually angled inward. On tests with such glass at 20 degrees to the vertical plane, hollow-point ammunition showed an average deflection of 16 degrees from the original trajectory (range, 13.2 to 19.9 degrees), with separation of the jacket from the core in half the tests. Lead bullets showed an average 10.7 degree deflection.

Pseudo-Powder Tattooing

Missile fragments, fragments from intermediate targets, postmortem insect bites, hemorrhage into hair follicles, and medical manipulation of a wound may all produce marks on the skin surrounding a gunshot wound which simulate powder tattoo marks. Differentiation of such artifacts from powder tattooing is usually but not always relatively easy.

The pseudo-tattoo marks most likely to cause confusion with powder tattooing are those produced by fragments of intermediate targets such as glass, wood or rock, or fragments of a bullet that has broken up after striking a hard surface. If a bullet passes through a sheet of glass, pseudo-tattoo marks may be produced by the fragments of the glass. This is seen most commonly in individuals seated in automobiles and shot through a side window that is made of tempered glass. The glass marks on the skin tend to be larger and more irregular with greater variation in size when compared with powder tattoo marks (Figure 4–33). They are also relatively more scant. Fragments of glass may be found embedded in the skin at these sites or adherent to the clothing. Examination of the recovered bullet with a dissecting microscope may reveal minute fragments of glass embedded in the tip.

Pseudo-tattooing can also be produced by fragments of the plastic casing used to enclose the shot in handgun shot cartridges. The fragment marks are usually very large and irregular (Figure 10–15).

High-velocity bullets striking glass may break up, showering the individual not only with glass fragments but also with fragments of lead from the core and metal jacketing. Thus, the pseudo-tattooing marks may be due not only to the glass but to the fragments of the bullet.

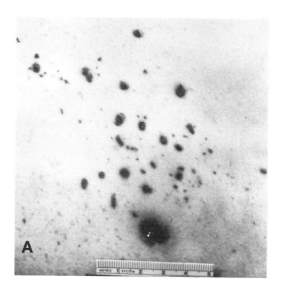

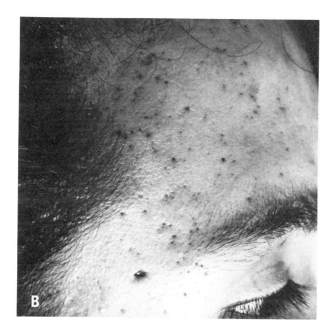

Figure 4–33 A. Irregular stippling of skin due to fragments of glass. **B.** Fine stipple marks due to fragments of glass.

A bullet ricocheting off a hard surface may result in the production of secondary fragments that may produce pseudo-powder tattooing of the skin. These marks can be due to fragments of wood or stone from the surface from which the bullet ricocheted or to metal fragments from the bullet itself. Such markings are usually larger, more irregular, and considerably more sparse than true powder tattoo marks. Fragments of wood or metal often will be found embedded in or adjacent to these markings. Bullets passing through wire screens may propel fragments of wire into the skin.

Occasionally individuals construct crude silencers, using steel wool as the packing material in the silencer. On firing the weapon, fragments of the steel wool may be projected out the end of the silencer, embedding themselves in the skin around the entrance. These markings are relatively sparse and fragments of the steel wool often can be found embedded in the skin.

Pseudo-tattoo marks may be produced in shotgun wounds by the packing used in some buckshot and birdshot loads. This will be discussed in more detail in Chapter 8.

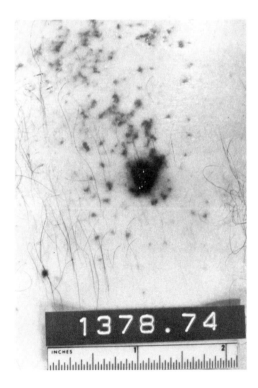

Figure 4–34 Postmortem insect bites around gunshot wound of entrance.

Postmortem insect activity may produce lesions on the skin that superficially resemble powder tattooing (Figure 4–34). Postmortem insect bites, however, are larger and more irregular and usually have a dry, yellow color to them. They often are arranged in a linear pattern, indicating the path of the insects across the body. Fresh wounds may ooze serosanguineous fluid that on drying forms a dark brown or black crust that may cause the insect bites more closely to resemble powder tattoo marks.

Gunshot wounds in hairy areas may result in hemorrhage in hair follicles. If the hair is shaved from the area of the wound, a cursory examination of the skin surrounding the entrance may cause the examiner to interpret the hemorrhage in the follicles as punctate powder tattoo marks (Figure 4–35). Closer examination, however, will reveal the true nature of the markings.

Occasionally surgical manipulation of a wound may produce markings that simulate powder tattoo marks. In the case illustrated, the wound was sutured closed by a surgeon (Figure 4–35). When the sutures were removed, the needle puncture marks were interpreted by a number of individuals as powder tattoo marks.

One of the more unusual cases of pseudo-powder tattooing encountered by the author involved a young boy who after shooting himself in the head survived a short time at a hospital. At autopsy, "tattoo marks" were seen on the flexor surface of the left forearm. Because the weapon was a bolt-action rifle, such tattooing could not have occurred. Subsequent investigation revealed that the deceased had had a tourniquet

Figure 4–35 Suture marks simulating powder tattoo marks.

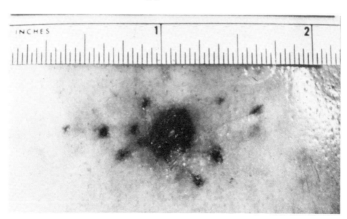

placed on his arm when seen in the emergency room. This tourniquet was never removed. Close examination of the markings on the skin, originally interpreted as tattoo marks, revealed them to be petechiae.

Pseudo-Soot

Just as various materials and body reactions can simulate powder tattooing, so can one have simulation of powder soot. There is usually no problem differentiating an oily material such as grease from soot. Problems can arise with material such as fingerprint dusting powder which may be deposited on the body at the scene.

One case that initially caused a problem involved an individual shot in the left chest just above the pocket of his shirt. On examination there appeared to be a large quantity of soot around the bullet hole. Witnesses at the scene, however, said that the deceased had been shot from several feet away. Subsequently it was discovered that the deceased habitually carried lead pencils in the pocket with the points directed upward. As he moved about, the graphite wiped off the tips of the pencils onto the shirt. When the bullet was fired through this area, the graphite was interpreted mistakenly as soot.

Another case that caused difficulty involved an individual shot at multiple times with a high-velocity rifle while lying on an asphalt parking lot. The bullets striking the asphalt reduced some of it to a fine black powder that coated the clothing and body. Other bullets then entered the body in these areas. The blackening from the asphalt was mistaken initially as powder soot associated with the gunshot wounds.

Subcutaneous hemorrhage may have a purple-black appearance and on superficial examination may appear to be soot. More commonly, cases are seen in which a gunshot wound has dried out, giving the edges a black appearance. An inexperienced pathologist may interpret this as soot and searing. Use of a dissecting microscope should differentiate soot from artifact. If there is any doubt as to the nature of the entrance, it should be excised and submitted for Energy Dispersive X-Ray (EDX) analysis. Alternatively, the suspected black deposit around an entrance wound can be swabbed with moistened (nitric acid) cotton swabs, and these can be analyzed by flameless atomic absorption. The soot itself is of course carbon and nonspecific, but primer residues (lead, antimony, and barium) will accompany the soot and can be detected in the sooty deposit.

Ricochet Bullets

For both solid surfaces and water there is a critical angle of impact (incidence) below which a bullet striking the surface usually will ricochet rather than penetrate. Bullets ricocheting off water invariably ricochet at angles greater than the impact angle, typically 2 to 3 times the impact angle.[8] This is in contrast to that for solid surfaces, where the angle of ricochet is usually smaller than the impact angle.[9]

Table 4–1 gives the approximate critical angle for some representative cartridges and bullet types in regard to ricocheting off water.[8] The critical angles listed are those at which the particular bullet just began to ricochet. As one can see, the critical angles are small (3 to 8 degrees). At an impact angle of 15 degrees, all the listed projectiles penetrated water. Not surprisingly, Haag found that bullets lose their gyroscopic stability after ricocheting from water.

Bullets ricocheting off solid surfaces usually ricochet at angles smaller than the impact angle.[9] Such bullets are unstable and will tumble. Table 4–2 gives the average ricochet angle for a number of cartridges whose bullets struck smooth stone at incident angles of 10, 20, and 30 degrees. In only one instance was the ricochet angle greater than the incident angle. This involved a full metal-jacketed M-1 carbine bullet. Haag believes that this was due to disintegration of the surface at the impact site and that the bullet actually departed from a surface that was dissimilar both in texture and in plane from the original one.

In addition to the tests shown in Table 4–2, Haag conducted some test firings on smooth, dry desert sand, using .30 carbine and .38 Special rounds.[9] Firings were at 20, 30, and 45 degrees. There was no appreciable ricochet for any of these.

Table 4–1 Approximate Critical Angles for Various Cartridges and Bullet Types: Water

Caliber	Bullet	Approximate critical angle (degrees)
.22 Short	29 gr solid point	8
	27-gr hollow-point	5
.22 Long rifle	40-gr hollow-point	7
	37-gr hollow-point	5
.38 Special	158-gr lead roundnose	6
	125-gr jacketed hollow-point	6
.380 Auto	90-gr full metal-jacket	7
.222 Remington	50-gr jacketed soft-point	3
.30 MI Carbine	110-gr full metal-jacket	5
.30-06	150-gr full metal-jacket	7

Source: Modified from Haag, reference 8.

Table 4-2 Average Richochet Angles on Smooth Stone at Impact Angles of 10°, 20°, and 30°

Caliber	Bullet[a]	Average ricochet angle (degrees) at impact angle of		
		10°	20°	30°
.22 Short	29 gr RN	1.04	1.58	1.88
	27 gr HP	0.99	1.56	1.26
.22 LR	40 gr RN	1.33	0.94	1.22
	36 gr HP	1.30	1.68	1.19
.38 Special	158 gr RN	—	0.86	1.38
	1.30 gr FMJ	—	—	2.48
.30 MI carbine	110 gr FMJ	1[b]	7.32[c]	27.7[c]
6.5 × 55	156 gr FMJ	1.6	—	—
	100 gr JHP	2	—	—

Source: Modified from Haag, reference 9.

[a] RN = lead roundnose; HP = lead hollow-point; FMJ = full metal-jacket; JHP = jacketed hollow-point.
[b] Bullet produced small crater.
[c] Bullet severely cratered stone.

Wounds of entrance produced by bullets ricocheting off hard surfaces tend to be larger and more irregular in shape than the round or oval-shaped wounds of entrance from an undeformed bullet. The edges of the entrance hole are usually ragged, with the surrounding zone of abraded skin large and irregular. The wounds produced are penetrating rather than perforating. There are two reasons. First, the bullet loses a significant amount of its velocity just by ricocheting off a hard surface (10 to 20% of impact velocity)[10]; second, the ricocheting bullet is deformed and rendered unstable before entering the body. Thus, when it does enter, it almost immediately tumbles end over end, losing all its velocity and kinetic energy in a short distance. In the case of lead bullets, the ricochet bullet when recovered from the body, has a flattened, mirror-like surface on one side (Figure 4-36). It is not uncommon to have the weave pattern of the clothing the deceased was wearing imprinted on one side of the bullet, as the bullet often will enter the body sideways. The weave pattern may also be on the base of the bullet, as the bullet may have entered backward. In Figure 4-36 the bullet ricocheted off a steel rail, passed through a screen door, and then struck the deceased. The pattern of the screen is on one side of the bullet.

Partial metal-jacketed bullets usually break up on striking a hard object peppering the body with fragments of jacket and lead core (Figure 4-37). These fragments are usually found embedded in or just beneath the skin.

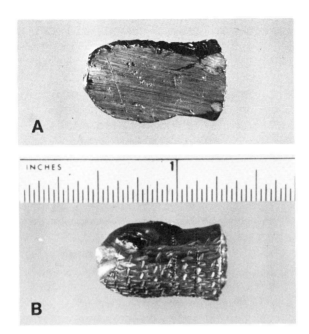

Figure 4–36 Ricochet lead bullet with mirror-like surface on one side and imprint of screen on other side.

Full metal-jacketed bullets can ricochet. The bullet may be flattened on one surface, with the jacket on occasion partly or completely stripped from the core, or it may be pancaked. The weave imprint of cloth may be present on the lead base or exposed core of such bullets.

A ricochet lead bullet should be suspected when an irregular wound of entrance is found in conjunction with shallow penetration of the body and recovery of a bullet with a flattened, smooth surface on one side. Shallow penetration of the body by a nonricocheting lead bullet that on recovery is flattened on one surface occurs if the bullet enters the body and strikes a large bone, flattening itself while ricocheting off the bone, i.e., an internal ricochet. Such internal ricochets almost invariably involve small-caliber low-velocity lead bullets, such as the .22 rimfire and a large, heavy bone such as the femur or humerus. The entrance in the skin will have a normal wound appearance. A nonricocheting full metal-jacketed bullet may strike a heavy bone such as the femur and either pancake or fragment. The jacket will be squeezed together and most of the lead core will be squeezed out the base. The bone may or may not be fractured. The author has seen this phenomenon in calibers from .25 to .45.

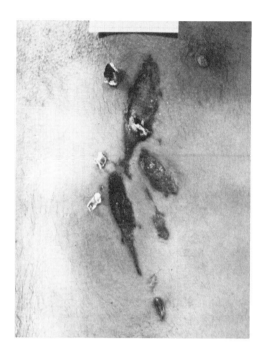

Figure 4-37 Fragment wounds of chest due to partial metal jacketed bullet that disintegrated on striking ground.

If an individual was close to the surface off which the bullet ricocheted, fragments of material from the surface as well as fragments of bullet torn off at the time of ricochet may impact around the wound of entrance, producing secondary missile wounds. These wounds are usually of a minor significance in that the fragments are usually of insufficient mass and velocity to cause any serious harm. The marks produced may on occasion be confused with powder tattoo marks. The marks, however, are larger and more irregular in shape than powder tattoo marks.

Occasionally a bullet that exits a body will strike a hard surface, flatten out, and rebound back into the clothing. The author has seen this in three instances. In two cases the individuals were leaning against concrete walls, and in the third the individual was lying on a concrete floor. The bullets were pancaked, having a thickness of less than a nickel.

Bone

Bone is a specialized form of dense connective tissue; it is composed of calcium salts embedded in a matrix of collagenous fibers. For a bullet to enter the surface of bone, a minimum velocity of 200 ft/sec is necessary.[11,12] Once penetration has been effected, the bullet's remaining velocity operates to effect deeper penetration in direct proportion to the square of the velocity and the sectional density of the bullet. As the bullet penetrates bone, it fragments the bone, creating a temporary cavity. The fragments initially are propelled toward the periphery of the cavity. As undulation of the cavity occurs, the fragments return to the center, where the majority remain.[12] A number of bony fragments, however, move forward in the direction of the bullet. These act as secondary missiles, causing further injury.

The direction in which the bullet was traveling when it perforated a bone can be determined by the appearance of the wound in the bone. When a bullet perforates bone, it bevels out the bone in the direction in which it is traveling. The entrance in the bone has a round to oval, sharp-edged, "punched-out" appearance (Figure 4–38b). The opposite surface of the bone—i.e., the exit side—is excavated in a conelike manner (Figure 4–38c). This difference in appearance of entrance and exit wounds is best seen in the flat bone of skull. As the bullet enters the skull, it creates a round to oval sharp-edged hole in the outer table of the skull, with a large, beveled-out hole on the inner table. When the bullet exits the cranial cavity, the inner table is the entrance surface and the outer table becomes the exit surface with the conelike exit wound.

Chips of bone can flake off the edge of an entrance defect, producing an effect resembling beveling. Such chipping of the edge of the wound of entrance is very superficial and usually does not lead to confusion with an exit hole, because it is not nearly as marked as the beveled surface. Rare exceptions do occur.

Coe has collected a number of cases (all but one involving contact wounds) that show partial or complete beveling of the outer table of bone at the entrance sites.[13] The beveling is of such a degree that it easily could be ascribed to an exiting bullet. Such entrances should not be confused with exits, as examination will show beveling of both the inner and the outer tables.

Differentiation of entrance versus exit often is not possible in the case of paper-thin bones such as the orbital plates or the temporal bones of children. In both instances the bone is too thin for creation of the funnel-shaped wound tract that makes differentiation of entrance versus exit possible.

When a bullet perforates bone, it often leaves a thin deposit of lead on the edges of the entrance hole. This thin gray rim should not be confused with the wider zone of powder blackening seen in contact wounds overlying bone. Examination of the entrance with a dissecting microscope will show the gray rim to consist of fragments of lead.

Teeth, like bone, show a sharp-edged, punched-out appearance on the entrance surface and beveling of the exit surface when a bullet perforates them.

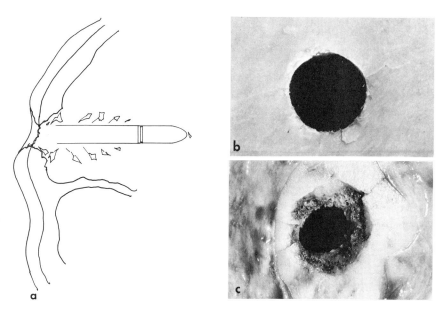

Figure 4–38 a. Bullet perforating bone. **b.** Entrance in bone. **c.** Exit in bone.

Bullet Wounds of the Skull

Tangential wounds of the skull have classically been called "gutter wounds."[14] In first-degree gutter wounds only the outer table of the skull is grooved by the bullet, with resultant carrying away of small bone fragments. In second-degree wounds pressure waves generated by the bullet fracture the inner table. In third-degree wounds the bullet perforates the skull in the center of the tangential wound. The outer table is fragmented, and there are depressed fragments of the internal table if not comminution and pulverization of both tables in the center of the wound track. After third-degree wounds come "superficial perforating wounds." Here there is production of separate entrance and exit wounds in the bone.

A low-velocity bullet may strike the skull at a shallow angle such that it does not penetrate but rather flattens out, forming a thin oval lead disk. The bullet may then slide along the surface of the skull beneath the scalp. This usually occurs with .22 Short bullets.

A bullet striking the skull at a shallow angle may produce a punched-out oval defect in the skull without the bullet actually entering the cranial cavity. The bullet may flatten out and be recovered from beneath the scalp or exit. The fragments of bone may be driven into the brain and can cause death.

Bullets striking the skull at a shallow angle may split into two fragments as they perforate the bone, with one fragment exiting from the opposite end of the entrance hole in the bone and the other fragment entering the cranial cavity. This creates in the skull a keyhole-shaped wound consisting of a combined wound of entrance and exit (Figure 4–39).[15] One end of this keyhole wound will have the sharp edges typical of a wound of entrance, whereas the other end will have the external beveling of a wound of exit.

Bullet wounds of the head may produce cerebral injury and death without entrance into the cranial cavity. Thus, the author has seen a case of a 65-year-old white male who shot himself in the ear with a .32 revolver. The bullet traveled through the petrous bone before coming to rest adjacent to the sella turcica. Although the bullet caused extensive comminuted fractures of the petrous bone, it did not enter the cranial cavity. The dura overlying the petrous bone was intact. Examination of the brain revealed extensive contusions of the ventral surface of the temporal lobe overlying the bone. No lacerations of the brain were present.

The production of secondary fractures of the skull in gunshot wounds of the head is dependent on two factors: the range at the time of discharge and the kinetic energy possessed by the bullet. The most common sites for secondary skull fractures are the paper-thin orbital plates. These are extremely sensitive to a sudden increase in intracranial pressure such as that produced by a bullet entering the cranial cavity.

Secondary fractures are very common in contact wounds of the head. This is due to the gas produced by discharge entering the cranial cavity, expanding, and contributing to the stress placed on the boney chamber by the temporary cavity. The more gas produced, the more that enters the skull and the more likely it is that the fractures will be produced. An extreme example of this is provided by contact wounds from a centerfire rifle or shotgun. These weapons cause explosive wounds of the head, with large fragments of bone and brain typically being blown from the head.

In distant wounds, gas plays no part in the production of fractures. These fractures are produced by the pressure built up in the skull as a result of temporary cavity formation. The size of this cavity is proportional to the amount of kinetic energy lost by the bullet in its passage through the head. The greater the amount of kinetic energy lost, the larger the cavity; the larger the cavity, the greater the pressure produced on the walls of the cranial chamber and the more likely a fracture is to occur. Thus, secondary skull fractures are rare with wounds inflicted by a low-energy .22 Short cartridge but are the rule with wounds from a centerfire rifle. Although secondary skull fractures are uncommon with

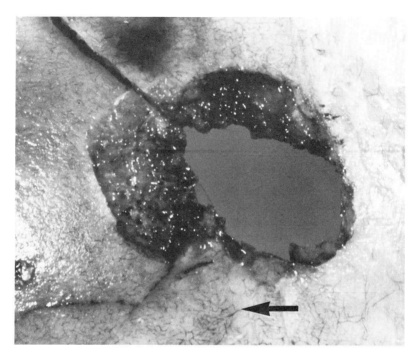

Figure 4–39 Keyhole wound of bone. **Arrow** indicates path of bullet.

.22 Short ammunition (even in contact wounds), .22 Long rifle cartridges usually produce secondary fractures in contact wounds and not uncommonly in distant wounds. With the .22 Short cartridge, fractures are usually if not invariably limited to the orbital plates; with the .22 Long Rifles cartridge, fractures not only of the orbital plates but the cranial vault can occur.

The fact that the fractures in a skull are due to temporary cavity formation was demonstrated by a series of experiments with skulls.[11] When skulls were empty, the bullets "drilled" neat entrances and exits without any fractures. When the skulls were filled with gelatin to simulate the brain, massive secondary skull fractures were produced.

On occasion one will be presented with what initially appears to be a perforating gunshot wound of the head but in fact is a penetrating wound. There will be both an entrance and an "exit" wound in the scalp. The autopsy reveals the bullet still to be in the head. What happens is that the bullet, after entering the head and perforating the brain, strikes the opposite side of the skull with sufficient force to fracture it and propel a piece of bone out through the scalp. The bullet itself has insufficient velocity to exit the head. In a variation of this involving semijacketed ammunition, the lead core exits while the copper jacket remains. Rarely, the jacket exits and the core remains. This again points out the need for x-rays in all gunshot wounds of the head.

Caliber Determination from Entrance Wounds

The caliber of the bullet that caused an entrance wound cannot be determined by the diameter of the entrance. A .38-caliber bullet can produce a hole having the diameter of a .32 caliber bullet and vice versa. The size of the hole is due not only to the diameter of the bullet but also to the elasticity of the skin and the location of the wound. An entrance wound in an area where the skin is tightly stretched will have a diameter different from that of a wound in an area where the skin is lax. Bullet wounds in areas where the skin lies in folds or creases may be slit-shaped.

Bullet Wipe

Bullet holes of entrance in the skin on occasion have a gray coloration to the abrasion ring. This gray rim around the entrance is very common and more prominent in clothing, where it is called "bullet wipe" (see Chapter 12). It should not be confused with powder soot from a contact wound. Bullet wipe has been said to be characteristic of revolver bullets, but it may be produced by full metal jacketed automatic pistol bullets as well. Bullet wipe consists principally of soot deposited on the surface of the bullet as it moves down the barrel. In the case of revolver bullets, some of this material may be lubricant as well.

References

1. Barnes, F.C., Helson, R.A. An empirical study of gunpowder residue patterns. J. Forensic Sci. 19(3): 448–462, 1974.
2. Adelson, L. A microscopic study of dermal gunshot wounds. Am. J. Clin. Pathol. 35: 393, 1961.
3. Peak, S.A. A thin-layer chromatographic procedure for confirming the presence and identity of smokeless powder flakes. J. Forensic Sci. 25(3): 679–681, 1980.
4. Thoresby, F.P., Darlow, H.M. The mechanisms of primary infection of bullet wounds. Br. J. Surg. 54: 359–361, 1967.
5. Von Beck, B. Cited by La Garde, L.A. Can a septic bullet infect a gunshot wound? N.Y. Med. J. 56: 458–464, 1892.
6. Light, F.W. Gunshot wounds of entrance and exit in experimental animals. J. Trauma 3(2): 120–128, 1963.

7. Thorton, J. The effects of tempered glass on bullet trajectory. AFTE Journal 15(3): 29 (Summary), July 1983.

8. Haag, L.C. Bullet ricochet from water. AFTE Journal 11(3): 27–34, July 1974.

9. Haag, L.C. Bullet ricochet: an empirical study and a device for measuring ricochet angle. AFTE Journal 7(3): 44–51, December 1975.

10. V.J.M. Di Maio and I. Stone, unpublished experiments.

11. Beyer, J.D. (ed.). *Wound Ballistics.* Washington, D.C.: Superintendent of Documents, U.S. Government Printing Office, 1962.

12. Amato, J.J., Billy, L.J., Lawson, N.S., Rich., N.M. High velocity missile injury. Am. J. Surg. 127: 454–459, 1974.

13. Coe, J.I. External beveling of entrance wounds by handguns. Am. J. Forensic Med. Pathol. 3(3): 215–220, September 1982.

14. La Garde, L.A. *Gunshot injuries,* 2nd ed. New York: William Wood and Co., 1916.

15. Dixon, D.S. Keyhole lesions in gunshot wounds of the skull and direction of fire. J. Forensic Sci. 27(3): 555–566, 1982.

Wounds from Handguns 5

Handguns are the most commonly used form of firearm in both homicides and suicides in the United States. Handguns are low-velocity, low-energy weapons having muzzle velocities generally below 1400 ft/sec. Advertised velocities of revolver cartridges traditionally have not been accurate because they are obtained in test devices that have no cylinder gap and have a barrel longer than is normally found in most revolvers. Advertised velocities for semiautomatic pistols are more accurate as there is no cylinder gap from which gas can escape. Even in well-made revolvers, the cylinder gap will cause a velocity loss of approximately 100 to 200 ft/sec, depending on initial velocities and pressures as well as the construction tolerances of the weapon. The length of the barrel also influences muzzle velocity. The longer the barrel, the greater the velocity. Table 5–1 gives the advertised muzzle velocities of some .22-caliber and .38 Special ammunition compared to the actual velocities determined in revolvers with 2-, 4- and 6-in. barrels. The velocity of .22-caliber ammunition in a rifle is also given.

The Remington Firearms Company has introduced a new method of measuring the performance of revolver ammunition to reflect ballistics results more truly as they appear in actual practice. The new method involves use of the vented test barrel. The technique takes into account the cylinder gap (controlled at 0.008 in.), barrel length (4 in.), powder position (horizontal), and production tolerances, as well as allowing for reasonable wear and tear.[1] Table 5–2 shows a comparison between the ballistics data that Remington previously published concerning its ammunition and the results of the new technique. Significant differences in the results can be seen.

Table 5-1 Advertised Muzzle Velocities Versus Actual Velocities

Cartridge	Advertised muzzle velocity (ft/sec)	Actual muzzle velocities (ft/sec)			
		2-in. barrel	4-in. barrel	6-in. barrel	Rifle
.22 Long Rifle	1255	916	1034	1052	1237
.22 Short	1095	851	861	960	1005
.38 Special	855	687	722	765	

Table 5-2 Conventional Test Barrel Ballistics Versus Vented Test Barrel Ballistics

Caliber	Bullet		Muzzle velocity: conventional test barrel (ft/sec)	Muzzle velocity: vented barrel (ft/sec)
	Wt(gr)	Style		
.38 Special	125	SJHP[a]	1028	945
	148	WC	770	710
	158	Lead RN	885	755
	200	Lead RN	730	635
.357 Magnum	125	SJHP	1675	1450
	158	SJHP	1550	1235
	158	Lead SWC	1410	1235

[a] SJHP = Semijacketed hollow point; WC = wad cutter; RN = Roundnose; SWC = Semiwad cutter.

Theoretically, the muzzle velocity in Saturday night special revolvers should be less than that in well-made revolvers because of greater tolerance differences in the Saturday night specials. Experiments, however, do not always substantiate this. The results of one such test can be seen in Table 5-3. There are no significant differences between the muzzle velocities of the Saturday night specials and those of well-made Smith & Wesson revolvers.

Handgun wounds can be divided into four categories, depending on the distance from muzzle to target. These are: contact, near contact, intermediate, and distant (see Chapter 4).

Contact Wounds

A contact wound is one in which the muzzle of the weapon is held against the body at the time of discharge. Contact wounds can be hard, loose, angled or incomplete. In contact wounds gas, soot, and metallic particles avulsed from the bullet by the rifling, vaporized metal from the

Table 5–3 Muzzle Velocities of .38 Special Cartridges Fired in Smith and Wesson and "Saturday Night" Revolvers of Various Barrel Lengths

	Muzzle velocity (ft/sec ± 1 s.d.)	
Barrel length	Smith & Wesson	R.G.
2 in.	687 ± 8	677 ± 11
4 in.	687 ± 15	722 ± 31
6 in.	765 ± 13	748 ± 18

bullet and cartridge case, primer residue, and powder particles all are driven into the wound track along with the bullet.

If the muzzle of the weapon is held very tightly against the skin, indenting it (hard contact) at the time of discharge, all the materials emerging from the muzzle will be driven into the wound, often leaving very little external evidence that one is dealing with a contact wound. Inspection of the entrance, however, usually will disclose searing and powder blackening (soot) of the immediate edge of the wound (Figure 5–1). Subsequent autopsy will reveal soot and unburnt powder particles in the wound track.

Hard contact wounds of the head from .22 Short or .32 Smith & Wesson Short cartridges are often difficult to interpret because of the small powder charge loaded into such cartridges. These wounds may appear to be distant because of our inability to detect the small amount of soot produced and to recover unburned powder grains in the wound track. Compounding this problem is the fact that in distant wounds from .22 Short and .32 S & W Short cartridges, drying of the edges can simulate the blackened and seared margins of hard contact wounds. In situations such as this as well as in cases of decomposition of a body, examination of the wounds with the dissecting microscope for soot and powder grains is of value.

In the author's experience with the dissecting microscope, soot is always present in contact handgun wounds, with powder particles identified in at least half the cases. Unfortunately, recognition of material as soot is to a certain degree subjective. Drying, hemolyzed blood, and decomposition can simulate or mask soot. In cases in which one is not sure whether a wound is contact and in which no powder particles can be identified by the dissecting microscope, the use of energy dispersive x-ray (EDX) or flameless atomic absorption (FAAS) should be employed. Using these devices, one can analyze for the vaporized metals from the bullet, cartridge case, and primer. The best results are obtained when the wound is excised and examined at leisure in a laboratory. If, because

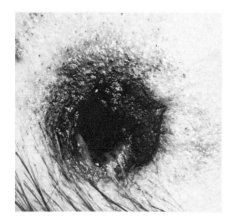

Figure 5−1 Close-up of hard contact wound of the head with a .38 revolver.

of the location of the wound, e.g., the face, it is desirous not to excise it, swabbing of both the skin around the entrance and the wound track with cotton-tipped swabs moistened by either saline solution or acid can be made, with submission of the swabs for FAAS. The analysis of material by EDX and FAAS will be discussed in greater detail in Chapter 12.

In contact wounds, muscle surrounding the entrance may have a cherry-red hue, due to carboxyhemoglobin and carboxymyoglobin formation from the carbon monoxide in the muzzle gas. Even if discoloration is not present, elevated levels of carbon monoxide may be detected on chemical analysis. Control samples of muscle always should be taken from another area of the body if such determinations are to be made. It should be realized that, whereas elevated carbon monoxide levels in the muscle are significant, the lack of carbon monoxide is not, as carboxyhemoglobin formation does not always occur. By using gas chromatography, carbon monoxide has been detected in wounds inflicted up to 30 cm from the muzzle.[2]

The presence of both powder particles and carbon monoxide in a gunshot wound would seem to leave no doubt that one is dealing with an entrance wound. In fact, on occasion both carbon monoxide and powder may be found at an exit. In the case illustrated in Figure 5−2, the deceased shot himself in the left chest with a .357 Magnum revolver. A perfect imprint of the muzzle was seen on the chest, thus indicating the contact nature of the wound. Examination of the exit in the back, however, revealed grains of ball powder in the exit wound and a cherry-red color in the adjacent muscle caused by carbon monoxide. The presence of carbon monoxide was confirmed analytically. To confuse even further the interpretation of the wounds in this case, the exit was shored. Thus, the exit was characterized by an abraded margin, powder grains, and carbon monoxide.

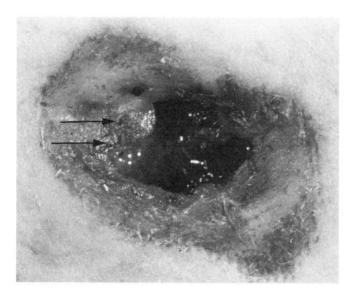

Figure 5−2 Shored exit wound of back with grains of ball powder in exit wound.

The author has seen a number of cases in which ball powder traveled through the body and was found at the exit. All cases involved contact wounds, with the entrances in both head and trunk. The weapons involved were of .22 Magnum, .38 Special, or .357 Magnum caliber. The author has never seen a case in which flake powder traveled completely through the body and was in or adjacent to the exit. He has knowledge, however, of one case involving cylindrical powder in which an individual shot himself in the head with a .44 Magnum handgun and cylindrical powder grains were present in the wound tract, through the brain, and at the exit in the scalp.[3]

Though carbon monoxide and powder may travel through a body and be found at the exit, this is never the case with soot. Soot is present only at entrances.

Contact Wounds over Bone

Contact wounds in regions of the body where only a thin layer of skin and subcutaneous tissue overlies the bone usually have a stellate or cruciform appearance that is totally unlike the round or oval perforating wounds seen in other areas (Figure 5−3). The most common area in which stellate wounds occur is the head. The unusual appearance of contact wounds over bone is due to the effects of the gas of discharge in this area. When a weapon is fired, the gases produced by the combustion of the propellant emerge from the barrel in a highly compressed state. In

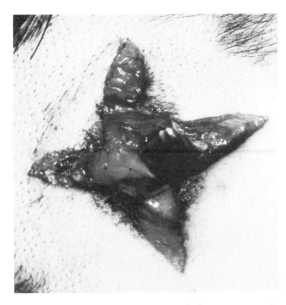

Figure 5–3 Stellate-shaped contact wound of temple from .38 Special revolver.

hard contact wounds they follow the bullet through the skin into the subcutaneous tissue where they immediately begin to expand. Where a thin layer of skin overlies bone, as in the head, these gases expand between the skin and the outer table of the skull, lifting up and ballooning out the skin (Figure 5–4). If the stretching exceeds the elasticity of the skin, it will tear. These tears radiate from the entrance, producing a stellate or cruciform appearing wound of entrance. Reapproximation of the torn edges of the wound will reveal the seared, blackened margins of the original entrance site. In some cases, instead of the classical stellate or cruciform wound, one finds a very large circular wound with ragged, blackened, and seared margins.

The presence of tearing of the skin as well as its extent depends on the caliber of the weapon, the amount of gas produced by the combustion of the propellant, the firmness with which the gun is held against the body, and the elasticity of the skin. Thus, contact wounds of the head with a .22 Short usually produce no tearing, whereas those due to a .45 automatic usually do. It must be stressed, however, that exceptions occur.

Ragged, irregular, and even cruciform or stellate wounds may occur in noncontact gunshot shootings, when the bullet enters over a bony prominence covered by a thin layer of tightly stretched skin (Figure 5–5). The supraorbital ridge, the cheek bone, and jaw are the most common sites. If the bullet is deformed or tumbles prior to striking the body, the tendency to produce cruciform or stellate wounds is accen-

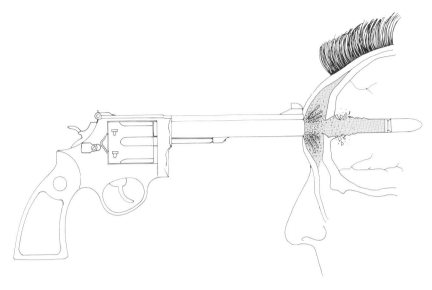

Figure 5-4 Contact wound of head showing dissection of gas between scalp and skull.

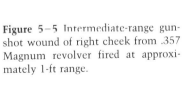

Figure 5-5 Intermediate-range gunshot wound of right cheek from .357 Magnum revolver fired at approximately 1-ft range.

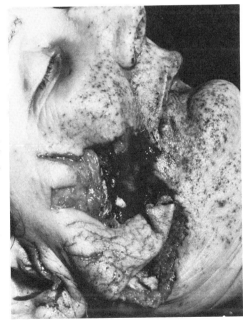

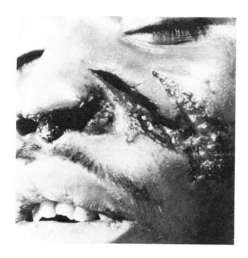

Figure 5-6 Tangential gunshot would of left check from 9-mm bullet.

tuated. A tangential gunshot wound of the face may also simulate a stellate contact wound (Figure 5-6).

In contact wounds of the head, if the skin and soft tissue are retracted, soot will usually be found deposited on the outer table of the skull around the hole of entrance (Figure 5-7). Soot may also be present on the inner table and even on the dura. Soot is usually not seen on bone when the wound is inflicted by either a .22 Short or a .32 Smith & Wesson Short cartridge.

Very rarely in contact wounds of the head caused by weapons of .38 Special caliber and above that fire cartridges loaded with ball powder,

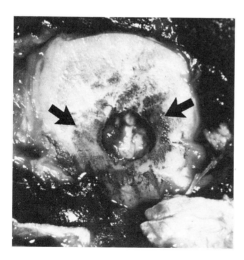

Figure 5-7 Powder soot deposited on outer table of skull around entrance site.

the large irregular or stellate wounds produced may appear to show neither soot nor powder. Careful searching with a dissecting microscope, however, usually reveals a few grains of ball powder.

In contact wounds of the trunk, stellate or cruciform entrances in the skin usually do not occur—even when the weapon and ammunition used produce large volumes of gas—because the gas is able to expand into the abdominal cavity, chest cavity, or soft tissue. Rarely, contact wounds of the chest overlying the sternum which are inflicted by handguns firing some of the new high-velocity pistol ammunition may produce extremely large circular wounds of entrance with ragged margins. These entrance wounds may initially be interpreted as close-range shotgun wounds. The extensive nature of these wounds is due to the large amount of gas produced by such ammunition. These large irregular wounds are almost always due to cartridges loaded with ball powder. In rare instances, there may be no visible soot or powder in spite of the contact nature of the wound. The reason for this is unknown.

In contact gunshot wounds over bone, the gas expanding in the subcutaneous tissue may produce effects other than tearing of the skin. The ballooned-out skin may slam against the muzzle of the weapon with enough force to imprint the outline of the muzzle on the skin (Figure 5–8). Such imprints may be extremely detailed. The more gas produced by the ammunition and weapon, the harder the skin will impact against the muzzle, and thus the greater the detail of the imprint.

Imprints of the muzzle of the weapon occur not only in regions where a thin layer of skin overlies bone but also in the chest and abdomen (Figure 5–9). In contact wounds of the chest and abdomen, the gas expands in the visceral cavities and adjacent soft tissue. Thus, instead of

Figure 5–8 Contact wound with muzzle imprint.

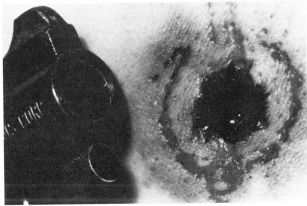

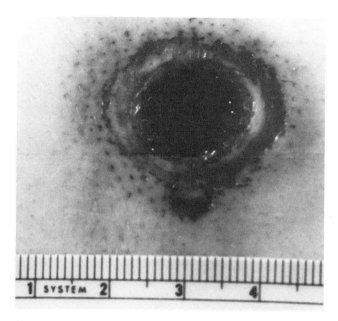

Figure 5−9 Muzzle imprint on chest from .38 Special Colt revolver.

just the skin flaring out against the muzzle, the whole chest or abdominal wall will bulge out.

In contact wounds in which there is a muzzle imprint, one may see an area or zone of abraded skin surrounding the bullet hole (Figure 5−10). This zone of abrasion is due to the skin rubbing against the muzzle of the weapon when, on firing, the skin flares back after firing, impacting and enveloping the muzzle. This zone is often interpreted incorrectly as being caused by searing of the skin by the hot gases of combustion. Differentiation is made on the basis of the fact that in seared zones, such as those seen in near-contact wounds, the area of seared skin is heavily impregnated with soot, whereas in this impact zone it is not. This zone is often wider than the diameter of the barrel because the skin has been bent back around the end of the barrel, totally enclosing it.

In most cases, instead of the aforementioned zone, one has a muzzle imprint. This is the classical imprinted abrasion around a wound of entrance, consisting of the outline of the end of the barrel and sometimes the outline of the front sight (Figures 5−8 and 5−9). In such instances the skin lying against the muzzle is not abraded except at the point where it flares out around the lateral edges of the muzzle of the barrel and the edges of the front sight.

A loose contact wound is produced if the muzzle of the weapon is perpendicular to and in very light contact with the skin at the time of

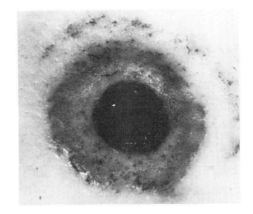

Figure 5-10 Hard contact wound of chest from 9-mm automatic. Abraded skin around entrance.

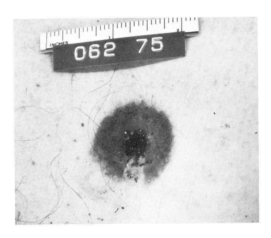

Figure 5-11 Loose contact wound with circular zone of soot around entrance.

discharge. The skin is not indented by the muzzle. In such a case, gas can escape from between the muzzle and the skin, producing a circular zone of soot around the wound of entrance (Figure 5-11). This zone of powder soot deposition can be easily wiped away. Particles of powder, vaporized metals, and soot will still be deposited in the wound track along with carbon monoxide.

Angled and incomplete contact wounds and their appearances have been discussed in detail in Chapter 4.

Near-Contact Wounds

These wounds and their characteristics have already been discussed in detail in Chapter 4. However, a number of additional points can be made. Small piles of clumps of unburned powder may pile up on the edges of the entrance in the seared zone of skin in such wounds. These collections of powder are most prominent in wounds inflicted by .22 Magnum handguns whose cartridges contain ball powder. Near-contact wounds with handguns usually occur at ranges less than 10 mm. There is some variation depending on caliber, ammunition, and barrel length.

Hair

Many textbooks in their descriptions of contact and near-contact wounds in hairy regions put great stress on the presence of burned hair. In actual practice, charred or seared hair is rarely seen, most probably because the gas emerging from the barrel blows away any charred hair. Even in seared zones of skin, however, unburned hairs are numerous. Occasionally, seared hair is seen when a revolver is discharged close to the head while long hair overlays the cylinder gap.

Gas Injuries

The gas produced by combustion of the propellant can produce internal injuries as severe as or more severe than injuries produced by the missile. Gas-produced injuries are most severe in the head because of the closed and unyielding nature of the skull. The skull, unlike the chest or abdominal cavity, cannot expand to relieve the pressure of the entering gases. In contact wounds of the head from high-velocity rifles or shotguns, large quantities of gas entering the skull produce massive blow-out fractures with extensive mutilating injuries. The top of the head is often literally blown off. Contact wounds of the head with handguns, while often producing secondary skull fractures, do not ordinarily produce the massive injuries seen in high-velocity rifles and shotguns. Fractures of the orbital plates are the most common fractures seen with contact handgun wounds of the head, but these fractures are routine with distant wounds as well.

Although massive injuries from contact handgun wounds of the head ordinarily do not occur, there are some exceptions. These pertain to some of the newly produced high-velocity .38 Special cartridges, some .357 Magnum loadings, and the .44 Magnum cartridge. These cartridges can inflict wounds that in their severity mimic contact wounds from rifles and shotguns. Such a wound is illustrated in Figure 5−12, where the deceased was an elderly white female who shot herself in the head with a .38 Special revolver. The ammunition used was Remington 125-gr, jacketed, hollow-point, and loaded with ball powder. Because of the severe nature of the wound, on the initial viewing of this body it was suspected that the woman had been shot with a shotgun.

Contact wounds of the abdomen and chest from handguns ordinarily

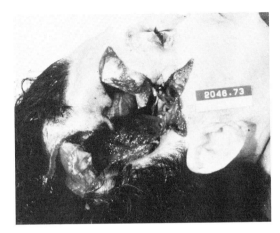

Figure 5-12 Contact wound of right temple from .38 Special revolver firing a high pressure load.

do not produce striking injuries of the internal viscera due to gas. Exceptions occur with the new high-velocity loadings, especially if the wound is inflicted over the heart or the liver.

Intermediate-Range Wounds

An intermediate-range gunshot wound is one in which the muzzle of the weapon is away from the body at the time of discharge yet is sufficiently close so that powder grains emerging from the muzzle along with the bullet produce powder tattooing of the skin; this is the sine qua non of intermediate-range gunshot wounds.

In addition to the powder tattooing, there may be blackening of the skin or material around the entrance site from soot produced by combustion of the propellant. The size and density of the area of powder blackening vary with the caliber of the weapon, the barrel length, the type of propellant powder, and the distance from muzzle to target. As the range increases, the intensity of powder blackening decreases and the size of the soot pattern area increases. For virtually all handgun cartridges, soot is absent beyond 30 cm (12 in.). For a more detailed discussion of powder soot, see Chapter 4.

Although soot usually can be wiped away either by copious bleeding or intentional wiping, power tattooing cannot. Tattooing consists of numerous reddish brown to orange-red, punctate lesions surrounding the wound of entrance (Figure 5-13). Powder tattooing is due to the impaction of unburned, partially burned, or burning powder grains onto and into the skin. Powder tattooing is an antemortem phenomenon and

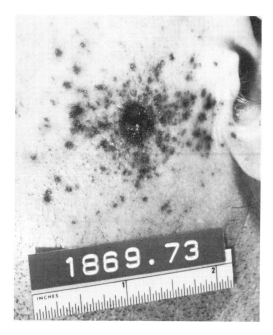

Figure 5-13 Powder tattooing from disk powder.

indicates that the individual was alive or at least that the heart was beating at the time the victim was shot. If an individual is shot at intermediate range after the heart has stopped beating, mechanical markings will be produced on the skin. These markings, however, will not have the reddish color, i.e., the vital reaction, of antemortem tattoo marks. Postmortem tattoo marks have a yellow, moist appearance. They are less numerous than markings produced in the living subject at the same range.

For handguns, forensic textbooks generally have stated that powder tattooing extends out to a maximum distance of 18 to 24 in. (45 to 60 cm) from the muzzle. Such statements are no longer accurate since the introduction of different physical forms of propellant powder. At present, all handgun cartridges are loaded with one of four forms of propellant: flake, spherical ball powder, flattened ball powder, and cylindrical powder (Figure 5-14). Flake powder is the most commonly used form of powder. Currently, ball powder is used mostly in high pressure loadings such as the .357 Magnum cartridge—because for consistent homogeneous ignition of ball powder, high pressure and thus high temperature conditions are necessary. In the past, ball powder was used for pistol loadings down to the .25 ACP. Some manufactures use uncoated ball powder for better ignition; these have a pale green color to the grains.

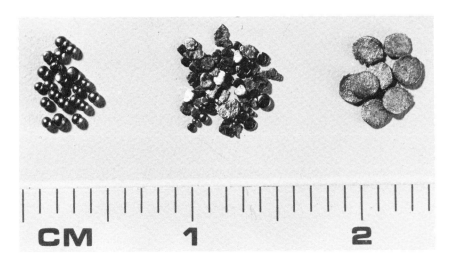

Figure 5–14 Ball, flattened ball, and flake (disk).

Flake powder usually is in the form of disks though some foreign manufactures have flake powder in the form of quadrangles. The circular disks of flake powder can vary greatly from a small to a large diameter and from thin to very thick. If the graphite coating is burned from such flakes they have a pale green translucent appearance.

Handgun cartridges loaded with cylindrical powder are uncommon. Norma sells centerfire handgun cartridges with such powder and one brand of .22 Magnum rimfire cartridge is loaded with cylindrical powder.

As a result of animal experiments, it appears that in a .38 Special revolver with a 4-in. barrel, cartridges with flake powder produce powder tattooing out to 18 to 24 in. (45 to 60 cm). Cartridges loaded with flattened ball produce tattooing out to 30 to 36 in. (75 to 90 cm), and while cartridges loaded with true or spherical powder produce tatooing out to 36 to 42 in. (90 to 105 cm) (Table 5–4).

In contrast, a .22 caliber revolver with a 2-in. barrel, firing .22 Long Rifle cartridges produces powder tattooing out to 18 to 24 in. (45 to 60 cm) with flake powder and 12 to 18 in. (30 to 45 cm) with ball powder (Table 5–5).

In the .38 Special caliber, powder tattooing extends out to greater ranges with ball powder (both spherical and flattened ball) than with flake powder, because of the shape of the powder grains. The sphere has a better aerodynamic form than a flake; thus, ball powder can travel farther with greater velocity, enabling it to mark the skin at a greater range. In the .22 ammunition the flake powder produces tattooing out to

Table 5−4 Maximum Range of Powder Tattooing from .38 Special Revolver with 4-in. Barrel

	Type of powder		
Range (cm)	Flake[a]	Flattened ball	Ball
30	+	+	+
45	+	+	+
60	+	+	+
75	0	+	+
90		+	+
105		0	+
120			0

[a]+ = tattooing. 0 = no tattooing.

Table 5−5 Maximum Range of Powder Tattooing from .22 Revolver with 2-in. Barrel Firing Long Rifle Ammunition

	Type of Powder[a]	
Range (cm)	Flake	Ball
15	+	+
30	+	+
45	+	+
60	+	0
75	0	0

[a]+ = Tattooing. 0 = No tattooing.

a greater distance than ball powder. The explanation is that the individual grains of ball powder used in the .22 Long Rifle ammunition are so fine that any aerodynamic benefit obtained from the shape is lost as a result of its lighter mass.

The maximum ranges for powder tattooing that have been given should be used only as a rough guide as these data are based on animal tests.[4] The maximum range at which tattooing occurs, as well as the size of the powder tattoo pattern, depends not only on the form of the powder but on a number of other variables, including the barrel length, the caliber, the individual weapon, and the presence of intermediate objects such as hair or clothing that will absorb some or all of the powder grains.

The greater the range, the larger and less dense the powder tattoo pattern. The increase in size of the pattern is due to gradual dispersion of the powder grains, with decreased density of the pattern resulting not only from dispersion but also from rapid loss of velocity of the individual grains; fewer grains reach the target and those that do may not have enough velocity to mark the skin. At the same range, a gun with a short barrel will produce a wider and denser tattoo pattern than a longer barrel weapon as more unburned particles of powder will emerge from the short barrel (Figure 5–15). Tattooing will, of course, disappear at a closer range with a short-barreled gun compared with a long-barreled gun.

Figure 5–15 Two intermediate-range gunshot wounds (range, 15 cm). Upper tattoo pattern produced by weapon with 6-in. barrel; lower pattern from weapon with 2-in. barrel.

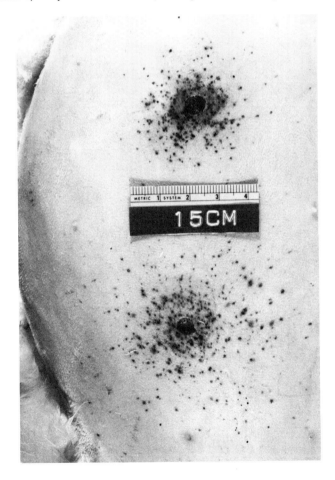

Silencers will filter out a great proportion of the soot and powder particles, thus making the range from muzzle to target appear greater than it actually was.

To a degree, hair and clothing prevent powder from reaching the skin. In centerfire cartridges, ball powder readily perforates hair and clothing at close range. In contrast, cartridges loaded with flake powder usually do not produce powder tattooing through clothing or hair, as the grains of flake powder have difficulty in perforating these materials. However, the author has seen occasional cases in which flake powder has perforated clothing and hair.

The influence of the type of powder on the extent and degree of powder tattooing and blackening was exhibited in a case in which an individual was shot with a .45 automatic loaded with Norma ammunition. Testing revealed that the maximum range of powder tattooing and blackening in this particular weapon with this particular ammunition was only 6 in.

Although powder tattooing extends out only to a maximum of 105 cm with a .38-caliber revolver, the individual powder grains can travel much farther. In an experiment using a .38 Special 4-in. barrel revolver firing Remington ammunition in which the bullet was a 158-gr lead missile and the powder was flake powder, individual flakes of powder were deposited on material out to a maximum of 6 ft from muzzle to target (Table 5−6).[5] A Remington cartridge loaded with a 125-gr semi-jacketed hollow-point bullet and ball powder discharged from the same weapon deposited powder grains on a target 20 ft. from the muzzle. This cartridge is no longer loaded with ball powder but now contains flake powder. Discharging some of this newer ammunition resulted in flake

Table 5−6 Maximum Distances Traveled from Muzzle to Target by Different Forms of Powder from Different Caliber Weapon (both with 4-in. barrels)

Caliber	Type of powder in cartridge case	Maximum distance traveled by powder grains (ft)
.38 Special	Ball	20
	Flake[a]	9
	Flake[b]	6
.357 Magnum	Ball	12
	Ball	15
	Flake	10

[a] High-velocity loading.
[b] Standard velocity loading.

powder grains being deposited on clothing out to a maximum of 9 ft. from the muzzle (Table 5-6).

Tests were carried out with a .357 Magnum revolver having a 4-in. barrel. Cartridges loaded with flattened ball powder deposited grains of powder out to a maximum of 15 ft. Cartridges loaded with flake powder deposited flake powder out to a maximum of 10 ft. (Table 5-6).

In view of the fact that powder grains can travel such great distances, the presence of one or two unburned grains of powder around an entrance on the skin or clothing does not necessarily indicate an intermediate-range wound but, depending on the individual form of powder, can be produced by a weapon being discharged as much as 15 to 20 ft. from the victim. At these ranges, however, the powder has insufficient velocity to mark the skin.

In addition to soot and powder grains, other materials are deposited on the body when a weapon is discharged in close proximity to the body. These materials include: antimony, barium and lead from the primer; copper and zinc (sometimes nickel) vaporized from the cartridge case by the intense heat; fragments of metal stripped from or vaporized from previously fired bullets and deposited in the barrel; lead stripped or vaporized from the bullet that was fired; and grease and oil that had coated the barrel or bullet before discharge. The metallic particles can be detected on the body or on clothing by soft x-ray if they are large enough. Trace metal deposits of these metals can be detected by FAAS, EDX, and, with the exception of lead, neutron activation.

The appearance of powder tattoo marks on the skin depends on the physical form of the powder. Powder tattoo marks produced by flake and cylindrical powder are irregular in shape and reddish brown in color, and they show great variability in size (Figure 5-13). Such markings are usually relatively sparse compared to tattooing from ball powder. Slit-like tattoo marks due to flake powder grains striking on their side may be seen. Occasionally, fragments or intact flakes or both will be found embedded in the skin. More commonly, however, flakes will be found lying on the skin. The number of such flakes is relatively small. Flakes can on occasion penetrate into the dermis, in which case they may produce bleeding from these sites. Small blood clots at the points of penetration may give the appearance of a spray of dried blood. The author has seen a few cases involving flake powder where large numbers of flakes were embedded in the epidermis with some penetrating into the dermis. The flakes of powder were found to be very small, very thick yellow-green disks. The tattooing produced by these thick disks very closely resembles the tattooing of ball powder. Only recovery of disks or balls of powder make differentiation possible.

In contrast to flake powder, powder tattooing due to spherical ball powder is considerably more dense with numerous fine, circular, bright red tattoo marks, many containing a ball of unburned powder lodged in the center of the lesion (Figure 5−5; Figure 12−4 B). On seeing the powder tattoo marks from spherical ball powder, one is struck immediately by the resemblance to the petechiae of an intravascular coagulation disorder. Attempts at wiping away the ball powder grains are only partly successful, as many if not most of the little balls of powder are deeply embedded in the skin.

In powder tattoo patterns due to flattened ball, the number of markings produced is greater than in the case of flake powder but fewer than in the case of ball powder. The individual markings tend to be finer, more uniform and more hemorrhagic than flake, approaching those of ball powder. Powder grains are recovered embedded in the skin, but they are not nearly as numerous as in cases of true ball powder tattooing.

The previous descriptions of powder tattooing concerned centerfire handguns. Powder tattooing from .22 rimfire cartridges is different. Those cartridges are loaded with either small, thick disks or very fine ball powder (Winchester ammunition). Ball powder produces extremely fine but faint tattooing, whereas flake powder produces a larger, more prominent tattoo pattern. These markings more closely resemble those of centerfire flattened ball powder than those of traditional flake powder. In some instances flake or parts of flakes have penetrated into the dermis.

The author has never seen powder tattooing of the palms of the hands from powder exiting the muzzle of a gun, even though it is not uncommon for an individual to have one hand in front of the weapon at the time of discharge. The author has seen cases in which grains of powder were embedded in the palms. The vital reaction known as tattooing was absent, however (Figure 4−9). Lack of tattooing in the palms is probably due to the greater thickness of the stratum corneum protecting the dermis from any trauma. The author has seen one case where there appeared to be some four to five faint powder tattoo marks on the palm. In this particular case, because of the nature of the entrance wound, this powder would have had to have come out the cylinder gap. Therefore, it is possible that the marks on the palm were not tattoo marks, but marks due to fragments of lead coming out the cylinder gap.

The size of the powder tattoo pattern present on the body around the wound of entrance can be used to determine the range at which the weapon was discharged. To do this, however, the same weapon and a lot of ammunition must be used. Selection of ammunition used for test firings is extremely important because different brands and lots of ammunition contain different powders and quantities of propellant. Cartridges of the same manufacturer, design and bullet weight may contain different powders, as the manufacturer may change the powder from one lot of ammunition to another. Therefore, ideally, unfired cartridges recovered from the gun or cartridges that came from the same box of ammunition that the fired ammunition came from should be used in the tests.

If a weapon is discharged at intermediate range when the barrel is at an angle to the skin, the resultant tattooing generally will be present predominantly on the side from which the bullet came. If it is on both sides, the tattooing will be more intense on the side from which the bullet came and diffuse and sparse on the opposite side (Figure 5–16).

Muzzle-to-victim range determinations from powder tattoo patterns on the skin are made by firearms examiners, using measurements of the tattoo pattern obtained by the pathologist. The distance at which a test pattern identical to the powder tattoo pattern on the body is produced is assumed to be the range at which the gun was fired at the individual. Test patterns generally are produced on white blotting paper. Unfortunately, experiments have indicated that powder tattoo patterns on paper are consistent with skin tattoo patterns only up to 18 in. of range.[4] At ranges greater than 18 in., there is no correlation between the size and density of the tattoo pattern produced on the body and the pattern produced on blotting paper.

Another problem with range determinations that are based on the size of powder tattoo patterns is a simple one of variation in measuring. Different individuals measuring the same powder tattoo pattern may produce different measurements.[4] This is due to the fact that some individuals measure the whole tattoo pattern, whereas others measure the main area of the pattern, excluding occasional "flier" tattoo marks.

Figure 5–16 Angled intermediate gunshot wound with powder tattooing on side from which the bullet came. **Arrow** indicates direction of bullet.

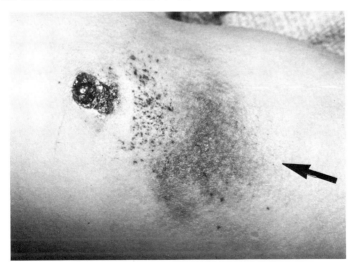

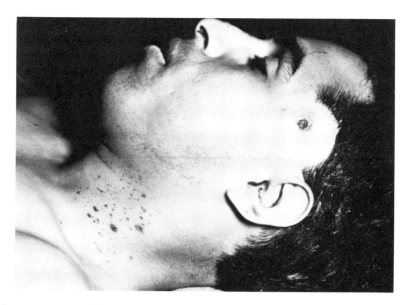

Figure 5–17 Suicidal contact wound of left temple with powder tattooing and lead fragment stippling of left side of neck. The larger areas of hemorrhage are due to the lead fragments.

Cylinder Gap

When a revolver is fired, gas, soot, and powder emerge not only from the end of the muzzle but also from the gap between the cylinder and the barrel. This material emerges at an approximate right angle to the long axis of the weapon. If the revolver is in close proximity to the body at the time of discharge, powder escaping from the cylinder gap may produce tattooing of the skin. This tattooing will be relatively scant.

If the cylinder of the revolver is out of alignment with the barrel, as the bullet jumps from the cylinder to the barrel, fragments of lead may be sheared off the bullet. These fragments can produce marks on the skin that resemble powder tattoo marks. Such marks, however, are larger, more irregular, and more hemorrhagic than traditional powder tattoo marks. In addition, fragments of lead usually are seen embedded in the skin. These fragment wounds often are intermingled with the true powder tattooing produced by powder escaping from the cylinder gap (Figure 5–17).

Distant Wounds

In distant gunshot wounds, the muzzle of the weapon is held sufficiently far from the body so that there is neither deposition of soot nor powder tattooing. For centerfire handguns, distant gunshot wounds begin beyond 24 in. (60 cm) from muzzle to target for cartridges loaded with flake powder and beyond 42 in. (105 cm) for cartridges loaded with ball powder. The exact range depends on the particular weapon and ammunition and can be determined exactly only by experimentation with the specific weapon and ammunition.

All these figures presuppose the lack of clothing. Clothing will absorb soot and powder, in some cases making intermediate-range wounds appear to be distant by examination of the body alone. This points out the need for examination of the clothing in conjunction with the autopsy. The presence of isolated powder particles on either the clothing or the body does not necessarily signify that one is dealing with an intermediate range wound, as individual powder particles may travel considerable distances before deposition on the body.

Whether powder perforates clothing to mark the skin depends on the nature of the material, the number of layers of cloth, and the physical form of the powder. With handguns, ball powder can readily perforate one and even two layers of cloth to produce tattooing of the underlying skin (Figure 5-18). Rarely, ball powder will perforate three layers; the author has never seen it perforate four layers and produce tattooing. Flake powder usually does not perforate even one layer of cloth, though he has seen it do so on rare occasions in weapons ranging in caliber from .22 to .38. In these instances, the powder was usually small thick disks.

Range determinations cannot be made for distant gunshot wounds. Bullets fired from 5, 50, or 500 ft will produce identical entrances. Gunshot wounds of entrance are identified by the presence of a reddish zone of abraded skin (the abrasion ring) around the entrance hole. This zone becomes brown and then black as it dries. The abrasion ring is due to the bullet rubbing raw the edges of the hole as it indents and pierces the skin. Occasionally, entrance wounds due to jacketed or semijacketed handgun bullet such as the .357 Magnum will not have an abrasion ring that is observable either by the naked eye or dissecting microscope (Figure 5-19).

Addendum: Centerfire Handgun Cartridges

There are scores of centerfire handgun cartridges. A few of the more common ones will be described.

.25 Auto (ACP) (6.35 mm)

The .25 Auto, the smallest of the currently manufactured centerfire handgun cartridges, was introduced in the first decade of the twentieth century. The cartridge generally is loaded with a 50-gr full metal-

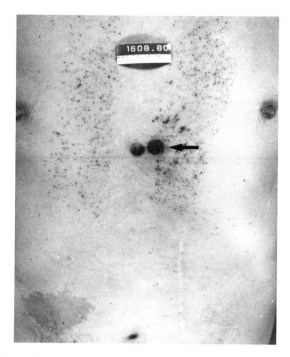

Figure 5–18 Unusual ball powder tattoo pattern resulting from shirt. The powder passed through the shirt, except for the center facing, where there were four layers of cloth rather than one. **Arrow** indicates entrance. Circular mark medial to entrance is imprint of button.

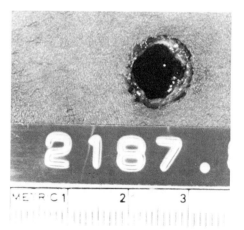

Figure 5–19 Entrance wound of back showing absence of abrasion ring. The bullet was a semijacketed .357 Magnum.

jacketed bullet. Muzzle velocity is around 810 ft/sec. A limited production run of cartridges loaded with a hollow-point jacketed bullet was made by Winchester in the early 1970s. All these cartridges were loaded with ball powder. These bullets as a general rule do not expand in the body. In 1981, Winchester-Western introduced a cartridge loaded with a 45-gr expanding-point projectile. The bullet is lead; it is not jacketed but is coated with a copper Lubaloy finish. The bullet has a hollow point filled with one No. 4 steel birdshot pellet. The projectile without the shot weights approximately 42.6 gr.

.32 Auto (ACP) (7.65 mm)

The .32 Auto was introduced in 1899 by Fabrique Nationale for the first successful semiautomatic pistol ever manufactured. It is used extensively in Europe. Czechoslavakia manufactured a submachine gun for it, the Scorpion. The cartridge is semirimmed and will chamber and fire in a .32 revolver. Bullet weight is generally 71 gr, with a muzzle velocity of 905 ft/sec. Winchester markets a cartridge loaded with a 60-gr aluminum-jacketed hollow-point bullet. Muzzle velocity is 970 ft/sec.

.32 Smith & Wesson and .32 Smith & Wesson Long

The .32 Smith & Wesson and .32 Smith & Wesson Long cartridges were introduced in 1878 and 1903, respectively. They are revolver cartridges. The .32 S & W is loaded with an 85-gr lead roundnose bullet. Muzzle velocity is 680 ft/sec. The .32 S & W Long is loaded with a 98-gr lead roundnose bullet. Muzzle velocity is 705 ft/sec. These cartridges have been used extensively in cheap weapons of the Saturday night special design.

.38 Smith & Wesson

The .38 Smith & Wesson revolver cartridge was introduced in 1877 with a black powder loading. In Britain it is called the .380/200. The cartridge is usually loaded with a 145-gr lead bullet. Muzzle velocity is 685 ft/sec. A 200-gr loading with a muzzle velocity of 630 ft/sec used to be available. The .38 S & W is essentially an obsolete cartridge.

.38 Special

Introduced in 1902, the .38 Special is the most popular handgun cartridge in the United States. The standard loading for more than 50 years was a 158 gr round nose lead bullet having a muzzle velocity of 755 ft/sec. Since the mid-1960s numerous high velocity semi-jacketed hollow point and soft point loadings have been introduced. Bullet weights are generally 95, 110, 125, and 158 gr in these new loadings. Muzzle velocity (vented) ranged from 950-1175 ft/sec. Any weapon chambered for the .357 Magnum cartridge will chamber and fire the .38 Special cartridge.

.357 Magnum

Introduced in 1935 by Smith & Wesson, the .357 Magnum is the .38 Special cartridge case lengthened about 1/10 in. so that it will not chamber in the .38 Special revolver. Standard loading was a 158-gr lead semiwadcutter bullet with a muzzle velocity of 1235 ft/sec. New semi-jacketed loadings are generally 110, 125, and 158 gr with muzzle velocities ranging from 1235 to 1450 ft/sec.

.380 Automatic (ACP) (9-mm Kurz; 9-mm Corto)

The .380 Automatic cartridge was introduced in the United States in 1908 by Colt and in Europe in 1912 by Fabrique Nationale. It has never equaled the popularity of the .32 ACP in Europe. Standard loading is a full metal-jacketed, 95-gr bullet with a velocity of 955 ft/sec. Semi-jacketed hollow-point loadings are commercially available.

.38 Colt Super Auto

The .38 Colt Super Auto cartridge was introduced in 1929 as an improved version of the .38 Colt Auto cartridge introduced in 1900. It never really gained much popularity and is essentially obsolete. Standard loading is a 130-gr full metal-jacketed bullet with a muzzle velocity of 1275 ft/sec. A 125-gr jacketed hollow-point version with a muzzle velocity of 1245 ft/sec is available.

9-mm Luger (Parabellum)

Introduced in 1902, the 9-mm Luger is the most widely used military handgun cartridge in the world. All modern submachine guns are chambered for this cartridge. The typically military cartridge is loaded with a 115-gr full metal-jacketed bullet and has a muzzle velocity of 1140 ft/sec. Cartridges loaded with lighter weight hollow-point bullets are available; the muzzle velocity of these rounds is higher. This caliber is considered by most American shooters as inferior to the .45 ACP. Studies by both the military and a number of civilian government agencies as well as studies by some private individuals have shown that this is incorrect; there is no appreciable differences in the effectiveness of the 9-mm and the .45 ACP cartridge.

.45 ACP

The .45 ACP cartridge was adopted as the official military caliber of the United States in 1911. It has never been popular outside the United States. Adoption was based on a series of wound ballistics tests by the U.S. Army prior to its adoption. It was considered a great "man stopper," but more recent testing has shown it no more effective than the 9-mm Luger cartridge. Standard military loading is with a 230-gr full metal-jacketed bullet that has a muzzle velocity of 850 ft/sec. Semijacketed hollow-point cartridges are available. This cartridge should not be confused with the .45 Colt cartridge introduced in 1873 by Colt for their Peacemaker single-action revolver. This latter cartridge, originally a black powder one, was loaded with 40 gr of black powder. A 255-gr lead bullet was propelled at a muzzle velocity of 810 ft/sec.

.44 Smith & Wesson Magnum

The .44 Smith & Wesson Magnum is the most powerful commercially successful handgun cartridge produced. It was introduced in 1955. Not only are a number of revolvers chambered for this cartridge but also a number of carbines. The cartridge is loaded with either a 240 gr lead soft-point bullet or a semi-jacketed hollow-point bullet. Muzzle velocity is 1180 ft/sec.

References

1. Remington Ammunition Catalogue, 1982.
2. Menzies, R.C., Scroggie, R.J., Labowitz, D.I.: Characteristics of silenced firearms and their wounding effects. J. Forensic Sci. 25(2): 239–262, 1981.
3. Patrick Besant-Matthews, M.D. Personal communication.
4. DiMaio, V.J.M., Petty, C.S., Stone, I.C. An experimental study of powder tattooing of the skin. J. Forensic Sci. 21(2): 367–372, 1976.
5. DiMaio, V.J.M., Norton, L. Unpublished experiments.

Wounds from .22 Caliber Rimfire Weapons

6

The most popular and most commonly fired caliber in the United States is the .22 rimfire. It is estimated that over 4 billion rounds of this ammunition are produced each year in the United States. The three most common forms of .22 rimfire ammunition are the .22 Short, the .22 Long, and the .22 Long Rifle (Figure 6–1). The .22 Magnum (Winchester Magnum Rimfire) is a very distant fourth in popularity (Figure 6–1).

The Flobert BB cap was the ancestor of the .22 rimfire cartridge. It was developed in 1845 by necking down a percussion cap and inserting a lead ball. The primer was the sole propellant. Subsequent development by Smith & Wesson resulted in the .22 Short cartridge. Introduced in 1857, this is the oldest commercial metallic cartridge. It was loaded with a 29-gr, conical-shaped lead bullet with a diameter the same as that of the case and with outside lubrication. A heel was put on the back of the bullet, so that it could be inserted into the case. The case then was crimped into the bullet. The cartridge originally was loaded with 4 gr of black powder.

The .22 Long cartridge appeared in 1871. This consisted of a lengthened case (the current .22 Long Rifle case), loaded with the 29-gr Short bullet. Five grains of black powder were used as a propellant. This cartridge, which is less accurate than either the Short or the Long Rifle cartridge, has outlived its usefulness. It still is sold in small quantities, however.

The .22 Long Rifle cartridge appeared in 1887. It consisted of the .22 Long case loaded with a 40-gr bullet and 5 gr of black powder. This is the most useful and most accurate of the rimfire cartridges.

In the years after the introduction of these three rimfire cartridges, a number of significant evolutionary changes followed. Smokeless pow-

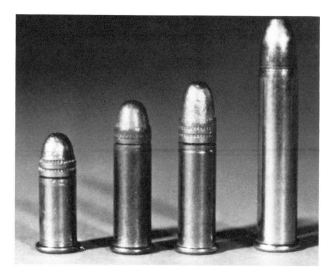

Figure 6−1 From left to right, .22 Short, .22 Long, .22 Long Rifle, and .22 Magnum.

der and the hollow-point design appeared in the 1890s; noncorrosive priming was introduced by Remington in 1927. In 1930, the first high-velocity loadings appeared. In these loadings, bullets of the same weight are propelled at higher velocities than the standard loadings.

The introduction of the .22 Magnum (Winchester Magnum Rimfire-WMR) occurred in 1959. It was developed as a rimfire cartridge that would possess a velocity close to that of a centerfire. It fires either a 40-gr jacketed hollow-point bullet or a 40-gr full metal-jacketed bullet. Both handguns and rifles are chambered for this cartridge. The .22 Magnum has a larger cartridge case diameter than the other rimfire cartridges and will not chamber in weapons chambered for the standard .22 rimfire cartridges. The .22 Short, Long, and Long Rifle cartridges will fit loosely in a weapon chambered for the Magnum cartridge. They ordinarily will not fire; if they do, the cases will split.

The .22 Magnum cartridge is loaded with an 0.224-in. bullet compared with the 0.223-in. bullet used in the other .22 rimfire cartridges. Some rimfire revolvers have interchangeable cylinders designed so that one cylinder is for the ordinary .22 rimfire cartridges and the other is for the .22 Magnum. The barrel has a groove diameter of 0.224 in., i.e., that of the Magnum bullet. When fired down these barrels, the 0.223-in lead bullet expands, as a result of gas pressure, to fill the rifling.

One additional rimfire cartridge should be mentioned: the 5-mm Remington Magnum. Introduced in 1970, this is the only modern necked rimfire cartridge. The bullet has a diameter of 0.2045 in., weighs

38 gr, and is of a jacketed, hollow-point design. Muzzle velocity is 2100 ft/sec, and rifles and handguns were made for it. This round was not a success and is obsolete.

.22 Short, Long, and Long Rifle Cartridges

The .22 Short, Long, and Long Rifle cartridges can be fired in both handguns and rifles. The term "Long Rifle" as it is applied to the most powerful of these three cartridges does not indicate that the cartridge is intended exclusively for rifles.

Rifles and handguns chambered for the .22 Long Rifle cartridge will fire the Short and Long cartridges as well. In the case of semiautomatic weapons, however, the weak recoil generated by the Short and Long cartridges is generally insufficient to work the action. A few semiautomatic rifles can fire .22 Short, Long, and Long Rifles interchangeably.

Repeated firing of .22 Short cartridges in a weapon chambered for the Long Rifle cartridge may cause leading of the firing chamber, with subsequent difficulty in inserting Long Rifle cartridges. Some handguns and rifles are designed to use Shorts only and will not chamber the longer cartridges.

Weapons chambered for the .22 rimfire cartridge have an 0.223-bore diameter with a 1 in 16 (1/16) twist. Optimum velocity is said to be obtained from a 14- to 16-in. barrel. No notable reduction in velocity occurs until the barrel reaches 8 in. in length.[1] Table 2–1 (see Chapter 2) gives the rifling characteristics of the more commonly available .22 rimfire rifles. Marlin uses Micro-Groove® rifling in the rifles they manufacture. There are 16 lands and grooves in Marlin rifles chambered for the .22 Short, Long, and Long Rifle cartridges and 20 lands and grooves in their .22 Magnum rifles. Recovery of a bullet with Micro-Groove® rifling indicates that the individual was shot with a rifle since such rifling is not found in handguns (Figure 6–2).

Figure 6–2 .22 Long Rifle bullets with Micro-Groove rifling.

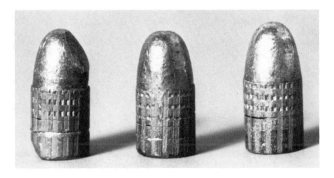

The .22 Short, Long, and Long Rifle cartridges are available in either standard-velocity loadings designed for target shooting, short-range hunting, and plinking or high-velocity loadings more suitable for hunting small game. High velocity cartridges contain the same bullet that is loaded in standard velocity cartridges but are loaded to a higher velocity. All three cartridges are loaded with unjacketed lead bullets. A small number of full metal-jacketed, .22 rimfire bullets were produced for the military during World War II. These are now rare. Tracer Long Rifle rimfire cartridges have been manufactured by the French.

There are four major manufacturers of .22 rimfire ammunition in the United States and probably hundreds in the world. The major manufacturers in the United States are:

Remington-Peters

Winchester-Western

Federal

CCI (Omark Industries)

The head stamp imprinted on the flat base of every U.S.-made .22-caliber rimfire cartridge will identify the manufacturer. Current symbols used by the manufacturers are shown in Figure 6–3. All Remington ammunition will henceforth have the inscription "Rem" on the base. These four ammunition companies sell their ammunition not only under the company name but also under secondary brand names. Thus, ammunition manufactured by Remington-Peters is sold under the Remington, the Peters, and the Mohawk brands. Winchester-Western sells their ammunition under the names Winchester, Western, and Wildcat. Some large chain stores, e.g., Sears, sell ammunition under a

Figure 6–3 .22 Headstamps. *Top row (from left to right)*: Federal, Winchester, Winchester, Winchester and Winchester. *Lower row (from left to right)*: Remington, CCI, CCI, Remington, and Winchester.

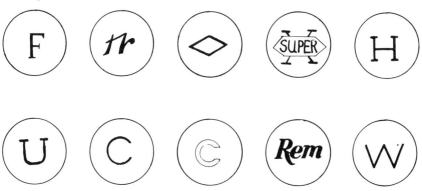

house brand. The head stamps on these cartridges, however, often show who the manufacturer is.

.22 rimfire ammunition, like all other ammunition, is made in batches called "lots". A lot is a large quantity of one type of ammunition that is manufactured under the same conditions and with materials as nearly identical as possible. Each lot is assigned a number, which is stamped on the box.

We shall now consider the three rimfire cartridges separately.

.22 Short Cartridge

The .22 Short cartridge is available in both standard and high velocity loadings. The standard-velocity cartridge is generally loaded with a solid, all-lead, 29-gr bullet. The high velocity cartridges contain either a 29-gr solid lead bullet or a 27-gr hollow-point bullet. The one exception to this is the Federal hollow-point bullet, which weighs 29 gr. The high-velocity bullets produced by Winchester, Federal, and CCI and sold under their respective primary brand names have a copper plating, whereas the Remington round has a "gold" coat (copper and zinc). High-velocity ammunition sold under secondary brand names, e.g., Mohawk and Wildcat, does not have the copper coat.

.22 Long Ammunition

The .22 Long ammunition is produced by all four major manufacturers. The cartridge is loaded with a solid 29-gr bullet. The bullet is copper-plated or has a "gold" coat (Remington).

.22 Long Rifle Ammunition

The .22 Long Rifle ammunition is available in either standard-velocity or high-velocity loadings. It is manufactured by all four major companies and is probably the most popular rimfire cartridge. The cartridge is loaded with a 40 gr, solid lead bullet or a hollow-point bullet. The weight of the hollow-point bullet varies, depending on the manufacturer. The standard hollow-point bullet weighs 36 gr as produced by Remington, 37 gr by Winchester and CCI, and 38 gr by Federal. Winchester manufactured a special Long Rifle cartridge loaded with a 40-gr hollow-point bullet called the "Dynapoint." This round had a very shallow cavity at the tip of the bullet.

The high-velocity loadings, whether hollow-point or solid, have a copper coating when manufactured by Federal, Winchester, and CCI and a "gold" coat when manufactured by Remington. High-velocity ammunition sold under secondary brand names—for example, Mohawk and Wildcat—does not have the copper coat.

In addition to the regular Long Rifle cartridges with which most people are familiar, .22 Long Rifle shot cartridges are also available. As loaded by Federal, Remington, and Winchester, the cartridges have a crimped metallic mouth and contain approximately 25 gr of No. 12 shot. The cartridges loaded by CCI contain 165 No. 12 pellets in a plastic capsule. Muzzle velocity for this particular round is said to be 1047 ft/sec. CCI also manufactures a .22 Magnum shot cartridge in which the shot is also enclosed in a plastic capsule. Deaths due to .22 shot cartridges are rare. Both suicides and homicides have been reported.[2,3] The .22 Long Rifle shot cartridges will perforate the temporal bone out to a range of 5 in. (Figure 6–4A).[2] In areas of the skull where the bone is thicker or at a range of greater than 5 in., close range wounds with this cartridge produce depressed skull fractures (Figure 6–4B). Di Maio and Spitz observed an unusual amount of powder blackening with the Remington "birdshot" cartridges, with soot out to 18 in. of range.[2]

In late 1976, CCI introduced a special .22 rimfire cartridge called the "Stinger." This .22 rimfire cartridge is loaded with a 32-gr hollow-point bullet; it is intended principally for use in rifles. A velocity of 1687 ft/sec is claimed by the manufacturer, compared to 1370 ft/sec for the conventional high-velocity 37-gr hollow-point bullet. The Stinger has a pentagonal hole in the point to speed expansion. A heavier charge of slower burning powder developed especially for this cartridge is used. The cartridge case, which is nickel-plated, is approximately 1/10 in. longer than the standard .22 Long Rifle case. The overall length of the Stinger and the regular .22 Long Rifle cartridge are the same, however.

The Winchester-Western Company countered the Stinger with the "Expediter." This high-velocity .22 rimfire cartridge, which was introduced in 1978, was loaded with a 29-gr hollow-point bullet. Muzzle velocity was 1680 ft/sec from a 24-in. barrel. The cartridge case was nickel-plated and was somewhat longer than the .22 Long Rifle case. This cartridge could be fired in any weapon chambered for the .22 Long Rifle cartridge, except those with match chambers. Pressure limits were within those intended for the .22 Long Rifle ammunition. This cartridge was discontinued in 1982.

In 1979, Remington introduced their "Yellow Jacket" ammunition. This is a high-velocity .22 Long Rifle cartridge with a 33-gr hollow-point bullet. The muzzle velocity in a .22 rifle with a 24-in. barrel is 1500 ft/sec compared with 1200 ft/sec for the Remington .22 Long Rifle, 40 gr, high-velocity round. Muzzle velocity in a Ruger automatic pistol with a 4¾-in. barrel is 1269 ft/sec compared to a muzzle velocity of 1048 ft/sec for an ordinary 40-gr high-velocity, .22 rimfire cartridge. The Yellow

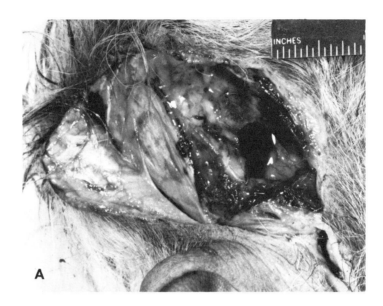

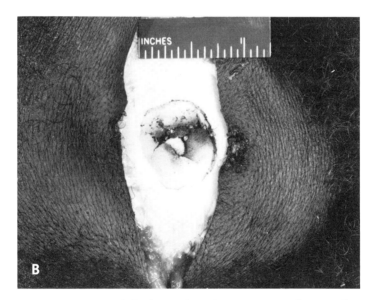

Figure 6–4 A. Contact wound of right temple with Remington .22 shot cartridge. Incised wound revealing soot deposited on outer table of bone. **B.** Distant gunshot wound of head from .22 shot cartridge. Wound incised revealing depressed fracture.

Jacket bullet is a truncated cone with a hollow point. Unlike the CCI Stinger and the Winchester Expediter, the cartridge case length is the standard Long Rifle length. Imprinted on the base of the cartridge case is the figure of a yellow jacket. A solid bullet version of the Yellow Jacket called the "Viper" appeared in 1982. The bullet weighs 36 gr and has a muzzle velocity of 1410 ft/sec in a rifle.

Federal introduced their high-velocity .22 Long Rifle cartridge, the "Spitfire," in January 1983. This round is loaded with a 33-gr lead hollow-point bullet. Muzzle velocity is 1376 ft/sec in a rifle with an 18½-in. barrel and 1506 ft/sec in a 24-in. barrel. With handguns, muzzle velocity is 1173 ft/sec in a 4-in. barrel.

CB and BB Caps

Both CCI and Winchester produce CB cartridges. Winchester produces only the .22 Short version, whereas CCI produces both .22 Short and Long versions. These cartridges are loaded with all-lead, 29-gr Short bullets. Reduced powder charges are used so that the muzzle velocity is 706 ft/sec for both the Short and Long CB cartridges compared to 865 ft/sec for the standard velocity Short cartridge (in 6-in. barreled weapons). BB caps imported from Europe consist of a case shorter than the Short case loaded with a lightweight lead bullet. The propellant is just the primer. BB caps are not manufactured in this country.

Frangible Ammunition

.22 frangible bullets were designed for use in shooting galleries and for stunning cattle for slaughter. The bullets consist of bonded fragments of iron or lead that disintegrate on striking a hard surface. Bullets composed of powdered iron show a slightly greater degree of fragmentation.

Although frangible bullets break up on striking a hard surface, such bullets readily penetrate the human body and have caused a number of deaths.[4] These bullets are of considerable forensic significance; when recovered from the body, they are unsuitable for ballistic comparison because of erosion of the bullet's surface. Both types of bullets show a fine particulate disintegration of the surface. At most, faint rifling marks unsuitable for ballistic comparison can be seen. The surface disintegration is due to the bonded fragment construction of the missile.

In a body, the iron bullets tend to break up into short cylinders or thick disks. An x-ray film of such a bullet in the body may be very characteristic. The iron gallery rounds can be identified easily by means of a magnet.

Wounds due to Rimfire Ammunition

Contact Wounds

.22 Short. Most contact wounds with .22 rimfire ammunition are self-inflicted wounds of the head. Hard contact wounds of the head inflicted with the .22 Short cartridge often present difficult problems of interpretation. The small amount of powder in the cartridge and the resultant small amount of soot and gas produced result in an absence of tears at the entrance as well as very little or no deposition of soot or powder in and about such a head wound. These wounds often are mistaken for distant wounds; however, close inspection of the entrance, usually shows some blackening and searing of the edges. Unfortunately, distant wounds can simulate this appearance if the edges of the entrance have dried out.

Internal examination of a hard contact wound of the head with the unaided eye often shows neither soot nor powder. Use of a dissecting microscopic may reveal some soot and less frequently powder. If on examination of a wound both externally and internally, using both the naked eye and the dissecting microscope, there is still no evidence of soot or powder and the wound is suspected of being contact, the wound should be examined by EDX or FAAS for metallic deposits from the primer, bullet, or cartridge case. Fortunately, such problems rarely arise. Often, with hard contact wounds from a .22 Short cartridge the problem is solved immediately by the observation of the imprint of the muzzle around the suspected contact wound of entrance.

Relative absence of soot and powder from a hard contact wound inflicted by a .22 Short cartridge will be even more pronounced if the weapon used is a rifle. The longer barrel length permits almost complete combustion of the propellant.

In contact wounds of the head from the .22 Short cartridge, there are generally no skull fractures, except perhaps of the orbital plates. The bullet rarely exits the cerebral cavity. Internal ricocheting with such a round is extremely common. When recovered, the bullet usually is severely mutilated.

Hard contact wounds of the body from a .22 Short cartridge can be identified more easily than those of the head. Because most of these wounds are through clothing, there is often a band of soot on the skin around the entrance. In all cases, the edges of these wounds are seared and blackened to a greater degree than is seen in head wounds. Soot and powder often can be seen using a dissecting microscope. These differences in comparison to head wounds may result because there is less "blow-back" of gas due to absence of bone to deflect back the gas.

.22 Long Rifle and .22 Magnum Cartridges. Hard contact wounds of the head with the .22 Long Rifle cartridge are large and usually circular in shape with ragged edges. True stellate wounds are the exception, not the rule. Soot, powder, and searing are prominent. Usually there is no difficulty in distinguishing a distant from a contact wound with the .22 Long Rifle cartridge. The use of a dissecting microscope will remove any doubts, as soot and powder can be seen readily in the subcutaneous tissue. Muzzle imprints are much more common than in wounds from the Short cartridge because of the greater gas volume produced. Secondary fractures of the skull in addition to fractures of the orbital plates are frequent. The bullet often exits the skull, though it may be found underneath the scalp, adjacent to the exit in the skull. X-ray of the head usually shows lead fragments at the entrance site and along the bullet track. However, the author has seen a number of instances of perforating .22 Long Rifle wounds of the head in which no lead was present on x-ray.

Hard contact wounds of the head with a .22 Magnum cartridge are noteworthy in that spherical ball powder, which is used in some brands of these cartridges, can transverse the head and be found at the exit. Contact wounds of the head with a .22 Magnum cartridge resemble .22 Long Rifle wounds in external appearance. Cruciform tears occur more frequently, however. .22 Magnum bullets almost invariably exit from the head.

Contact wounds of the body from the .22 Long Rifle cartridge show searing and blackening of the edges of the wound, often with a cuff of soot. Muzzle imprints are common. The bullet may perforate the body in contrast to .22 Short bullets, which virtually never perforate.

Wounds of the body caused by .22 Magnum bullets resemble .22 Long Rifle wounds. Muzzle imprints are common. If the weapon is a handgun, there are often piles of unburned ball powder at the entrance. Exit wounds of the trunk are usual.

Intermediate-Range Wounds

The appearance of individual powder tattoo marks, the size of the pattern, and the maximum distance out to which tattooing occurs depend on the physical form of the powder (flake, ball, or cylindrical), the range from gun to target, and the barrel length. .22 Magnum cartridges are loaded with either spherical ball or cylindrical powder. Winchester-Western .22 Short, Long, and Long Rifle cartridges are loaded with very fine ball powder. All the other manufacturers use flake powder.

Tattooing from .22 Short and Long Rifle ammunition loaded with ball powder is extremely fine. Animal tests, using a .22 handgun with a 2-in. barrel indicate that powder tattooing from Long Rifle cartridges loaded with ball powder extends out to a maximum of 18 in. (45 cm) from muzzle to target. Tattooing is absent at 24 in. (60 cm).

Cartridges loaded with flake powder produce fewer, larger, and more prominent powder tattoo marks. Flakes may penetrate into the dermis. Animal testing with a 2-in. barrel .22-caliber revolver revealed powder tattoo marks from Long Rifle cartridges loaded with flake powder extend out to a range of 18 to 24 in. (45 to 60 cm). Tattoo marks are gone by a range of 30 in. (75 cm).

.22 Magnum cartridges loaded with ball powder produces very dense tattooing more like the tattooing from centerfire cartridges. Cylindrical powder produces tattooing that resembles markings from flake powder.

Distant Wounds

Distant wounds of entrance from .22 rimfire bullets are generally circular to oval in shape. The circular wounds usually measure 5 mm in diameter, including the abrasion ring. In some areas of the body where the skin is very elastic and may be stretched when the bullet enters, e.g., the elbow, the entrance wound may be extremely small; in one case the complete diameter (including abrasion ring) was 3 mm. This wound initially was interpreted as a puncture wound and not a gunshot wound, as it was believed to be too small to be a gunshot wound. Distant wounds from .22 caliber bullets have been mistaken for ice-pick wounds and vice versa.

.22 Long Rifle hollow-point bullets fired from handguns do not as a general rule mushroom. If they strike bone, they can flatten out. Both solid-point and hollow-point bullets, rather than flattening out on striking bone, usually penetrate the bone. On recovery, they appear relatively intact and undeformed. Close examination, however, usually will show fine, brushlike scrape marks on their surface. Hollow-point bullets, fired from rifles, often mushroom without striking bone.

.22 Long Rifle bullet wounds of the head can produce linear fractures of the skull at a distant range whether the weapon used is a handgun or a rifle. These fracture involve the cranial vault and orbital plates for the most part and are due to temporary cavity formation.

References

1. Cochrane, D.W. Barrel lengths vs velocity and energy. A.F.T.E. 11(1):37−38, 1979.
2. DiMaio, V.J.M., Spitz, W.U. Injury by birdshot. J. Forensic Sci. 15(3): 396−402, 1970.
3. DiMaio, V.J.M., Minette, L.J., Johnson, S. Three deaths due to revolver shot shell cartridges. Forensic Sci. 4:247−251, 1974.
4. Graham, J.W., Petty, C.S., Flohr, D.M., Peterson, W.E. Forensic aspects of frangible bullets. J. Forensic Sci. 2(4): 507−515, 1966.

General References

Barnes, F.C. *Cartridges of the World*, 4th ed. Northfield IL: DBI Books Inc.

Lachuk, J. (ed.). *Wonderful World of the .22*. Los Angeles, CA: Peterson Publishing Co., 1972.

Annual ammunition catalogs published by Winchester, Remington, Federal, and CCI.

Wounds from Centerfire Rifles

7

Wounds caused by high-velocity centerfire rifles are markedly different from wounds caused by handguns or .22 rimfire rifles. Handguns and .22 rimfire rifles are relatively low-velocity weapons with muzzle velocities of between 650 and 1400 ft/sec; with the exception of the .357 Magnum and the .44 Magnum, muzzle energies are well below 500 ft-lb. The widely publicized .45 automatic has a muzzle velocity of only 850 ft/sec, with a muzzle energy of 370 ft-lb. In contrast, the muzzle velocities of modern high-velocity centerfire rifles range between 2400 and 4000 ft/sec (Table 7−1). The muzzle kinetic energy is never less than 1000 ft-lb; it is commonly in the 2000 range and may be as high as 5000 ft-lb of energy. Because of the low velocities and kinetic energies, injuries from both handgun and .22 rimfire rifle bullets are confined to tissue and organs directly in the wound path. In contrast, a high-velocity rifle bullet can injure structures without actually contacting them.

Before the mid-nineteenth century, most shoulder arms were smooth-bore with a caliber of .69 to .75. The projectiles they fired were soft lead spheres of from 484 to 580 gr. The propellant was black powder. Initial velocity was from 590 to 754 ft/sec.[1] Because of the low velocities possessed by these spherical balls, the injuries produced were confined to tissue and organs directly in the wound track.[2−4] The wound entrance was round and approximately the size of the bullet; it was surrounded by an extensive area of ecchymosis. The wound track through the tissue was greater than the diameter of the bullet. Musket balls usually lodged in the body. The exit wound, if present, was characteristically larger than the entrance wound. When such bullets struck bone, they often lodged in the bone or flattened against it. If the ball struck the bone at maximum velocity, it was capable of causing severe damage with exten-

Table 7-1 Ballistics of Various Handgun and Rifle Centerfire Cartridges

Cartridge	Bullet weight (gr)	Muzzle velocity (ft/sec)	Muzzle energy (ft-lb)
Handguns			
.25 Auto	50	810	73
.32 S&W	88	680	90
.38 Special	158	855	256
.357 Magnum	158	1410	696
9-mm	115	1155	341
.45 Auto	230	850	369
.44 Magnum	240	1470	1150
Rifles			
.223	55	3240	1282
.30-30	150	2390	1902
.30 Carbine	110	1990	967
.308	150	2820	2648
.30-06	150	2910	2820

sive comminution of the bone and displacement of bone spiculae along the wound track.

The 1850s saw the introduction of conical bullets (Minie bullets). These bullets ranged in caliber from .67 to .69. They had a conical shape, were made of soft lead, and weighed from 555 to 686 gr.[1] These bullets could be loaded in either smooth-bore or rifled weapons. The most significant difference from the spherical bullets was the sharp increase in velocity. Initial velocity with such ammunition ranged from 931 to 1017 ft/sec. The wounds caused by these bullets showed enormous destruction of tissue and were much more severe than injuries from the old round balls. The use of these weapons in combat—for example, the Civil War—brought about numerous accusations of the use of explosive bullets.[2-5] The increased wounding effectiveness of such ammunition was due to the fact that whereas the bullet weight was equal to or in many cases greater than that of the spherical bullet, the velocity was markedly increased. Thus, these conical bullets possessed significantly greater kinetic energy to inflict wounds.

Bone injuries from conical bullets were extremely severe. The term used to described them at the time was "explosive."[*,2,3] Pulpefaction of soft tissue secondary to fragments of bone and disintegrating particles from the bullet were described. Large wounds of exit were present.

In reviewing firearm wounds through the ages, one is struck by the recurrent use of the term "explosive" to describe wounds produced by newly introduced weapons or forms of ammunition. This term has been used to describe wounds produced by conical lead bullets, jacketed bullets, hunting bullets, and the M/16.

By the late nineteenth century, most rifles were generally of .40 to .50 caliber. The .45-70 cartridge adopted by the U.S. Army in 1873 is a typical example of the large-caliber black powder weapons in use. A typical loading for this cartridge was a 500-gr bullet with a muzzle velocity of 1315 ft/sec and muzzle energy of 1875 ft-lb.

The introduction of smokeless powder at the end of the nineteenth century lead to a general reduction of caliber so that most military weapons were of 6.5 to 8-mm caliber. Bullets used in these weapons were roundnosed and full metal-jacketed, weighed around 220 gr, and had a muzzle velocity of approximately 2000 ft/sec. Wounds produced by these bullets were believed by some authorities to be less severe than those due to the conical lead bullets.[2-4] Such observations were probably correct. These new bullets, being full metal-jacketed, tended to pass through the body without any deformation, thereby losing less kinetic energy than the conical lead bullets, which, being easily deformed in the body, lost large amounts of kinetic energy.

Almost immediately after the introduction of the roundnose ammunition, full metal-jacketed Spitzer (pointed) bullets were introduced. These bullets, averaging 150 gr, had muzzle velocities of approximately 2700 ft/sec. Soon after the appearance of these new high-velocity loadings, the observation was made that the wounds produced by these cartridges appeared to be "explosive."[2-4] The external signs of injuries were slight, with small entrance and exit sites combined with extensive disruption and laceration of the internal viscera and soft tissue. These injuries not uncommonly involved structures distant from the actual bullet path. The extensive nature of these injuries is now known to be due to the temporary cavity formation described in Chapter 3. These wounds were felt to be less severe than those due to lead conical bullets such as those used in the American Civil War.[3,4]

Discussion of rifle wounds in the medical literature is concerned almost exclusively with injuries from military ammunition. Wounds encountered by pathologists and medical examiners, however, almost always involve hunting ammunition. The design and construction of hunting ammunition are radically different from that of military ammunition. Because of these differences, the wounds produced by hunting ammunition are much more devastating.

Before discussing rifle wounds from high-velocity centerfire cartridges, one has to decide what a high-velocity centerfire rifle cartridge is. For the purpose of this discussion, it is defined as any cartridge with a centrally located primer intended to be fired in a rifle of caliber .17 or greater whose bullet is propelled at a velocity of more than 2000 ft/sec. The .30-caliber M-1 Carbine cartridge is neither a rifle nor a handgun cartridge. It has a muzzle velocity just below 2000 ft/sec. Wounds produced by the full metal-jacketed .30 Carbine bullet more closely resemble those from a Magnum pistol bullet than those from a centerfire rifle, whereas the wounds produced by soft-point or hollow-point .30 Carbine ammunition are much too extensive to be ascribed to pistol cartridges and most closely resemble in severity those seen with a rifle cartridge. Thus, the .30 Carbine cartridge lies in a transition zone between rifle and pistol cartridges in terms of wounding. The construction of the bullet loaded in the cartridge case determines whether the wound is pistol-like or rifle-like.

Research by the military has revealed that the feature of a bullet's interaction with soft tissue that contributes most to the severity and extent of the wound is the size of the temporary wound cavity (see Chapter 3). The size of this cavity is directly related to the amount of kinetic energy lost by a bullet in the tissue. Rifle bullets, by virtue of high velocities, possess considerably more kinetic energy than pistol bullets. Table 7 – 1 illustrates the muzzle velocities and kinetic energies of some typical pistol and rifle bullets. The marked contrast in the kinetic energy possessed by rifle bullets in comparison to pistol bullets is evident.

The severity and extent of a wound, however, are determined not by the amount of kinetic energy possessed by a bullet but rather by the amount of this energy that is lost in the tissue. The major determinants of the amount of kinetic energy lost by a bullet in the body are (1) the kinetic energy possessed by the bullet at the time of impact with the body, (2) the shape of the bullet, (3) the angle of yaw at the time of impact, (4) any change in the presented area of the bullet in its passage through the body, (5) construction of the bullet, and (6) the biological characteristics of the tissues through which the bullet passes.

By virtue of high velocities and thus higher kinetic energies, rifle bullets have the potential to produce extremely severe wounds. For military ammunition, velocity is the most important determinant of the severity of the wound, as military bullets have a full metal jacket that prevents deformation of the bullet. In contrast in hunting ammunition, bullet construction plays a role equal to or greater than that of velocity in determining the extent and severity of the wound. A hunting bullet is designed to deform in its passage through the body, producing an increase in its presenting area; this trait, plus a tendency to shed fragments of lead core, results in greater kinetic energy loss and thus greater tissue injury.

The two types of wound tracks produced when a bullet passes through tissue are the permanent wound track and the temporary cavity. As a bullet moves through the body, the tissue adjacent to the bullet's path is flung away in a radial manner, creating a temporary cavity. The size of this cavity is directly related to the amount of kinetic energy absorbed by the tissue. This cavity may be as much as 6 in. in diameter for high-velocity rifle bullets. The cavity undulates for 5 to 10 msec before it comes to rest as a permanent wound track. The pressure in the temporary cavity in the case of high-velocity rifle bullets can be tremendous, with shock waves of up to 100 to 200 atm. Organs struck by these bullets may undergo partial or complete disintegration. The pressures generated are sufficient to fracture bone and rupture vessels adjacent to the permanent wound track but not directly struck by the bullet.

The severe nature of wounds from high-velocity rifles is due to the large temporary cavities produced, exceeding the limits of elasticity of the tissue and organs. Body organs can absorb only a certain amount of kinetic energy and therefore a certain size of temporary cavity before the limits of their elasticity are exceeded and the organs shatter (pulpify). The severely destructive properties of rifle bullets are not possessed by pistol or .22 rimfire rifle bullets. The low velocity of such bullets, with resultant low kinetic energy imparted to the tissue, results in small temporary cavities that do not exceed the elastic limits of organs.

Centerfire Rifle Bullets

High-velocity centerfire rifle bullets differ in construction from handgun bullets in that rifle bullets have to have either full or partial metal jacketing. This is necessary because of the high velocities at which rifle bullets are propelled down a barrel. If the bullets were lead or lead alloy, these high velocities would result in the lead being stripped from the surface of the bullet by the rifling grooves. Some handloaders will load high velocity rifle cartridges with cast lead bullets. In such cases, however, they reduce the powder charge so that the muzzle velocities produced are generally below 1600 ft/sec. These bullets may or may not have a gas check. They are easily recognized by their long length and deep cannelures for lubricants (Figure 7−1).

Rifle bullets can be divided into four general categories on the basis of their configuration and construction. First is the full metal-jacketed bullet. This is the standard form of ammunition used by the military. The bullet has a lead or steel core, covered by an outside jacket of cupro-nickel or gilding metal. This metal jacket completely encloses the tip of the bullet, preventing it from expanding when it reaches its target. The tip of the bullet may be either pointed or rounded (Figure 7−2). The core is exposed at the base.

Soft-point rifle bullets have a lead core with a partial metal jacketing that is generally closed at the base (Figure 7−3). The lead core is exposed at the tip so as to facilitate expansion when the bullet strikes. The tip of the soft-point bullet may either taper to a point or have a rounded, blunt end. Expansion of soft-point bullets can be facilitated further by scallop-

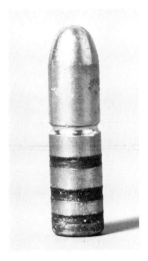

Figure 7−1 Cast rifle bullet with deep cannulures filled with grease.

ing the mouth of the jacket or cutting five or six notches around the jacket mouth. These modification allow uniform peel-back of the jacket when the bullet strikes the target. Soft-point bullets are the most widely used form of hunting ammunition.

Hollow-point rifle bullets are a variant of soft-point bullets. They are partial metal-jacketed hunting bullets that have a cavity at the tip of the bullet to facilitate expansion when the bullet strikes game. Hollow-point bullet are used for hunting and competitive shooting matches (Figure 7−3).

Figure 7−2 Full metal-jacketed military bullets. (a) 162-gr roundnose; (b) 150-gr Spitzer, and (c) 150-gr boat-tail.

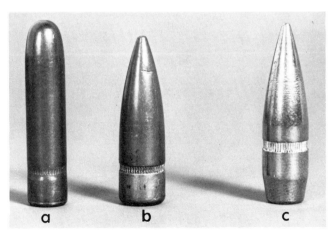

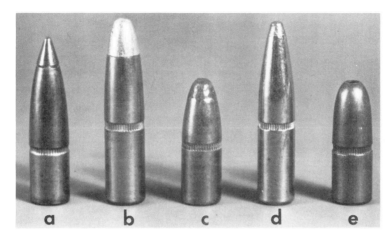

Figure 7-3 Hunting bullet. (a) Bronze-point®, (b) Silvertip®, (c) soft-point, (d) soft-point, and (e) hollow-point.

The fourth category of rifle bullets is a miscellaneous one of controlled expansion projectiles. This group includes Silver-Tip® ammunition by Winchester and the Bronze-Point® by Remington. The Silver-Tip® bullet is in reality a soft-point bullet whose lead tip is protected by a thin jacket of aluminum alloy (Figure 7-3). This aluminum sheath extends back under the jacket almost to the cannelure. The purpose of the aluminum jacket is to protect the exposed lead core so as to delay expansion slightly. The Remington Bronze-Point® has a pointed, wedge-shaped nose in the forward part of the jacket so that the lead is not exposed. A small cavity underlies this wedge. When the bullet strikes the target, the wedge is driven back into the bullet, expanding it.

From this discussion, we can see that hunting bullets differ from military ammunition in that the former are designed to expand or mushroom so as to transfer energy more efficiently to the target and to kill game more effectively. Ammunition manufacturers control the rate and extent of expansion of hunting ammunition by controlling the bullet velocity and the physical characteristics of the bullet. Thus, the degree of expansion can be controlled by the thickness and hardness of the jacket, the location of the bullet cannelure, the amount of lead exposed, the shape of the bullet, the composition of the lead core, and the design characteristic of the bullet.

Military bullets, by virtue of their full metal jackets, tend to pass through the body intact, thus producing less extensive injuries than hunting ammunition. Military bullets usually do not fragment in the body or shed fragments of lead in their paths. Because of the high velocity of such military rounds as well as their tough construction, it is possible for such bullets to pass through more than one individual before coming to rest. These bullets may be almost virginal in appearance after recovery from the body.

One exception to these observations is the 5.56-mm M-16 cartridge. This particular cartridge has gained widespread notoriety in both the lay press and the medical literature. The wounds inflicted often are described as explosive in nature. The bullet has been described as exploding in the body. Such statements are, of course, nonsense. The 5.56-mm round does not explode in the body; it does, however, have a tendency to tumble and fragment, with lead core "squirted" out the base. Because it does fragment, it tends to lose considerable amounts of kinetic energy, thus producing relatively severe wounds for the amount of muzzle energy that it possesses. The wounds produced by the 5.56-mm round are, in fact, less severe than those produced by lower velocity hunting ammunition such as the .30-30.

When full-metal jacketed 5.56 mm bullets break up in the body, the tip of the bullet tends to break off or bend at the cannelure (Figure 7−4). The tip remains relatively intact, while the lead core and the rest of the jacket tend to shred. The triangular shape of the tip of the bullet often can be seen on x-ray (Figure 7−4). Another round that has a tendency to tumble in the body is the 7.62 × 51 mm NATO cartridge.

High-Velocity Rifle Wounds

Wounds from high-velocity rifles may be classified as contact, intermediate, or distant. Contact wounds of the head are the most devastating, producing a bursting rupture of the head (Figure 7−5). Large irregular tears in the scalp radiate from the entrance site. Powder soot and searing are typically present at the entrance site. On occasion in hard contact wounds, virtually no soot will be present.

In some hard contact wounds of the head, the entrance may be difficult to locate because of the massive destruction. Large pieces of the skull and brain are typically blown away, with pulpification of the residual brain in the cranial cavity. Pieces of scalp may be sheared off. The skull shows extensive comminuted fractures. Such wounding effects appear to be due partly to the large quantities of gas produced by combustion of the propellant. This gas begins to expand as soon as it emerges from the muzzle of the weapon. If the gun is held in contact with the head, this gas follows the bullet into the cranial cavity, producing an effect that can only be described as explosive. That the massive wounds produced are due partly to the gas can be deduced from cases of suicides in which the weapon used was equipped with a flash suppressor. This device is attached to the muzzle of military weapons so as to break up the "ball of fire" occurring when an individual discharges a

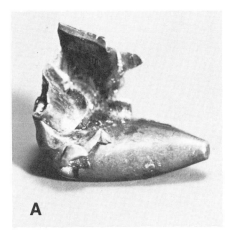

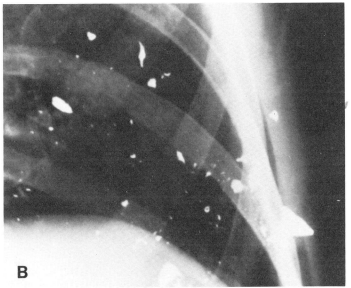

Figure 7–4 A. Full metal-jacketed .223 bullet bent at cannulure. **B.** "Lead snowstorm" resulting from full metal-jacketed .223 bullets. .223 bullet bent at cannulure can be seen on x-ray.

weapon at night. The purpose of this device is to make soldiers firing weapons at night less susceptible to enemy counterfire. It disperses the gas emerging from the barrel through a number of slits in the sides of the flash suppressor. If an individual shoots himself with a flash suppressor-equipped weapon so that the end of it is in contact with the head, the flash suppressor will divert most of the gas emerging from the barrel before it has an opportunity to enter the cranial cavity. Thus, the wound

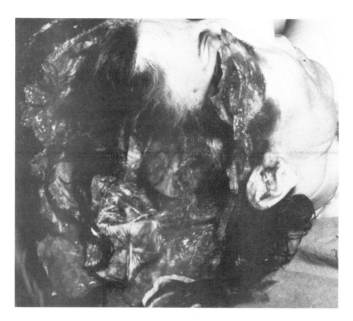

Figure 7 – 5 Homicidal contact wound of right temple from .30-30 rifle.

produced by a weapon with a flash suppressor will be less severe than a wound produced by the same weapon without a flash suppressor. In contact wounds, the gas diverted by the flash suppressor may produce a characteristic pattern of searing and soot deposition (Figure 4 – 13).

If the muzzle of a rifle is inserted in the mouth, massive wounds from the gas and the temporary cavity occur. An explosive blowout type of wound may occur with superficial linear lacerations in the nasolabial folds as well as radiating from the corners of the mouth (Figure 7 – 6).

Contact wounds of the chest and abdomen do not have the dramatic external appearance of such wounds in the head. There is no tearing of the skin due to gas. The wound of entrance is typically circular in shape. Usually, it will be larger in diameter than those due to pistol bullets. The edges of the wound are seared from the effect of the hot gases of combustion. Powder soot is deposited in and around the wound. The amount of soot, however, is less than that seen with most pistols. The imprint of the muzzle of the weapon is commonly present (Figure 7 – 7). Such imprints are due to the gas of combustion entering the chest or abdominal cavities, expanding in them, and slamming the chest or abdominal wall into the muzzle of the weapon. The fact that the whole wall is flung against the muzzle of the weapon by the gas, rather than just the skin as in head wounds, accounts for the fact that the skin is not torn. The outward moving chest or abdominal wall may envelop the muzzle to such a degree that the imprint of the front sight will be

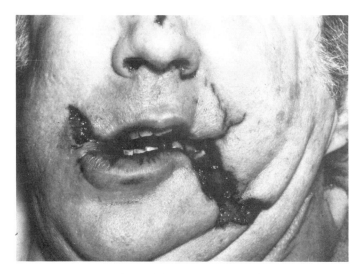

Figure 7–6 Tears at corners of mouth from intraoral gunshot wound.

Figure 7–7 Contact wound of chest from .30-30 rifle with muzzle imprint. (From DiMaio, V.J.M. Wounds caused by centerfire rifles. Clin. Lab. Med. 3:257–271, 1983. Published with permission.)

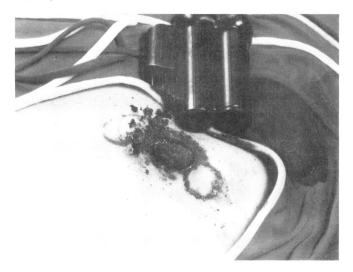

muzzle to such a degree that the imprint of the front sight will be impressed on the skin even though the front sight is recessed a half inch from the muzzle of the weapon. In lever-action weapons with a magazine under the barrel, the imprint of the end of the magazine may be imparted to the skin (Figure 7–7).

In contrast to their benign external appearance, contact high velocity rifle wounds of the chest and abdomen produce massive internal injuries. The severe nature of these wounds, due to both the effects of the gas and temporary cavity, literally pulpify organs, such as the heart and liver. In contact wounds of the thorax or abdomen, the musculature surrounding the entrance may show a cherry-red coloration due to the presence of large amounts of carbon monoxide in the propellant gases. This carbon monoxide may follow the missile through the body and may also be present in the muscle adjacent to the exit. In one case seen by the author, the concentration of carboxyhemoglobin in the muscle was greater at the exit than at the entrance.

In intermediate-range gunshot wounds, powder tattooing is present around the wound of entrance. Intermediate range and distant head wounds, show a wide range in the degree of severity, depending on the style of bullet and the entrance site in the head. Anything that tends to produce instability in the bullet as it enters the head results in more extensive injuries. Thus, bullets entering through the thick occipital bone cause greater injuries than those entering the temporal area. Intermediate and distant range wounds of the head can be just as devastating as contact wounds (Figure 7–8). This is especially true for hunting ammunition. As the hunting bullet rapidly expands, large quantities of kinetic energy are lost in the cranial cavity. This produces a large temporary cavity with resultant high pressure, all within the rigid framework of the skull. The pressure produces extensive fracture of the skull, large lacerations of the scalp, and ejection of fragments of bone and brain tissue. Location of entrance and exit wounds may require extensive reconstruction of the skull, with careful realignment of the edges of the scalp and bone. Sometimes the entrance in the skin cannot be determined with absolute certainty.

Gunshot wounds with full metal-jacketed ammunition are generally not as devastating. If for some reason, however, the bullet begins to tumble, extensive wounds just as devastating as those due to hunting ammunition can be produced.

Distant wounds of entrance in areas overlying bone—e.g., the head— may have a stellate appearance suggestive of a contact wound (Figure 7–9). This is probably due to the temporary cavity ballooning out skin that is tightly stretched over bone, with resultant tearing of the skin.

Distant entrance wounds of the trunk inflicted by high velocity rifle bullets are similar to those produced by pistol bullets. The only poten-

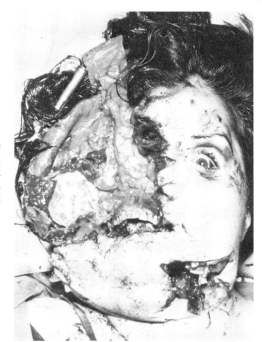

Figure 7–8 High-velocity rifle wound of right half of head from .30-30 rifle. Bullet entered in back of head. Ejected cartridge case can be seen in hair. Second gunshot wound of left side of neck.

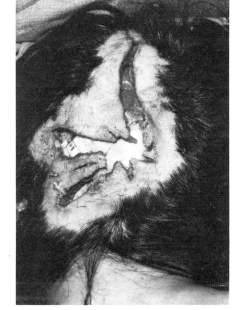

Figure 7–9 Large stellate distant wound of entrance in back of head from .30-30 rifle. (From DiMaio, V.J.M. Wound caused by centerfire rifles. Clin. Lab. Med. 3:257–271, 1983. Published with permission.)

tial differences are that the abrasion ring around the rifle wound of entrance is narrower than that seen in a pistol wound and that multiple small (less than 1 mm) micro-tears radiate outward from the edges of the perforation. *In some instances no abrasion ring is present*, just a round or oval punched-out perforation with micro-tears (Figure 7−10).

Distant entrance wounds of the lateral aspect of the thorax from approximately the milk line to the posterior axillary line may be unusually large. Like most distant wounds they are circular in shape, but the diameter of the entrance perforation can be up to 1 in. (25 mm) in diameter. The cause of this is unknown.

Internal injuries of the trunk due to high-velocity rifle bullets, fired at intermediate and distant ranges are extremely devastating, with massive destruction and pulpification of the organs. These are due to temporary cavity formation, with its high-pressure effects. In distant wounds of the chest and abdomen, the thoracic or abdominal wall may be propelled outward by the temporary cavity with such force that imprints of clothing or objects lying against the skin will be imparted to it (Figure 7−11).

Whatever the range, exit wounds of the chest and abdomen from high-velocity rifle bullets all have the same appearance. They are larger and more irregular than the entrance wounds, with the majority of exit wounds 25 mm or less in diameter. The largest exit wound in the trunk that the author has seen measured 75 × 40 mm.

Powder Tattooing

The range out to which powder tattooing occurs from centerfire rifles depends on the physical form of powder in the cartridge cases. Two forms of powder are used in centerfire rifles cartridges: ball and cylin-

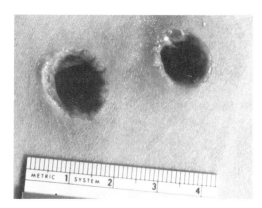

Figure 7−10 Two distant entrance wounds of back from centerfire rifle. Note absence of abrasion ring and presence of microtears.

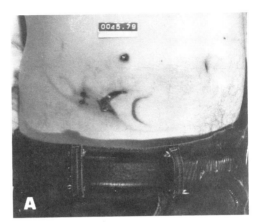

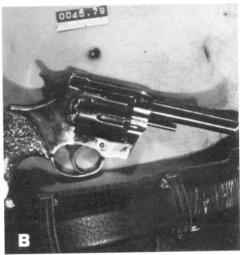

Figure 7–11 A. and **B**. Entrance wound from 7-mm Magnum rifle with patterned abrasions due to revolver tucked in waistband.

drical powder (Figure 7–12). A series of tests were carried out by the author on live anesthetized rabbits. The chest and abdomen were shaved and the remaining hair was removed by depilatory cream. The rabbits were shot in the chest and abdomen at varying distances, using a Winchester Model 94 .30-30 rifle and a Remington 788, caliber .223, with a 24-inch barrel. Two brands of ammunition were used in each rifle. One was loaded with cylindrical powder, and the other had ball powder. The tests indicated that the maximum range at which powder tattooing occurs is different for the different forms of powder. For the .30-30 rifle, cartridges loaded with cylindrical powder produced heavy powder tattooing with deposition of soot at a range of 6 in. (15 cm). By 12

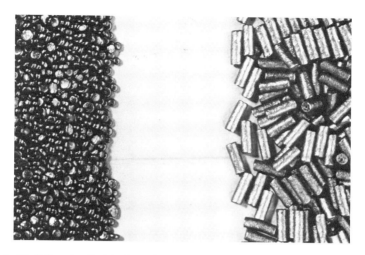

Figure 7–12 Ball and cylindrical powder.

in. (30 cm) only a few scattered powder tattoo marks were present. No tattooing occurred at 18 or 24 in. (45 or 60 cm). Powder tattooing with ball powder extended out to 30 in. (75 cm), at which range it was present in moderate density. At a range of 36 in. (90 cm), ball powder no longer produced any tattooing (Table 7–2).

For the .223 rifle, cartridges loaded with cylindrical powder produced rare tattooing out to 12 in. (30 cm). By 18 in. (45 cm), no powder tattooing was present. Powder tattooing caused by ball powder was heavy at 18 in. (45 cm) and scattered at 36 in. (90 cm). At 42 in. (105 cm) it was gone (Table 7–2).

Powder tattooing at greater ranges for ball powder compared with cylindrical powder is due to the shape of the powder grains. A sphere has a better aerodynamic form than a cylinder. Ball powder grains can travel farther with greater velocity, enabling them to mark the skin at a greater range.

The powder tattoo marks produced by these two different forms of powder have different appearances. The markings from ball powder tend to be small, circular, and hemorrhagic, occurring in great numbers (Figure 7–13). Tattoo marks produced by cylindrical powder are larger, more irregular in shape and size, and relatively sparse in number compared with ball powder tattooing. Examination of such markings reveals that a number of them have a linear configuration (Figure 7–13). The number of tattoo marks from cylindrical powder at 6 in. was less than the number of powder tattoo marks produced at 24 in. by ball powder.

The skin of rabbits is thinner and more delicate than that of humans. Therefore, powder tattooing should theoretically occur out to greater

Table 7–2 Maximum Range Out To Which Tattooing Presents

Range (cm)	Cylindrical powder	Ball powder
Caliber: .30-30		
15	+++[a]	–
30	+	–
45	0	–
60	0	++
75	–	++
90	–	0
Caliber: .223		
15	+++	–
30	+	–
45	0	+++
60	–	–
75	–	++
90	–	+
105	–	0

[a] – = not tested. 0 = no tattooing. + = rare tattoo marks. ++ = moderate tattooing. +++ = dense tattooing.

maximum distances for rabbits than for humans. Thus, the data provided by these experiments should be considered only as a guide to the extreme maximum distances at which powder tattooing can occur.

X-rays

X-rays of individuals shot with hunting ammunition usually show a characteristic radiologic picture that is seen almost exclusively with this form of rifle ammunition. This is the so-called "lead snowstorm."[6] As the expanding bullet moves through the body, fragments of lead break off the lead core and are hurled out into the surrounding tissues. Thus, an x-ray shows scores of small radioopaque bullet fragments scattered along the wound track (the lead snowstorm) (Figure 7–14). Such a picture is not seen with pistol bullets, nor, with one exception, with full metal-jacketed rifle bullets. The sole exception is the 5.56-mm cartridge, whose propensity to fragment as been previously discussed (Figure 7–4). Although the snowstorm appearance of an x-ray almost always indicates that the individual was shot with high velocity rifle hunting ammunition, absence of such a picture does not absolutely rule out this possibility. The lead snow-storm from hunting ammunition is dependent on the velocity of the bullet. If a rifle bullet is fired at low velocity or if it has been slowed by passing through various other targets before striking an individual, x-rays will not show a lead snow-storm.

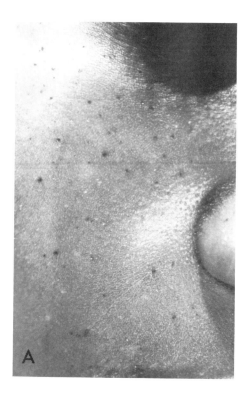

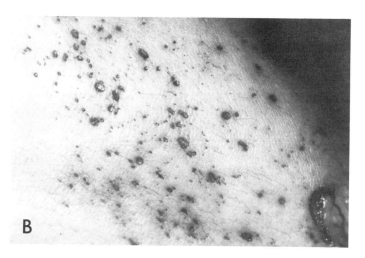

Figure 7-13 A. Ball powder tattooing of face. **B.** Tattooing of arm from cylindrical powder. (From DiMaio, V.J.M. Wounds caused by centerfire rifles. Clin. Lab. Med. 3: 257-271, 1983. Published with permission.)

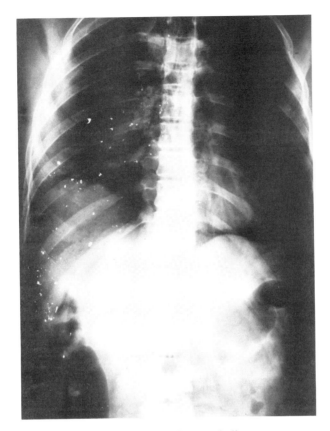

Figure 7–14 "Lead snowstorm" from .30-30 hunting bullet.

Perforating Tendency of Centerfire Rifle Bullets

Full metal-jacketed rifle bullets with rare exceptions invariable exit if the deceased is the primary target and is within a few hundred yards of the muzzle of the weapon. The 5.56-mm round is the only full metal-jacketed round that has a tendency to stay in the body. Most hunting bullets also exit the body. Of a total of 34 high-velocity rifle wounds from hunting ammunition reviewed by the author, in all but 7 instances the bullet exited.[6]

Intermediary Targets

If a rifle bullet passes through an intermediate target, such as a metal plate or glass, before striking an individual, the severity of the wound produced may be much greater than that from a primary wound cause by the same bullet. This is due to the fact that the severity of a wound is directly related to the amount of kinetic energy the bullet loses in the body. If the bullet is deformed or rendered unstable—that is, tumbles as a result of striking an intermediate target—when it strikes the victim, it will more readily lose kinetic energy, thus increasing the severity of the wound. This is true even though the bullet has lost kinetic energy in piercing the intermediate target. This phenomenon is more marked in hunting ammunition. If multiple intermediate targets are perforated, the bullet may lose so much kinetic energy in these intermediate targets that the wound no longer has the characteristics of a high-velocity wound but rather those of a handgun wound.

In passing through an intermediate target, the bullet, whether it be full metal-jacketed or hunting, may break up at least to some degree. If the individual is close to the intermediate target, he or she may be struck by multiple fragments of bullet and intermediate target. Even if the main mass of the bullet is intact, the skin around the entrance site may be "peppered" with fragments of metal broken off the bullet as it perforated the intermediate target or by fragments of the target itself (Figure 7–15). This latter material can consist of metal, glass, wood, or even bone if the intermediate target was an extremity. The entrance wound will be large and irregular because of tumbling or deformation of the bullet. The bullet may also carry large fragments of an intermediate target into the body. Figures 7–16 and 7–17 illustrate the case of an individual shot through an automobile car door with a .30-30 hunting rifle. The main mass of the bullet remained intact, penetrating into the chest and causing death. A small fragment of lead core also penetrated, with another fragment producing a superficial wound of the skin. In exiting the door, the bullet carried with it a large piece of steel, which in turn inflicted a fourth, penetrating wound. This piece of steel was recovered from the muscle of the side, not having penetrated into the chest cavity.

Addendum: Rifle Calibers

At present, at least 50 different caliber rifle cartridges are being manufactured in the United States. Some of these cartridges have been introduced recently, whereas others are almost obsolete with no weapons currently manufactured for them. Obsolete cartridges no longer manufactured are sometimes available from overseas sources as well as being manufactured by home reloaders or small specialized companies. Rifle cartridges that are not popular in the United States but are popular in other countries can be obtained from overseas sources. A few of the more common centerfire rifle calibers will be described.

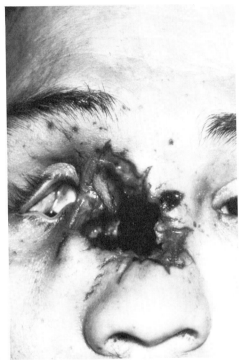

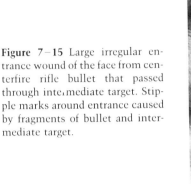

Figure 7–15 Large irregular entrance wound of the face from centerfire rifle bullet that passed through intermediate target. Stipple marks around entrance caused by fragments of bullet and intermediate target.

.222 Remington

The .22 Remington cartridge was introduced by Remington in 1950. It is intended for varmints and small game. Commercially, this cartridge is loaded with a 50-gr soft-point bullet or a 55-gr full metal-jacketed bullet. The full metal-jacketed bullet is rarely encountered. Muzzle velocity is 3140 to 3020 ft/sec.

.223 Remington

The .223 Remington cartridge was introduced in the Armalite AR-15 assault rifle in 1957. It is the standard rifle caliber of the U.S. Army and is now widely used overseas by other countries. The cartridge is loaded with a 55 gr bullet of either soft point or full metal jacket design. The civilian version is the soft point bullet; the full metal jacketed design, the military. This round is used for varmint and small game hunting. Muzzle velocity is approximately 3200 ft/sec, depending upon the barrel length.

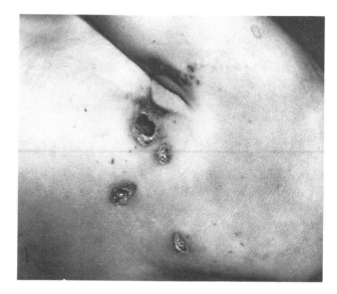

Figure 7–16 Bullet and shrapnel wounds of left side of chest from .30-30 rifle bullet that passed through car door.

Figure 7–17 X-ray of chest showing bullet in midline with steel fragment in left side of chest.

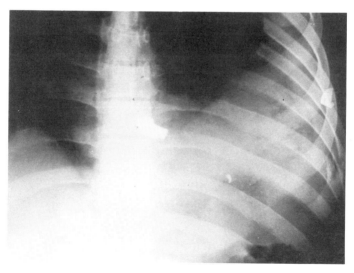

.30-30 Winchester

The .30-30 Winchester was the first small-bore smokeless powder sporting cartridge. It was introduced in 1894 for the Winchester Model 94. This round is essentially a deer cartridge. It is loaded with either 150- or 170-gr hunting bullets. This is probably the most popular hunting round in the United States. It is a relatively low-velocity centerfire cartridge with muzzle velocities ranging from 2400 to 2200 ft/sec.

.30-06 Springfield

The .30-06 Springfield cartridge was adopted in 1906 as the official military cartridge of the U.S. Armed Forces. It was replaced by the .308 Winchester in the early 1950s. Hunting bullets loaded in it weigh 110, 125, 150, 180, and 220 gr. Full metal-jacketed military cartridges are available. Muzzle velocities range from 3370 to 2400 ft/sec, depending on the weight of the bullet.

.270 Winchester

The .270 Winchester round was first marketed in 1925. It is the .30-06 cartridge necked down to .270 caliber. Commercial cartridges are loaded with 100-, 130-, and 150-gr hunting bullets. The performance is approximately that of the .30-06. Muzzle velocity ranges from 3480 to 2900 ft/sec.

.308 Winchester

The .308 Winchester round was introduced in 1952. It is the official NATO cartridge and is used in American machine guns. It loaded with 110-, 125-, 150-, 180-, and 200-gr hunting bullets. Military bullets are full metal-jacketed and usually weigh 150 gr. In ballistic performance it is approximately equal to the .30-06 cartridge. Muzzle velocities range from 3180 to 2450 ft/sec.

.243 Winchester

The .243 Winchester round was introduced in 1955. It is the .308 Winchester case, necked down to 6 mm. The round is intended for both varmints and deer hunting. It is loaded commercially with either an 80-gr or a 100-gr soft-point or hollow-point bullet. Muzzle velocity ranges from 3350 to 2960 ft/sec.

.30 M-1 Carbine

The .30 M-1 Carbine cartridge is neither a rifle cartridge nor a pistol cartridge. The round was originally developed for the U.S. military M-1 Carbine. Commercially, this round is loaded with a 110-gr soft-point or hollow-point bullet. The military round is loaded with a 111-gr full metal-jacketed bullet. Muzzle velocity is around 1990 ft/sec. The M-1 Carbine should not be confused with the M-1 Rifle (the Garand), which was chambered for the .30-06 cartridge.

References

1. Butler, D.F. *United States Firearms. The First Century 1776–1875.* New York: Winchester Press, 1971.
2. La Garde, L.A. *Gunshot Injuries.* New York: William Wood & Co, 1916.
3. Longmore, T. *Gunshot Injuries.* London: Longmans Green and Co., 1895.
4. Scott, R. *Projectile Trauma. An Inquiry into Bullet Wounds.* New York: Crown.
5. Edwards, WB. Civil War Guns. The Stackpole Co., Harrisburg, Penn., 1962.
6. DiMaio, V.J.M., Zumwalt, R.E. Rifle wounds from high velocity centerfire hunting ammunition. J Forensic Sci. 22(1): 132–140, 1977.

Wounds from Shotguns

8

Shotguns differ from rifles and handguns in construction, ammunition, ballistics, and use. Rifle and handguns fire a single projectile down a rifled barrel. Shotguns have a smooth bore; although they can fire a single projectile, they usually are employed to fire multiple pellets. Barrel lengths of shotguns range from 18 to 36 in.; 26, 28, and 30 in. are the usual lengths. United States federal law requires a minimum barrel length of 18 in. Barrels 18 and 20 in. in length traditionally have been used only for police riot guns. With modern powders, barrels lengths greater than 18 and 20 in. produce only insignificant increases in velocity.[1] Longer barrels are really just a matter of tradition, styling, and balance or a desire for a longer sighting radius.

The usual shotgun barrel does not have a rear sight. It possesses only a small rudimentary front sight consisting of a small brass bead. With the increased use of shotguns in deer hunting, manufacturers are now producing shotgun barrels 20 and 22 in. long that are equipped with rifle sights.

A shotgun barrel is divided into three areas: the chamber, the forcing cone, and the bore.[1,2] The chamber is the portion of the barrel that encloses the shotgun shell. It is slightly larger in diameter than the bore. The chambers are cut to the exact full length of the unfolded (fired) cartridge case. Between the chamber and the bore, there is a short, tapering section called the forcing cone. This section constricts the charge as it emerges from the shotgun shell, enabling the pellets to be pushed smoothly into the bore.

The archaic term "gauge" is used to describe the caliber of the shotgun.[1,2] This term refers to the number of lead balls of the given bore diameter that make up a pound. In 12-gauge for example, it would take 12 of the lead balls to make 1 lb. The only exception to this nominclature is

the .410, which has a bore 0.410 in. in diameter. The actual diameters of
the most common gauges are as follows:

Gauge	Bore diameter (in.)
10	0.775
12	0.729
16	0.662
20	0.615
28	0.550
.410	0.410

These are, of course, the nominal bore diameters, as there can be a
variation of a few thousands of an inch due to mechanical operations. As
the bore size of the shotgun increases, so does the number of pellets that
can be loaded in the shot shell. This increase is important to a hunter, as
the effectiveness of the shotgun depends on the accumulative effects of
several pellets hitting an animal rather than on a single wound by a
single pellet. The most popular gauge in the United States is the 12
gauge.

Most shotgun barrels have some degree of "choke," that is, partial
constriction of the bore of a shotgun barrel at its muzzle end so as to
control shot patterns. Choke constricts the diameter of the shot
column, increasing its overall length. The outer layers of shot are given
inward acceleration as they pass through the area of constriction (the
choke). This holds the shot column together for a greater distance as it
moves away from the muzzle.

Different degrees of choke will give different spreads for a particular
shotgun charge. The tighter the choke, the smaller the pattern of pellets.
The usual degrees of choke in descending order are full, modified,
improved cylinder, and cylinder. The degree of choke is based on the
percentage of pellets that will stay inside a 30-in. circle at 40 yd. The
only exception to this is the .410 shotgun, in which the pattern of shot is
determined at 25 yd in a 20-in circle. In determining the spread of the
shot patterns whether on paper or on the body, one must exlude "fliers,"
i.e., pellets deformed in the bore that stray from the main pattern.

The following table gives the percentage of shot that can be expected
in the various choke borings:

Choke	Percentage at 40 yd in 30-in. circle
Full choke	65−75
Modified choke	45−55
Improved cylinder	35−45
Cylinder	25−35

If one examines the table, one sees that a full-choke weapon is supposed to deliver a 65 to 75% pattern.[1] In fact, with modern ammunition, it may actually deliver a higher percentage of shot in a 30-in. circle, because of improvements in shot shell design. Plastic wads, redesign of composite wads, and plastic envelopes for shot have resulted in an increase in percentage of shot delivered to the 30-in. circle, i.e., "a tighter" grouping of pellets. In a full-choke weapon, large shot sizes such as BBs or No. 2 shot may give 75 to 85% shot patterns.[2] This improvement in pattern performance is true for all chokes. It decreases with small shot sizes, however, so that for a No. 9 shot there is no improvement in patterning.

Chokes may start anywhere from 1 to 6 in. from the end of the barrel. They may end flush with the barrel or ½ to 1 in. before it. The amount of constriction, i.e., choke, is relative to the actual bore diameter of the gun, which, as mentioned, may vary a few thousands of an inch. In a 12-gauge shotgun with a 0.729-in. diameter, a full choke barrel has a diameter at the muzzle of approximately 0.694.[2]

In theory, the cylinder bore has no choke. In practice, however, gun companies put some degree of choke in these barrels because a true cylinder bore throws patterns that are irregular in density and shape and have "holes" in them. Addition of 0.003 to 0.005 in. of constriction will make the pattern round with a more even density of shot.

Unlike rifles or pistols, many shotguns have barrels that are easily removable, so that an individual may have one shotgun but a number of barrels of different choke. Over-and-under and double-barrel shotguns usually have a different choke for each barrel.

Some shotguns are equipped with polychokes. These devices are installed at the end of the barrel and permit an individual to go from one choke to another simply by turning a sleeve. Winchester manufactures a shotgun in which one can screw different collars into the muzzle end of the barrel, changing the choke.

There is one common area of confusion concerning gauge and choke. No matter what the gauge, weapons of identical choke produce approximately the same size patterns at the same range. The pattern will differ only in density. A full-choke barrel, whether 12-gauge or 20-gauge will put 65 to 75% of the pellets in a 30-in. circle at 40 yd. The only difference is that the 12-gauge shell with its greater number of pellets will put more of these in the same area. Thus, assuming the same barrel length, choke, pellet size, and range, there should be no difference in the size of the patterns thrown by weapons of different gauges (with the exception of the .410).

Shotgun Ammunition

From the late nineteenth century until fairly recently, shotgun shells were constructed basically the same way. They consisted of a paper body (the tube), a thin brass or brass-coated steel head, a primer, powder, paper, cardboard or composite wads, and lead shot (Figure 8–1A).

The wads were of four types (Figure 8–1B). First was the base wad which was compressed paper or other material inside the shotgun shell at its base. Its purpose was to fill up the space in the shell not occupied by the propellant powder. This wad was not expelled on firing. The overpowder wad was between the propellant and the filler wads. The overpowder wad was a disk of cardboard that acted as a gas seal and prevented contamination of the powder by grease from the filler wads. The filler wads lay in between the overpowder wad and the shot. The fill wads acted to seal the bore when the shotgun was fired, keeping the gas behind the pellets. In addition, they cushioned the shot against the blast of hot gases, preventing deformation, fusion, and melting of the pellets. Filler wads were greased so that they would lubricate and clean the bore as they moved down it. The mouth of the shotgun tube was closed by a thin cardboard disk—the over-shot wad—with the edge of the mouth turned down over this wad in what was called a "rolled crimp."

The brass head of the shotgun had a rim on it. This rim aided in extraction and head spacing of the shell. In the latter function it prevented the case from moving too far forward into the shotgun chamber.

Until 1960 the shotgun tube was made of paper. In 1960, Remington introduced their SP shell (Figure 8–2a).[3] This shell has a polyethylene tube, a brass-plated steel head, and a nonintegral base wad, made from an asbestos-like material molded to shape under pressure. In 1972, Remington introduced their plastic RXP shell, which has a solid head section, i.e., an integral base wad that is continuous with the tube wall.[3] This round is used in the Remington skeet and trap loadings (Figure 8–2b).

Winchester introduced two types of plastic shot shells in 1964.[3] One was a shell with a corrugated or ribbed tube surface and a nonintegral base wad. This shell was subsequently phased out. The other plastic hull was produced by a combination of injection molding and die forming. There is no separate base wad, with the head section being of solid plastic and continuous with the walls (Figure 8–2c).

The Federal Ammunition Company introduced plastic tubes in 1965.[3] Although most shotgun shells are now made with plastic tubes, some major shotgun shell manufacturers still produce shells with paper tubes. In fact, some competative skeet and trap shooters prefer such paper tube shells.

Standard shot shells in 12, 16, 20, and 28 gauges are 2 ¾ in. long. This

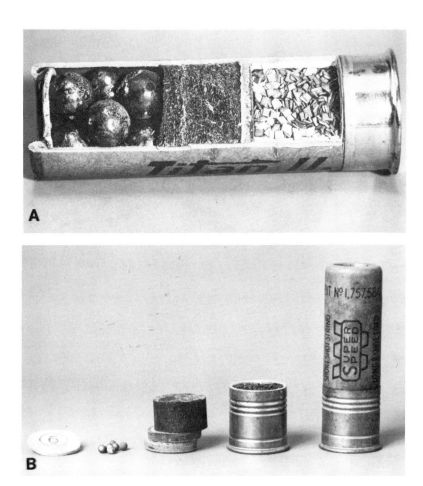

Figure 8–1 A. Traditional shotgun shell with paper tube, brass head, powder, cardboard over-the-powder wad, filler wads, shot, and an over-the-shot wad. **B.** Disassembled traditional shotgun shell showing wadding.

measurement is taken when the case has been fired, i.e., with the crimp unfolded. Unfired, the shells are approximately ¼ in. shorter. Magnum shotgun shells in 12, 16, and 20 gauges come in the standard 2¾-in. length as well as a 3-in. version in the case of 12 and 20 gauge. The standard-length Magnums can be fired in strong modern guns, whereas the 3-in. type is usable only in guns especially chambered for these rounds. The standard length shell for the 10 gauge is 2⅞ in. with 3½-in. being the Magnum round. There is no Magnum shell for the 28 gauge. The .410-gauge shells come in 2½ and 3 in. length. The longer shell contains a little more extra shot. It is not called Magnum, however.

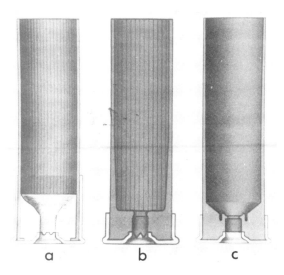

Figure 8-2 (a) Remington SP shell; (b) Remington RXP shell; and (c) Winchester shot shell.

The term "Magnum" implies a large cartridge with a high muzzle velocity. When speaking of Magnum shotgun shells, this is only partly true. Magnum shotgun shells may or may not be longer, but they do not produce higher velocities. Rather, these shells contain more shot. The additional shot is combined with a heavier powder charge, and so this is delivered at standard velocities.

In 1961, Federal began the introduction of color coding of its shotgun shells.[3] At present, Federal shotgun shells are red in 12 gauge, yellow in 20 gauge, and purple in 16 gauge. Remington and Winchester-Western color code their 20-gauge shells yellow; this color coding is done prevent using the wrong gauge ammunition in a weapon. Use of a 20-gauge shell in a 12 gauge is particularly dangerous; if a round is inserted, it will slide down into and lodge in the barrel. If a 12-gauge round is inserted into the weapon and the gun is fired, the 20-gauge round will blow up in the barrel.

Shotgun shells often are spoken of as being either low-brass or high-brass, depending on how high the brass head extends up the length of the tube (Figure 8-3). Whether a shogtun shell is high or low brass is no indication of the volume or strength of a shell.

Currently manufactured shotgun shells have brass or brass-plated steel heads. It is possible to produce all-plastic shotgun shells without a metal head. In fact, such shells have been marketed, though unsuccessfully. Winchester states that its compressioned plastic hull is strong

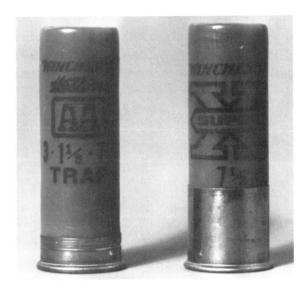

Figure 8-3 Low-brass and high-brass shotgun shells.

enough to be fired without the metal head, though they do not recommend this.[3]

By virtue of its design, the traditional shotgun shell had a number of defects. On firing, some of the hot gases from burning powder were able to bypass the over powder and filler wads and reach the shot charge. Here the hot gases partially melted and fused together a number of pellets. In addition to this problem, the rapid acceleration of the shot charge caused pellets at the bottom of the charge to be "welded" together by the pressure into small clumps. Furthermore as the charge moved down the barrel, pellets on the outer edge of the charge that were in direct contact with the barrel were flattened, as a result of both pressure and friction. Thus, by the time the pellets emerged from the barrel, only the central core of pellets, excluding those at the base, were round and undamaged. These undamaged pellets flew "true" toward the target, whereas the damaged pellets and clumps of pellets veered off at varying angles. These are the "fliers" seen in all shotgun patterns.

Another impairment to a good pattern was the overshot wad. This was supposed to slide off to one side of the shot column as it emerged from the barrel. This did not always happen, and the overshot wad sometimes fell into the shot column, disrupting it.

In an attempt to overcome these defects, ammunition manufacturers introduced a number of innovations. The first major change in shotgun shell design was the elimination of the rolled crimp and the overshot

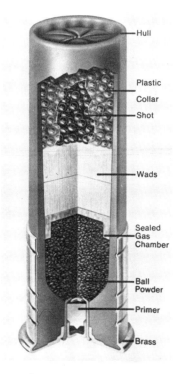

Hull

Plastic

Collar

Shot

Wads

Sealed
Gas
Chamber

Ball
Powder

Primer

Brass

Figure 8-4 Cross-section of present-day Winchester birdshot shell. (Courtesy of Winchester-Western.)

wad.[3] This was accomplished by introducing the "pie" crimp. In this procedure, closure of the paper shot shell was accomplished by having the tube folded in a number of equal segments and compressed inwardly to cover the shot column. Thus, the overshot wad was no longer necessary.

The second innovation was the introduction by Winchester of the "cup" wad. This was a type of overpowder wad whose cupped surface faced the powder. On ignition of the powder, the gas produced drove the lips of the cup outward, producing a gas-tight seal against the inner wall of the tube. Some shotgun shells had two cup wads. The second wad was at the base of the tube overlying the base wad. This cup wad was perforated in the center to let the flame from the primer reach the powder. The cup wad was so effective that it became possible to reduce the charge powder in the shotgun shells yet obtain the same ballistic performance. Cup wads are used in most of the shotgun ammunition loaded by Winchester-Western®.

In 1962, Winchester introduced the shot protective sleeve, or plastic shot collar.[3] This consists of a rectangular strip of plastic surrounding the shot charge. The collar acts to eliminate the abrasive-type damage that occurs as the pellets move down the barrel. The use of such a shot collar eliminates lead fouling of the bore and increases the density of shotgun patterns. Plastic shot collars are used in most Winchester

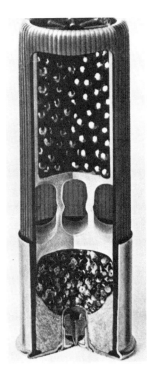

Figure 8-5 Cross-section of present-day Remington birdshot shell.

shotgun shell loadings. Figure 8-4 illustrates the present-day Winchester field load.

The traditional filler wads were made of felt or composition products. They overlay the thin cardboard overpowder wads. In 1963, Remington introduced the Power Piston®.[3] The Power Piston® is a one-piece plastic assemblage that provides a cup wad for sealing, a resilient spring center to cushion acceleration of shot and a polyethylene cup to prevent the shot from rubbing against the inner wall of the barrel (Figure 8-5). The Powder Piston® eliminates the overpowder wads, the filler wad, and the need for a shot collar. On firing, the gas of propulsion expands the lips of the cup-shaped base outward, providing a gastight seal against the inner wall of the shot shell case. The gas moves the cup wad forward, compressing the plastic spring members between the cup wad and the shot. The Powder Piston® and the shot begin to move forward, breaking the seal at the mouth of the shotgun shell. The shot charge is accelerated down the barrel, protected from contact with the barrel wall by the polyethylene cup and cushioned against the acceleration by the central spring section. The Power Piston® has four longitudinal slits the length of the shot container, dividing the walls of the container into four sections or "petals." As the wad assemblage containing the shot emerges from the barrel, the air pressure acts on the petals, bending them backward and releasing the shot (Figure 8-6). The wad then quickly falls away.

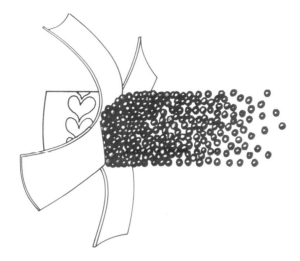

Figure 8–6 Power-Piston® opening up on leaving barrel.

Plastic wads similar to the Powder Piston® now are produced by all the major shotgun shell and shotgun shell component manufacturers. One slightly different approach is the wad assemblage of the Federal Ammunition Company. In 1968, they introduced the Triple-plus® wad column (Figure 8–7).[3] This consists of an all-plastic assemblage, made up of a gas-sealing overpowder wad with an integral plastic pillar that acts as a shock absorber. The pillar crushes on firing to cushion recoil and reduce the formation of shock. This assemblage is combined with a plastic shot cup that is separate from the plastic wad. Winchester uses a Powder-Piston-like all-plastic wad with a collapsible central portion in its trap and skeet loads.

Figure 8–8 shows the wadding used in most shot shells manufactured by Winchester, Federal, and Remington. This wadding is not used in buckshot or slug loadings.

In 1963, Winchester-Western began loading their buckshot shells with buckshot packed in granulated white polyethylene filler (Figure 8–9).[3] This filler cushions the shot pellets on firing, reducing shot distortion and improving the shot pattern. Remington soon followed Winchester's lead. In the late 1970s Winchester, Remington, and Federal began loading Magnum birdshot shells with granulated white filler for these aforementioned reasons. At close range this filler material can cause marks on the skin that can be mistaken for powder tattooing. This phenomenon will be discussed subsequently.

The white filler used in Winchester ammunition is polyethylene, whereas that in Remington is polypropylene. Federal uses both polyeth-

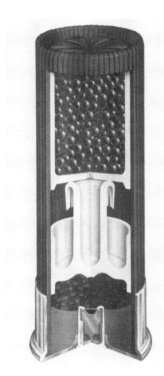

Figure 8-7 Cross-section of Federal birdshot shell.

Figure 8-8 Wadding used in (**a**) Winchester, (**b**) Federal, and (**c**) Remington birdshot loads.

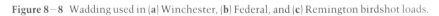

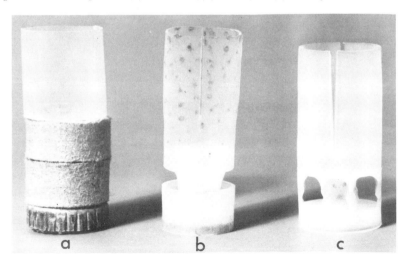

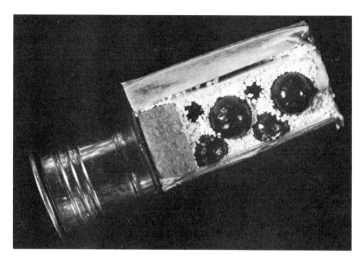

Figure 8-9 Winchester buckshot load showing buckshot packed in granulated white polyethylene filler.

ylene and polypropylene, with the latter the most widely used at present.

In spite of all the new designs in shotgun shells, traditionally constructed shells containing felt or composition filler wads and shells with overshot wads still are manufactured and marketed. In addition, many shells manufactured years ago are still around and may be encountered.

Examination of a box of shotgun ammunition and sometimes individual shot shells will reveal a series of three numbers such as $3\frac{3}{4}-1\frac{1}{4}-7\frac{1}{2}$. The last number, e.g., $7\frac{1}{2}$, refers to the size of the individual shot pellets; the middle number, e.g., $1\frac{1}{4}$, indicates the weight of the shot charge in ounces. The first number indicates the "dram equivalent" of the particular shell. This is an obsolete term that indicates the comparative power of a shotgun shell loaded in relationship to black powder loads. When black powder was used in shotgun shells, the relative power of the shell was indicated by listing the number of drams of black powder loaded in each shell. The more drams loaded, the more powerful the loading. Modern smokeless powder is rated in dram equivalents. Thus, a certain loading of a shotgun shell will be said to have a dram equivalent value of 3. This indicates that the charge of powder in this shell will drive the charge of shot to approximately the same velocity as 3 drams of black powder. The dram equivalent rating bears no relation to the amount of smokeless powder in the shotgun shell; thus, two shotgun shell cartridges loaded with the same weight and size shot can have the same dram equivalent rating with different quantities of smokeless powder.

Shot

Three general types of shot have been made: drop or soft shot, which is essentially pure lead; chilled or hard shot, which is lead hardened by the addition of antimony; plated shot. The latter is lead shot coated with a thin coat of copper or nickel to minimize distortion on firing, thereby maintaining a good aerodynamic shape and increasing the range. Winchester-Western sells this shot and cartridges loaded with it under the trade name of Lubaloy® shot. A fourth type of shot is now available: steel shot. This was produced because of recent government regulations prohibiting lead shot for migratory bird hunting in some areas. These pellets are made of softened steel. Individual steel pellets weigh less than comparably sized lead pellets and thus have less range.

Shotgun pellets fall into two general categories: birdshot and buckshot. Birdshot is used for birds and small game; buckshot is used for large game such as deer. Shot size ranges from No. 12 to 00 Buck. The smaller the shot number, the greater the pellet diameter. Table 8–1 gives the diameter, weight, and number of pellets per ounce for various birdshot pellet sizes.

Birdshot

The smallest bird shot is No. 12, which has a diameter of 0.05 in. (1.27 mm); the largest is BB shot, with a diameter of 0.18 in. (4.57 mm) (Table 8–1). BB shot should not be confused with the copper-coated steel BBs used in airgun. Airguns BBs have a diameter of 0.175 in. (4.44 mm).

The size of the shot in a shotgun shell usually is printed on the side of the tube. In shells where there is an overshot wad, the size of the shot may be printed upon this wad. Some shells are also marked with the

Table 8–1 Standard Shot: Sizes and Weights

No.	Diameter (in.)	Average weight of pellets		Approximate number/oz
		Grains	Milligrams	
12	.05	.18	11	2385
11	.06	.25	19	1750
9	.08	.75	49	585
8½	.085	.88	57	485
8	.09	1.07	69	410
7½	.095	1.25	81	350
6	.11	1.95	126	225
5	.12	2.58	167	170
4	.13	3.24	210	135
2	.15	4.86	315	90
BB	.18	8.75	567	50

weight of the shot charge and the dram equivalent. The number of pellets in such a shell can be determined easily by consulting a table such as Table 8−1. Thus, a shell loaded with 1 oz of No. 7½ shot contains approximately 350 pellets.

Theoretically, a shot shell loaded with No. 7½ shot should contain only pellets of this size. However, if one cuts open enough of these shells, one will find an occasional shell containing a few pellets of a different size, either one shot size larger or one size smaller. The vast majority of the pellets, however, will be 7½.

Buckshot Ammunition

There are three major manufacturers of buckshot ammunition in the United States: Remington-Peters, Winchester-Western, and Federal. These companies produce approximately 13 different loads in 12, 16, and 20 gauges. Smith & Wesson produced shotgun buckshot shells for a short time in the early 1970s.

Buckshot is usually manufactured in six sizes, ranging from No. 4 (0.24 in.) to 000 (0.360 in.). With buckshot ammunition, the number of pellets loaded into the shell is stated rather than the weight of the charge. Table 8−2 gives the diameter and weight of various sizes of buckshot pellets.

In 1963, Winchester-Western began loading their shotgun shells with buckshot packed in a white, granulated, polyethylene filler material (Figure 8−9). This filler cushions the shot on firing, reducing shot distortion and improving patterns. The shot and filler material are enclosed in a plastic shot collar. The end of the tube is closed with a "pie" crimp. Current Winchester buckshot loads contain the filler, the plastic shot collar, filler wads, and a cardboard cup wad.

In 1967, Remington began loading their shells with buckshot packed in a black, granulated polyethylene material. In October 1978, however, Remington buckshot began appearing loaded with a white poly-

Table 8−2 Buckshot: Sizes and Weights

No.	Diameter (in.)	Average weight of pellets	
		Grains	Milligrams
4	.24	20.6	1330
3	.25	23.4	1520
2	.27	29.4	1910
1	.30	40.0	2590
0	.32	48.3	3130
00	.33	53.8	3490
000	.36	68.0	4410

ethylene filler similar to that of Winchester. Current buckshot loads by Remington-Peters contain a white polypropylene filler material plus a plastic H wad used in the overpowder position. It is cupped on both ends, so that the filler wadding can expand the upper skirt for a secondary gas seal.

Federal buckshot loads ordinarily do not contain a packing material, nor are they closed with the now standard pie crimp. Instead they have the traditional filler wads and a thin plastic disklike over-the-shot wad. This design is preferred by some police agencies, as, if a shotgun is carried around in a car, the constant stop-and-go action of the vehicle can cause the buckshot to force open a "pie" crimp. This results in the granulated filler material coming out, entering, and possibly jamming the shotgun action. Federal buckshot ammunition can be obtained on special order with white filler, this filler is usually polypropylene.

The granulated filler is of interest to the forensic pathologist in that on firing ammunition loaded with filler, the filler accompanies the shot toward the target and can produce stipple marks on the skin identical in appearance to powder tattoo marks (Figure 8−10). Marks from the filler can vary from large and irregular, to small and regular, depending on the size and shape of the individual polyethylene granules. The white filler in Winchester shells has changed in form over the years. Older shells contain large coarse granules that produce large irregular marks on the skin (Figure 8−11). These should not be mistaken for powder tattooing under usual circumstances. Newer ammunition contains fine white granules that produce marks virtually identical to powder tattooing. The black filler formerly used in Remington 12-gauge buckshot shells was very fine and produced marks similar to powder. Because the filler

Figure 8−10 Buckshot pellets traveling through air, accompanied by white polyethylene filler.

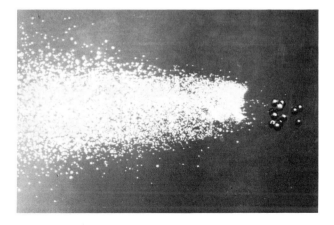

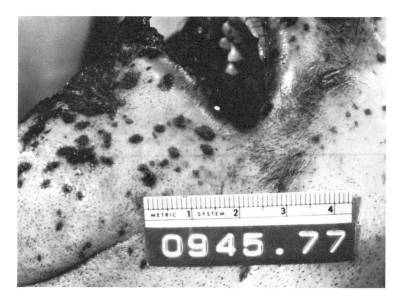

Figure 8-11 Large, irregular stipple marks of face caused by coarse white polyethylene filler loaded in early Winchester buckshot loads.

was black, it was mistaken for powder by the unwary. Remington always loaded their 20-gauge buckshot with white filler, possibly because of the translucent hull shells for 20 gauge. All Remington buckshot is now loaded with finely granular white material. Special-order Federal buckshot has similar packing material.

Smith & Wesson for a time produced 12-gauge buckshot loads. These shells were loaded with what appears to be chopped up blue plastic casing material. The marks produced by it are relatively large and irregular.

Winchester, Remington, and Federal now load Magnum birdshot loads with polyethylene or polypropylene filler. In all shells seen by the author the filler has consisted of fine white granules.

Animal experiments have shown that with a 12-gauge shotgun, stippling caused by filler extends out to a greater distance than powder tattooing. Although tattooing can extend out to a maximum of 1 m, stippling from filler material can extend out to 2 to 3 m of range. The white filler can be deposited on a body out to a maximum of 6 to 8 yd.

The most popular buckshot load in this country is a 12-gauge 2¾ shell loaded with 9-00 Buck pellets. Some police agencies, however, have begun using No. 1 and No. 4 Buck, as they feel that these loadings give a denser and more even pattern with a greater probability of a hit.

Shotgun Slugs

Shotgun slugs are used for deer and bear hunting in heavily populated areas where the slug's rapid loss of velocity allegedly affords greater protection from shooting mishaps. Three types of shotgun slugs are on the market: the American Foster; the European Brenneke slug and the sabot slug (Figure 8–12).

The Brenneke slug was developed in Germany in 1898. It has a pointed nose with felt and cardboard wads attached to the base by a screw. Approximately 12 angled ribs are present on the surface of the slug. The longer profile provided by the wad allegedly decreases tumbling and improves accuracy. Brenneke slugs are uncommon in the United States. Nominal slug weights, including felt and cardboard wads, are 491 gr in 12 gauge, 427 gr in 16 gauge, and 364 gr in 20 gauge. The advertised muzzle velocity ranges from 1593 ft/sec in 12 gauge to 1513 ft/sec in 20 gauge. The weight of the slug will vary somewhat depending on the country of manufacture. The diameter of a slug in 12 gauge, measuring from the top of one rib to the other, is 18.47 mm (0.727 in.); it is 16.13 mm (0.635 in.) from groove to groove.

The Foster slug is the traditional American shotgun slug. It is a roundnose soft lead projectile, with a deep, concave base, and has anywhere from 12 to 15 angled, hellical grooves cut into its surface. Since 1982, Winchester, Remington, and Federal all have introduced hollowpoint shotgun slugs. Slugs manufactured by Federal have a plastic insert in the hollow base to preclude entry of the wad into the cavity on firing.

The purpose of the grooves on the surface of a slug is to cause the slug to rotate on its long axis when it leaves the barrel. This slow rotation, combined with the balance created by a heavy nose and a hollow base, results in greater accuracy than would be the case with a solid, nongrooved projectile.

Figure 8–12 Shotgun slugs. (a) Foster, (b) Brenneke, and (c) Smith & Wesson sabot.

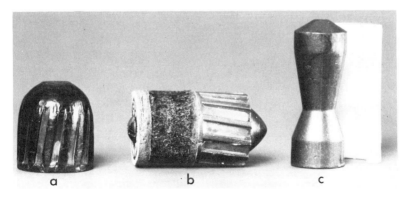

Foster slugs are made in 10, 12, 16, 20, and .410 gauges. In diameter, the slugs are equal to or smaller than the tightest choke. On firing, the slugs expand and fill the bore. The weight of the slugs has traditionally been 1 oz (437 gr) in 12 gauge, ⅘ oz (350 gr) in 16 gauge, ⅝ (273) gr in 20 gauge, and ⅕ oz (870 gr) in 0.410 gauge. Heavier slugs in 12 and 20 gauge are available.

The sabot slug was introduced to the United States by Smith & Wesson. They no longer manufacture shotgun ammunition, however. This slug was made only in 12-gauge. It had an hourglass configuration with a hollow base in which there was a white plastic insert. This slug lay in a sabot consisting of two halves of high-density polyethylene plastic. The slug, encased in the sabot made a projectile of 12-gauge diameter. On firing, the sabot with the enclosed slug moved down the barrel as one unit. The sabot contacted the bore, not the slug. On exiting the muzzle, the sabot fell away.

Sabot slugs were made in police and civilian versions. Both slugs had a nominal weight of 440 gm. The advertised muzzle velocity of the police round was 1450 ft/sec. The diameter at the front and rear was 0.50 in.

The police slug was loaded into a blue, ribbed plastic case on whose side "Police" was lettered in white. The tip of the slug and the end of the sabot were visible at the mouth of the shotgun shell. The sabot was of white plastic. The civilian slug was in a similar shotgun tube, except that there was no white lettering. Again, the tip of the slug and the sabot were visible. The sabot in the civilian slug was made of black plastic.

Both police and civilian shells were closed with a rolled crimp. In both shells, the sabot rested on a cardboard wad, which in turn rested on a white plastic wad.

At close range the plastic sabot will enter the body or may inflict surface injuries to the skin. In a sawed-off shotgun in which the end of the barrel has not been smoothed out, slivers of steel may project into the bore. If a sabot slug is fired in such a weapon, the spicules of steel may mark the plastic sabot so as to make ballistic comparison possible. This may also occur with plastic wads such as the Power Piston.®.

The police version of the sabot slug was intended to be fired in weapons having only a cylinder or modified choke. Firing in weapons of greater choke could cause the slug to snap at the hourglass waist. The civilian slug of softer lead could be fired in weapons of any choke. Sabot slugs now are manufactured by Ballistic Research Industries of California.

The wound of entrance from an American Foster shotgun slug is circular in shape, with a diameter approximately that of the slug. The edge of the wound is abraded just as for a bullet wound. Determination of the gauge from the diameter of the entrance wound is not possible. At close range the wad may either enter the entrance wound or strike adjacent skin, producing a wad mark. Shotgun slugs produce massive internal injuries comparable in severity to those produced by a high-velocity rifle bullet. As a Foster slug moves through the body, it tends to "pancake" and usually remains in the body. The slug may come to rest as a flattened lead disk or may break into a few large pieces. X-rays often show a central disk of lead with 2 to 4 comma-like pieces of lead adjacent to or surrounding the disk. These comma-like pieces of lead break off from the edge of the pancaked slug (Figure 8−13). Slugs do not produce the x-ray picture of the "lead snowstorm" seen with high-velocity hunting rifle bullets.

Some years ago, people in rural areas who did not wish to expend money on the purchase of slugs made their own jury-rigged slugs from birdshot shells. They would cut a deep groove around the circumference of the birdshot shell just above the metal head. They hoped that on firing, the tube would separate at this cut. With plastic tubes separation usually does not occur. If separation occurs, the tube and its contained load of shot leave the barrel and travel to the target as one mass. In such a case, pellets, wads, and the cut-off portion of hull will be recovered from the body. Figure 8−14 illustrates such a case. The deceased was shot twice in the head with a 12-gauge shotgun firing birdshot. Recovered from the head was the plastic tube from a shell that had been cut in front of the metal head to create a homemade slug.

A second case involved a plastic hull in which separation did occur, but the pie crimp at the end of the shell was also forced. Thus, the shot exited the barrel normally, but the cut portion of the shell was deposited in the barrel. On the next firing of the weapon, an unaltered buckshot

Figure 8−13 X-ray of body showing breakup of slug.

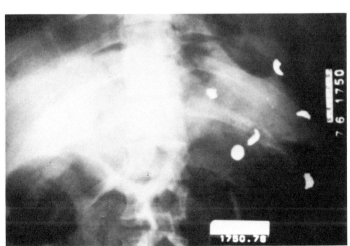

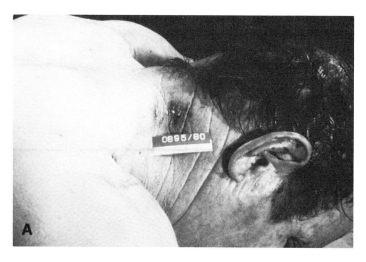

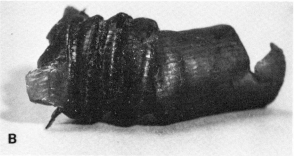

Figure 8–14 A. Entrance wound of right side of back of neck. **B.** Recovered portion of hull from wound.

shell was used. The buckshot swept the deposited hull out the barrel into the body. Thus, at autopsy buckshot, wads, and the distal two-thirds of a birdshot tube were recovered from the body.

Wound Ballistics of the Shotgun

At close range, the shotgun is the most formidable and destructive of all small arms. The severity and lethality of a shotgun wound depend on the organs struck by the pellets as well as the amount of kinetic energy the pellets lose in these organs. Unlike bullets, shotgun pellets rarely exit the body. Therefore, the kinetic energy of wounding in shotguns is usually equal to the striking energy. This striking kinetic energy is proportional to the number, weight, and velocity of the pellets that strike the body. In rifled weapons, the weight of the bullet does not change no matter how great the distance. In contrast, in shotguns, as the range increases there is dispersion of shot with resultant decrease in the number of pellets that strike the target.

Although velocity does decrease with range in rifled weapons, the decrease is very little at the short ranges at which most killings occur. However, the unfavorable ballistic shape of the shotgun pellet, combined with the lack of stabilizing spin, causes a rapid fall-off in velocity and thus kinetic energy. Thus, in contrast to rifled weapons, in shotguns the range from muzzle to target is extremely important in determining the velocity and kinetic energy possessed by the pellets and thus the severity of the injury.

The range in muzzle velocity in shotguns of different gauges is not very great. There is only a small degree of variation in velocity, depending on the size and weight of the pellet charge. All that a larger gauge or Magnum load does is provide more pellets, producing a denser pattern and not a greater velocity. The larger sized shot is, however, more effective at longer range because it retains its velocity better than the smaller shot.

The devastating effect of the shotgun at close range is shown by the following data. A 12-gauge shotgun shell loaded with No. 7½ shot and traveling at 1220 ft/sec has a total muzzle energy of 1771 ft-lb, almost that of a .30-30 rifle. A 12-gauge shotgun shell with nine 00 Buck pellets and a muzzle velocity of 1325 ft/sec has a muzzle energy of 211 ft-lb per pellet, or a total muzzle energy of 1899 ft-lb. This is the energy of a .30-30 rifle bullet. Unlike rifle bullets, however, shotgun pellets rarely exit the body. Therefore, when one is shot with a shotgun, all the kinetic energy is transferred to the body as wounding effects. A 12-gauge shotgun slug is so effective, because of the transfer of kinetic energy. The slug, which weighs approximately 402 gr, has a muzzle velocity of 1600 ft/sec and a muzzle energy of 2485 ft-lb. This muzzle energy can be compared to 1282 ft-lb of energy for a 5.56-mm cartridge and 1902 ft-lb for a .30-30. As a shotgun slug usually stays in the body, the devastating effect of this projectile is easy to understand.

Shotgun Wounds

Figure 8–15A–D show the sequence of events that occur at the muzzle on firing a shotgun. Note the large gas cloud that is partly responsible for the severe nature of the wounds at contact range.

Contact shotgun wounds of the head are among the most mutilating firearms wounds there are. Bursting ruptures of the head are the rule rather than the exception. These are the wounds of which an individual is said to have "blown his head off." In some cases, this is almost literally true. The skull may be largely fragmented and the brain pulpe-

184

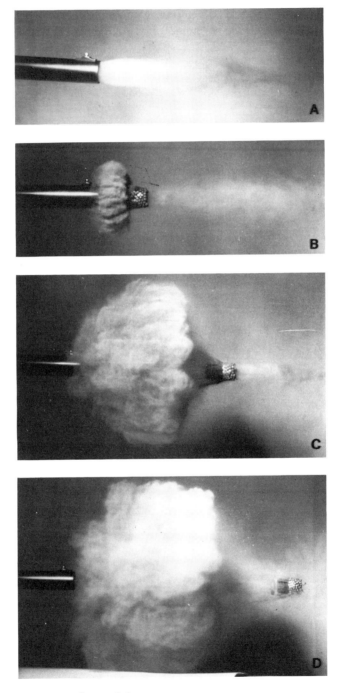

Figure 8–15 A–D. Discharge of shotgun.

fied. Large fragments of the cranial vault and both cerebral hemispheres are often ejected from the head. The scalp is extensively lacerated.

Such severe injuries in contact wounds of the head are due to two factors: The first is the charge of shot entering the skull, which expends its energy and produces severe internal pressure. The second is the gas from combustion of the propellant (Figure 8−15D). This gas, entering the closed chamber of the head, begins to expand rapidly, producing pressure on the bony framework of the skull. The only way for the skull to relieve the pressure produced is to shatter.

Most contact shotgun wounds of the head are suicidal in origin. The most common site of entrance for contact shotgun wounds of the head are the temporal regions. Most right-handed individuals shoot themselves in the right temple. When they do so, they use the right hand to push the trigger and the left hand to steady the muzzle against the head. Because of this, powder soot may be present on the left hand (Figure 8−16). Even if there is no visible powder residue, primer residue may be present on the back or palm of the left hand. Soot or primer residue or both are virtually never found on the hand that was used to fire the weapon. If a compensator was present at the end of the muzzle, a gridlike pattern of soot deposition may be present on the palm of the hand holding the muzzle (Figure 8−17).

Most contact shotgun wounds of the head from weapons of 10, 12, 16, or 20 gauge, result in evisceration of the supratentorial portion of the brain. This is true whether the entrance is in the temple or the mouth. The great bulk of the pellets and the wad will exit in such cases. An x-ray of the head may show only 3 or 4 remaining pellets from a shell that held hundreds.

Figure 8−16 Soot deposit on hand used to cradle muzzle end of shotgun.

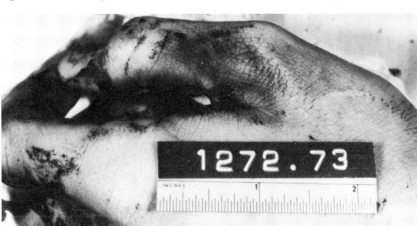

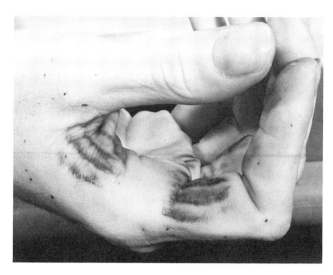

Figure 8-17 Patterned soot deposit due to compensator.

Although massive injuries of the head with evisceration of the brain are the rule, they are not inevitable. The author has seen numerous cases in which an individual shot himself in the head with a shotgun and no pellets exited. Almost invariably, such wounds are inflicted in the mouth or under the jaw and not the temporal region. Even though no pellets exited, there are massive fractures of the skull and pulpification of the brain. The weapons in these cases ranged from .410 gauge to 12 gauge.

Occasionally, people shooting themselves in the mouth tilt the head too far backward before firing. This results in their "shooting off" the face and sometimes the frontal lobes (Figure 8-18). In such instances, death may not be immediate. The author has seen individuals survive weeks with such wounds.

In the typical contact wound of the head, the entrance site is easy to locate, as large quantities of soot will be found at it. The edges of the wound will be seared and blackened (Figure 8-19). In wounds of the temporal region, the entrance is often bisected by large lacerations extending across the top of the head. Fragmentation of the skull usually occurs. The exit site of the pellets may not be found because of missing fragments of bone and the massive comminuted fractures of the skull.

In intraoral gunshot wounds, soot is present on the palate, the tongue, and sometimes the lips. Stretchlike striae or superficial lacerations of the perioral skin and nasolabial folds often occur because of the sudden transient "bulging out" of the face, caused by the temporary cavity and the gas (Figure 8-20).

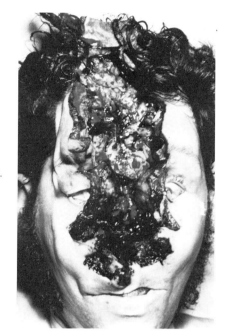

Figure 8–18 Intraoral shotgun wound.

Figure 8–19 Contact wound of right temple with evisceration of brain. Note large amount of soot at entrance site.

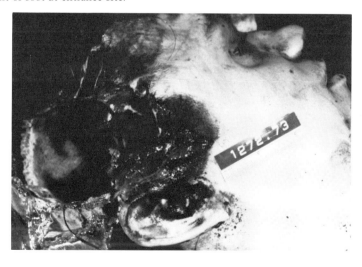

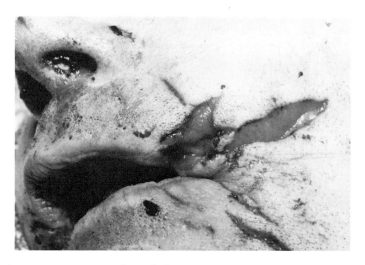

Figure 8–20 Tears at corner of mouth due to intraoral shotgun wound.

Although soot is seen around the entrance in most contact wounds of the head, this is not absolute. The author has encountered a number of cases in which no soot was seen either externally or internally (Figure 8–21). All cases involved Winchester ammunition loaded with ball powder. In all but one of these cases, ball powder grains were readily identified in the wound. The most disturbing case involved an individual who shot himself in the temporoparietal region with a 12-gauge shotgun firing Winchester birdshot. The suicide took place in front of scores of witnesses. The head injury was massive, with evisceration of the brain. Neither powder nor soot could be found on or in the head. Since not all the cranial contents were recovered from the scene, it is possible that a more diligent search would have revealed at least powder grains.

Intermediate-range and close-range shotgun wounds of the head are almost as mutilating as contact wounds because pellets are still traveling in a single mass. This is especially true if they strike the skull at a relatively shallow angle and then exit. Large gaping tears of the scalp are present. Careful reapproximation of the scalp and examination of the edges will reveal the entrance site, which will be indicated by the abrasion ring. Stretch-like striae may radiate from the entrance as well. The exact site of the exit of the pellets, however, is often not apparent. Reconstruction of the shattered skull may help in discovery of the entrance and exit.

Contact wounds of the trunk appear relatively innocuous when compared with the massive destruction produced by such wounds in the head. The wound of entrance will be circular in shape and will have a

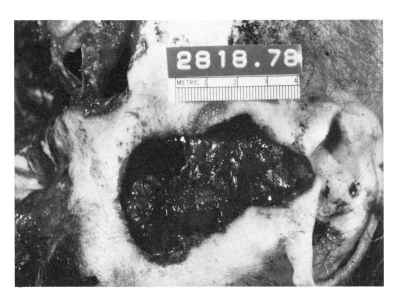

Figure 8–21 Contact wound of right temple with 12-gauge shotgun. Note absence of soot. Ball powder was recovered from entrance.

diameter approximately equal to that of the bore of the weapon Figure 8–22. In hard contact wounds, no soot surrounds the entrance site. The edges of the wound will be seared and blackened by the hot gases. The skin will not be split, as in head wounds, because the gases disperse in the underlying soft tissue and visceral cavities. These gases, however, will cause the chest or abdominal wall to flare out abruptly, impacting the muzzle of the weapon with great force. This often will result in a detailed imprint of the muzzle of the shotgun. In double-barrel weapons, the imprint of the unfired barrel often will be present. The chest and abdomen may flare out to such a degree and with such force as to have impressed on them the outline of the hand holding the barrel or even a chain or medal that was present around the neck (Figure 8–23). The flared-out chest or abdomen may envelope the end of the barrel so that an imprint of the front sight may be present, even though the sight is 1 in. from the muzzle end.

The wound of entrance may be surrounded by a wide zone of raw, abraded skin caused by flaring out of the skin of the chest or abdominal wall around the muzzle at the time of discharge. The mechanical action of the skin rubbing against the end of the barrel causes abrasion of the superficial layers.

If the muzzle of a shotgun is held in loose contact or near contact with the body, there will be a circular area of soot deposited on the skin

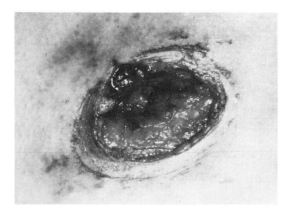

Figure 8-22 Contact wound of chest with muzzle imprint. No soot present at entrance site.

Figure 8-23 Contact wound of abdomen with imprint of wrist and hand. Note the watchband around wrist.

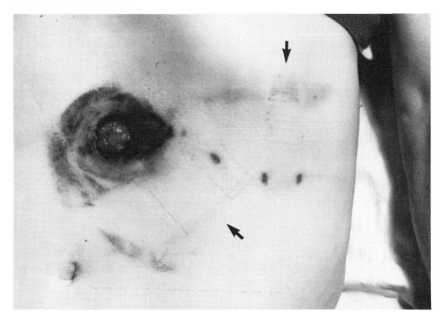

surrounding the entrance hole. As the range increases, the diameter of the soot deposit increases, but the density decreases. Deposition of soot continues out to a range of approximately 30 cm.

If the skin is reflected from around a contact wound of entrance, the underlying muscle will have a cherry red hue from carboxyhemoglobin formation, with the source of the carbon monoxide (CO) being the gases of combustion of the gunpowder. CO is not necessarily confined to the immediate adjacent muscle but can spread 15 cm or more from the entrance. CO also may accompany the shot in its path through the body; if a large mass of shot lodges subcutaneously in the back, CO may produce a cherry red hue to the adjacent muscle.

As the range increases beyond 1 to 2 cm from muzzle to target, powder tattooing will occur (Figure 8–24). Powder tattooing from a shotgun is less dense than the tattooing a handgun produces at the same range. This is due to more complete consumption of powder caused by the greater barrel length. The maximum range out to which powder tattooing occurs from a shotgun depends to a great degree on the type of powder, i.e., ball or flake. In shotgun shells loaded with flake powder and fired in a 28-in. barrel 12-gauge shotgun with a modified choke, powder tattooing was present out to 24 in. (60 cm) but disappeared by 30 in. (75 cm). Using the same weapon and firing cartridges loaded with ball powder, definite tattooing was present at 30 in. (75 cm), with a very few marks present at 36 in. (90 cm), but was absent by 40 in. (125 cm). Just as in handguns, ball powder produces fine powder tattoo marks and can readily go through clothing (Figure 8–24).

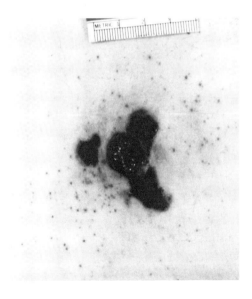

Figure 8–24 Intermediate-range .410 shotgun wound of chest with ball powder tattooing. The deceased was shot through flannel pajamas.

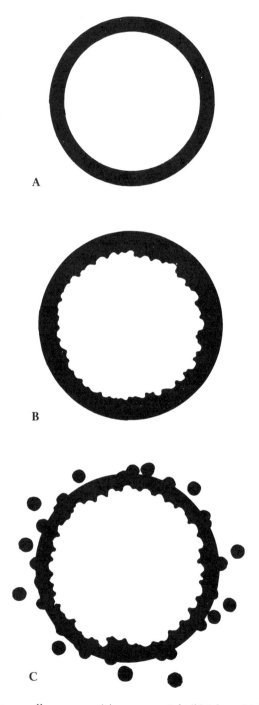

Figure 8-25 Shotgun pellet patterns. (a) contact to 2 ft, (b) 3 ft, and (c) 4 ft.

All these data are based on tests done in rabbits, whose skin is thinner than that of humans; therefore, these figures should be considered only as maximum ranges out to which powder tattooing will occur in humans. In addition, other factors such as barrel length, also have an effect on the maximum range and density of powder tattooing.

As the muzzle of the shotgun is moved farther from the body, the diameter of the circular wound of entrance increases in size until a point is reached where individual pellets begin to separate from the main mass (Figure 8−25). From contact to 2 ft, birdshot fired from a shotgun, independent of its gauge (excluding the .410), produces a single round entrance wound approximately ¾ in. to 1 in. in diameter. By 3 ft, the wound widens out to approximately ⅞ in. for a barrel with modified choke to 1¼ in. for a cylinder bore weapon. The edges of the wounds will have scalloped margins (Figure 8−26). By 4 ft, the modified choke barrel produces an entrance hole approximately 1 in. in diameter with the cylindrical bore barrel producing an entrance 1¾ in. in diameter. Scattered satellite pellet holes are present around entrances at this range (Figure 8−27). By 6 to 7 ft, there is a definite cuff of satellite pellet holes around a slightly irregular wound of entrance for a shotgun with a modified barrel (Figure 8−28). For a cylindrical bore weapon, the wound is ragged with a prominent cuff of pellet holes around the entrance. Beyond 10 ft, there is great variation in the size of the pellet pattern depending on the ammunition used, the choke of the gun and most important, the range. At the same range (beyond 10 ft), the pattern for different guns and brands of ammunition may vary from a central

Figure 8−26 Shotgun wound of chest with scalloping of margins (range, approximately 3 ft).

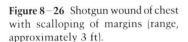
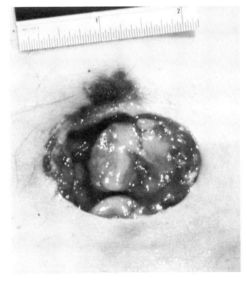

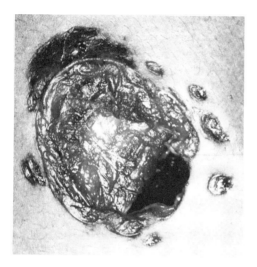

Figure 8-27 Entrance wound with scattered satellite pellet holes (range, approximately 4 ft).

irregular perforation with numerous satellite wounds to a pattern of multiple individual pellet wounds.

In all deaths from shotgun wounds, the size of the shot pattern on the body should be measured so that the range can be determined accurately. There have been many formulas published to determine the range at which a shotgun has been discharged, but none of these formulas is reliable. The wound measurements given in the previous para-

Figure 8-28 Slightly irregular wound of entrance surrounded by pellet holes (range estimated at 5 to 7 ft).

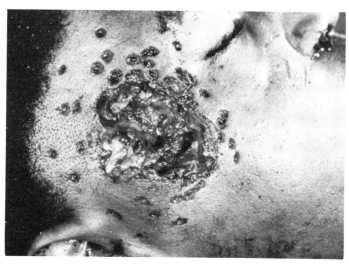

graph should be used only as a rough guide in estimating range. The only reliable method of determining range is to obtain the actual weapon and the same brand of ammunition used and then conduct a series of test shots so as to reproduce on paper the pattern of the fatal wound on the body. It must be stressed that identical weapons of the same choke may produce different patterns; thus, the actual weapon used in the killing must be used. A fact that is not often appreciated is that ammunition plays a great part in the size of the pattern. Different brands of ammunition, even when loaded with the same shot size, produce different patterns at the same range.

Another factor that is often not considered and that can cause errors in range determination involves the measurement of the shot pattern on the body. Different individuals measure the same pattern differently. The occasional flier should be ignored, and only the main mass of the pellet pattern should be measured.

At close range, when there is only a single large wound of entrance, the wad from a shotgun shell will be found inside the body. If the shell contained a plastic Power Piston® wad or plastic shot cup, as the wad enters the body, the individual arms or "petals" that have peeled back in flight may produce a patterned abrasion around the wound of entrance (Figure 8–29). In 12, 16, and 20 gauges, one will have a circular wound of entrance in the center of a Maltese Cross abrasion. In .410 gauge the shot cup has only three petals; thus, three equally spaced rectangular abrasions radiate from the entrance rather than four (Figure 8–30).

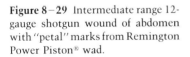

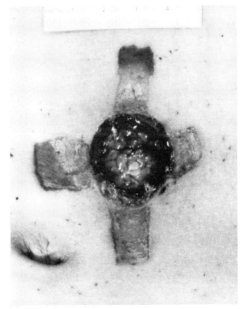

Figure 8–29 Intermediate range 12-gauge shotgun wound of abdomen with "petal" marks from Remington Power Piston® wad.

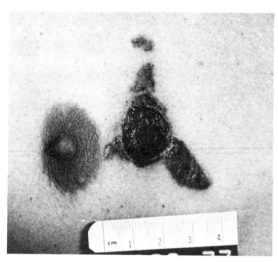

Figure 8–30 .410 shotgun wound of chest. Note the three equally spaced "petal" marks characteristic of the .410.

In the author's experience, petals marks from plastic shot cups have always been accompanied by powder tattooing of the adjacent skin if the skin is bare. Petal marks are seen at ranges between 1 and 3 ft. Before 1 ft of range, the petals have not folded back sufficiently to mark the skin. By 1 ft, they have opened sufficiently to produce the Maltese Cross pattern. The increasing air resistance bends the petals back so that after 3 ft they are generally flush with the sides of the wad base, and no petal marks are produced. Sometimes not all the petals bend back uniformly, and one finds a circular wound of entrance with only one petal mark (Figure 8–31).

As the range increases, the wads gradually fall behind and separate from the main shot mass. At still relatively close range the wad may impact the side of the wound of entrance before sliding into the body. Thus, one will have a circular entrance surrounded by a symmetric abrasion ring with a large, irregular area of abraded margin on one side where the wad impacted. As the range increases (5 to 8 ft), however, the wads will drift laterally until they impact on the skin adjacent to the entrance site and do not enter (Figure 8–32). At this time the wad will leave a circular or oval imprint on the skin. In shotgun shells loaded with both an over-the shot wad and a plastic shot cup, one may get two sets of wad markings. As the range from muzzle to target increases still farther, the wads will miss the body or strike with so little energy that they will not leave a mark on the skin. The maximum range out to which wads will produce patterned abrasions on the body is unknown. Filler

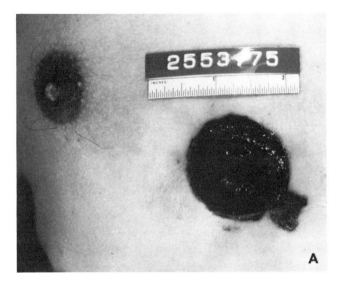

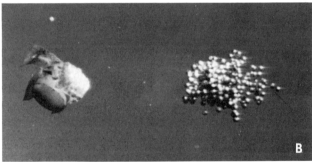

Figure 8–31 A. 12-gauge entrance wound of chest with single "petal" mark. **B.** Plastic wad falling behind shot. Note that three of the four petals have folded back, with one still protruding.

wads have produced marks at least out to 15 ft, and plastic wads out to 20 ft.

In some instances, for unknown reasons, the shot cup or Power Piston® does not open to release the shot. Thus, the mass of shot travels to and through the body in one compact mass. In the case illustrated, this happened to a limited degree (Figure 8–33). Most of the pellets stayed in the Power Piston® and exited with it. Some pellets, however, did emerge from the wad as it moved through the body.

Shot charges may strike an intermediate target such as a pane of glass, a screen, or an arm before striking the body. This intermediate target will cause an increase in the dispersion of the shot. Estimates of the

198

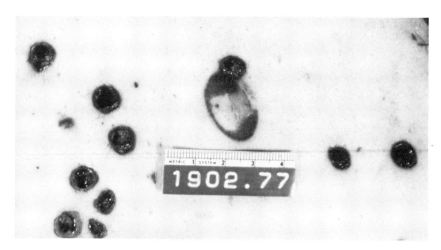

Figure 8–32 Circular abrasion of skin from composite wad.

Figure 8–33 Perforating shotgun wound of chest. Note the small number of pellets present. The circular mark in the upper left-hand corner of the picture indicates where the pellets entered.

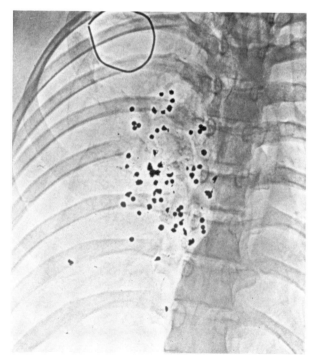

range from the pattern on the body in such cases will be erroneous. The only way to determine the range correctly is to interpose a similar intermediate target when test firing. Breitenecker believes, and the author agrees, that even heavy clothing can act as an intermediate target, thus producing an entrance wound in the skin larger than that in the outer garment.[4]

In the case of a young boy accidently shot with a 12-gauge slug, his hand—specifically, a finger—acted as an intermediate target. The slug fragmented the bone and soft tissue of the finger, propelling it against the deceased's chest, where these fragments produced irregular areas of abrasion (Figure 8–34).

On occasion, when bodies have been burned or are markedly decomposed, authorities have attempted to use the size of the shotgun pattern within the body as determined by x-ray for estimation of range. However, experiments have revealed that this methods is completely unreliable. Both close-range wounds and wounds of several yard's distance can give similar patterns on x-ray because of the "billard-ball" effect of the pellets on entering the body in close range shotgun wounds[4,5] In such wounds, the pellets are bunched when they strike the victim. Because of this, they strike one another, bouncing off at various angles.

Internal injuries, due to shotgun pellets are extremely variable, depending on the range at which an individual is shot. In contact wounds, where one is dealing with the effects of both the pellets and the gas, there may be near disintegration of organs. Close-range wounds, in which the pellets enter in a relatively compact mass, can also result in pulpification of organs. As the range increases, and the pellets enter the

Figure 8–34 Entrance wound of chest from 12-gauge slug. The irregular abrasions around the entrance are due to fragments of the victim's finger.

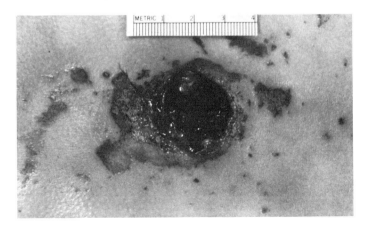

body separately, the wounds produced will resemble those from a low-velocity handgun bullet.

Perforating wounds of the trunk from shotgun pellets are uncommon. Most shotgun pellets expend all their energy in the victim. When they do occur, exit wounds usually result from a tangential wound; contact wounds in an extremely thin person, and contact or close-up wounds from shells loaded with buckshot. The wound of exit produced may vary from a large, irregular, gaping wound caused by a mass of pellets exiting to a single slitlike exit wound produced by one pellet. Only very rarely will one see exit wounds of the trunk from a direct hit with birdshot. Such cases may be due to the welding together of a number of shot at the time of firing so that these pellets move through the body as a single mass.

In all shotgun deaths, the size of the pattern on the body should be measured and recorded. Photographs of the wound pattern are recommended. These can be used for subsequent range determinations. Shot and wads should be recovered and retained. Examination of the wad will give the gauge of the shotgun and the make of the ammunition. Measurements of the pellets will give the pellet size. On rare occasions, irregularities at the end of the muzzle will impart scratch marks on plastic wads that are sufficiently distinctive to make positive ballistics comparison between the wad recovered from the body and a test wad fired from the suspect weapon. Such cases usually occur when the barrel of the shotgun has been sawed off, leaving jagged metal projections into the barrel. Such comparisons are also possible with the plastic sabot of shotgun slugs.

Window Screens as Intermediate Targets

At ranges from contact to 4 ft, discharge of a shotgun through a window screen will result in production of a square hole in the screen. This is independent of the gauge, choke, barrel length, type of wad, and shot size. The major factor in the production of a square hole is the distance from muzzle to screen. A square hole usually is produced at ranges from contact to approximately 4 ft. A perfect square is not produced all the time, as one side can have a rounded appearance. Examination of the square hole shows that the individual wires of the screen are broken and bent outward by the bullet. The wires tend to be longer in the corners and shorter on the sides. When the strands are bent back into place, a circular hole is formed.

As the range increases beyond 4 ft, the pellets start to spread and the hole takes on a circular appearance. At farther distances, individual pellet holes appear around the circular defect. Slugs produce square holes at all distances.

Wounds from Buckshot

The appearance of a wound resulting from buckshot depends principally on the range between the victim and the muzzle of the weapon. A contact wound will consist of a circular wound of entrance whose diameter is approximately the same as that of the bore of the shotgun. The edges of the wound will be seared and abraded. The wound of entrance often is surrounded by a wide zone of raw, abraded skin caused by flaring out of the skin around the muzzle at the time of discharge when the gas produced by the burning propellant enters the body. The mechanical action of the skin rubbing against the tip of the barrel causes the abrasion of the skin. If the weapon is held in loose contact with the skin, there will be deposition of soot surrounding the entrance. Deposition of soot continues out to a range of approximately 30 cm.

As the range from target to muzzle increases beyond a few centimeters, powder tattooing of the skin appears. Depending on the form of powder present, i.e., ball or disk, powder tattooing in a 12-gauge shotgun will extend out to a maximum range of approximately 90 to 125 cm for ball powder and 60 to 75 for flake powder. The ability of granulated filler in buckshot loads to simulate powder tattooing has been discussed previously.

As the range increases, the diameter of the entrance will increase gradually. At 3 ft, the edges of the wound will have a scalloped shape. At 4 ft, there will be separation of buckshot pellets from the main mass so that there will be a large gaping wound with a few satellite holes. At 9 ft, there will generally be individual pellet holes (Figure 8–35).

Figure 8–35 Wounds from 00 buckshot. Note the abrasions from wadding (arrows).

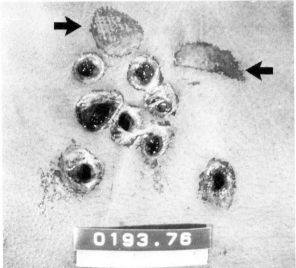

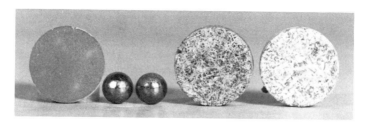

Figure 8–36 Disassembled Federal buckshot shell showing the thin plastic over-the-wad, 00 buckshot pellets, a composite cushion wad, and a cork wad.

At close range, when there is still one large perforation, the wad usually follows the buckshot into the body. As the range increases, the wad will move laterally from the main pellet mass path and will impact the skin either among or adjacent to the individual pellet holes, producing an oval or circular abrasion (Figure 8–35).

Federal buckshot cartridges contain a composite and a cork wad as filler wads (Figure 8–36). The cork wad overlies the powder. The author has seen a case of an individual shot in the chest at close range (approximately 1½ to 2 ft) with a shotgun loaded with Federal buckshot. The single large entrance was surrounded by a number of irregular abrasions in addition to some powder tattooing (Figure 8–37). No intermediate targets were present. Federal buckshot cartridges are closed with a thin plastic disk-like over-the-shot wad. This wad does not fragment on firing and is recoverable intact at the scene or from the body (Figure 8–38). Test firings revealed, however, that the cork wad fragmented on firing and that the fragments of cork were responsible for the skin markings.

In most cases in which an individual is shot in the trunk with buckshot, the pellets will remain in the body. On some occasions, usually in contact or close-up buckshot wounds, the pellets may exit.

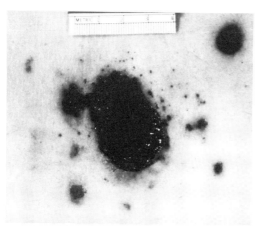

Figure 8–37 Intermediate-range shotgun wound of chest showing powder tattooing and large irregular areas of abrasion.

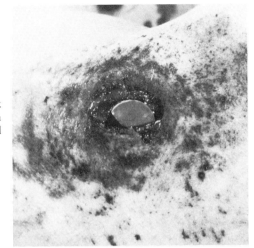

Figure 8–38 Shotgun wound of neck with a plastic over-the-shot wad from a Federal buckshot shell embedded in the entrance.

Sawed-Off Shotguns

Tests by the author of sawed-off shotguns at ranges of 21 ft or less have revealed that the barrel length of a cylinder-bore shotgun has no significant effect on the size of the pattern until the barrel has been sawed off to less than 9 in. At this point, the patterns produced by the shot begin to open up significantly.

In a sawed-off shotgun in which the end of the barrel has not been reamed out, slivers of steel may project into the bore. If plastic wads are fired in such a weapon, the spicules of steel may mark the wad, making ballistic comparison possible.

Shotgun Diverters

Recent technilogical advances have resulted in the development of shotgun diverters. This is a device attached to the end of the shotgun barrel that changes the normal circular pattern of shot to a controlled, predictable, rectangular pattern. This rectangular pattern is formed by the diverting ribs integral with the bore of the device coupled with compounded angles. The mass of shot is reformed after it leaves the barrel and enters the forward diverter section. The action of the gases on the walls of the diverter reorient the shot, so that a rectangular pattern is formed after exiting the muzzle. Shotgun slugs may be fired through the diverter. These slugs, however, will be deformed, having a rectangular shape.

Automatic Ejection of Fired Hulls

The author has seen a number of unquestionable cases of suicide utilizing a pump shotgun in which death was instantaneous, yet the pump shotgun used to commit suicide had an empty chamber and an ejected hull was present at the scene. Although these cases were suicide, such circumstances should arouse the suspicion of homicide. Some pump shotguns will automatically eject the fired case after discharge if the slide is not restrained in a forward position. Other pump shotguns will unlock and eject the fired case only partially. If this weapon falls to the ground, landing on its butt, enough momentum may be given the shotgun bolt to cause it to go backward, ejecting the fired case. Though ejection may occur in the aforementioned situations, there is never sufficient energy for the bolt to come forward and chamber a new round.

Shotgun Shells Exclusive of Buckshot

There are three major manufacturers of shotgun shells in the United States: Remington-Peters, Winchester-Western, and Federal. The shot shells they produce will be considered individually (Table 8–3).

Remington-Peters

Shotgun ammunition produced by Remington is designated as Express, Sure-Shot (Field), and RXP. All have plastic tubes, loaded with flake powder and closed with a "pie" crimp.

Express loads have plastic SP tubes and high brass heads. With the exception of .410 shells, all have plastic Power Piston® wads. The .410 uses a plastic shot container. Some Express birdshots loads have the pellets packed in white plastic material.

Sure-Shot shells have plastic SP tubes and low brass heads. The Power Piston wad is used in all shells except for a special 12-gauge Scatter Load loaded with No. 8 shot that contains a post wad to increase dispersion of shot.

RXP shells have plastic tubes with integral wads and low brass heads. They are loaded with a one-piece Power Piston® wad. RXP shells are intended for skeet and trap shooting.

Winchester-Western

Ammunition marketed by Winchester-Western is sold under the designations of Super-X, Upland, and AA Plus. All are loaded with ball powder. Virtually all shells are constructed with one-piece, compression-form plastic tubes. All the shells are closed with a pie crimp.

Super-X shells have a high brass head, an over-the-powder cup wad,

Table 8–3 Shotshell Loads (Winchester-Western, Remington-Peters, and Federal

Gauge	Length of shell (in)	Shot (oz)	Shot size
Magnum loads			
10[a]	3½	2¼	BB,2,4
10[a,b]	3½	2	BB,2,4
12	3	1⅞	BB,2,4
12[a,b]	3	1⅝	2,4,6
12[a,b]	2¾	1½	2,4,5,6
16	2¾	1¼	2,4,6
20	3	1¼	2,4,6,7½
20	2¾	1⅛	4,6,7½
Long-range loads			
10[a,b]	2⅞	1⅝	4
12	2¾	1¼	BB,2,4,5,6,7½,8,9
16	2¾	1⅛	4,5,6,7½,9
20	2¾	1	4,5,6,7½,9
28[a,b]	2¾	¾	6,7½,8
410[b]	2½	½	6,7½
410[b]	3	11/16	4,5,6,7½,8
Field loads			
12	2¾	1¼	7½,8,9
12	2¾	1⅛	4,5,6,7½,8,9
16	2¾	1⅛	4,5,6,7½,8
20	2¾	1	4,5,6,7½,8,9
Skeet and trap			
12	2¾	1⅛	7½,8
12	2¾	1⅛	7½,8,9
20	2¾	⅞	9
28[a]	2¾	¾	9
410[a]	2½	½	9
Buckshot			
10[c]	3½	—	4 Buck-54 pellets
12	3 Mag.	—	00 Buck-15 pellets
12	3 Mag.	—	4 Buck-41 pellets
12[b]	2¾ Mag.	—	1 Buck-20 pellets
12	2¾ Mag.	—	00 Buck-12 pellets
12	2¾	—	00 Buck- 9 pellets
12	2¾	—	0 Buck-12 pellets
12	2¾	—	1 Buck-16 pellets
12	2¾	—	4 Buck-27 pellets
12[a]	2¾ Mag.	—	000 Buck- 8 pellets
12[a]	3 Mag.	—	000 Buck-10 pellets
16	2¾	—	1 Buck-12 pellets
20	2¾	—	3 Buck-20 pellets

(continued)

Table 8–3 *(continued)*

Gauge	Length of shell (in)	Shot (oz)	Shot size
Rifled slugs			
10	3½	1¾	Slug
12[c]	2¾	1¼	Slug
12	2¾	1	Slug
16	2¾	⅘	Slug
20[b]	2¾	⅝	Slug
20[a,b]	2¾	¾	Slug
410	2½	⅕	Slug
Steel shot loads			
10[c]	3½	1⅝	BB,2
12[c]	2¾	1⅛	1,2,4
12[a,c]	2¾	1¼	BB,1,2,4
12[b]	3	1¼	1,2,4
12[b]	2¾	1⅛	1,2,4
20[c]	3	1	4

[a] Winchester-Western only.   [n] Remington-Peters only.   [c] Federal only.

composite filler wads, and a plastic collar. Some shells are loaded with copper-coated (Lubaloy) shot. Super Double-X shells use granulated plastic packing added to the shot column to protect the shot.

Upland shells have a low brass head, an overpowder cup wad, composite filler wads, and a plastic collar.

AA Plus shells are intended for skeet and trap shooting only. They have a low brass head and a one-piece plastic wad. Skeet and trap loads with paper hulls are also manufactured.

Federal Ammunition

Virtually all shotgun ammunition manufactured by Federal uses plastic hulls. Federal hulls are color coded: red for 12 gauge; purple for 16 gauge, and yellow for 20-gauge. Plastic hulls have a ribbed appearance and, with few exceptions, a pie-crimped mouth. Flake powder is used in the shells.

Federal shotgun shells use a wide variety of wad systems. The most common is the Triple-Plus wad. This is found in most Hi-Power and Field Loads.

Federal produces Premium Magnum shotgun shells in 10, 12, and 20 gauge. These shells are loaded with shot loaded in a granulated plastic filler.

Miscellaneous Shotgun Ammunition

Brass Shotgun Shells

Brass shotgun shells are now relatively uncommon in the United States. Remington, the last manufacturer of them, stopped production in 1957. Brass shotgun shells have been imported into the United States.

Winchester Tracer Rounds

Winchester tracer rounds were introduced in 1965 in 12 gauge only. The 12-gauge tracer load was intended for use by skeet and trap shooters so that they could see where the shot had gone. This round contains a spherical aluminum capsule with a short hollow tail. The capsule containing the tracer compound lies above the filler wads among the shot (Figure 8−39). The tracer is ignited by powder gases through an opening in the center of the wad column that communicates with the lumen of the tail. When fired, the tracer appears as a glowing dart of yellow-white flame.

Remington Modi-Pac

The Remington Modi-Pac refers to the Modified Impact Shotgun Shell. This round, which apparently was produced in the late 1960s, used an SP tube with a rolled crimp. It was intended by law enforcement agencies

Figure 8−39 Disassembled Winchester tracer round.

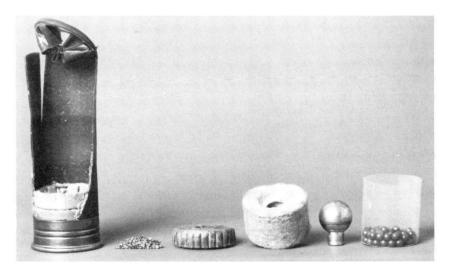

for riot control. Only 12-gauge shells were manufactured; these shells contain ¼ oz of 0.120-in.-diameter plastic pellets. Approximately 320 pellets per load were used. The muzzle velocity was 1600 ft/sec. Loss of velocity was extremely rapid because of light weight of the pellets. Thus, at 15 yd, muzzle velocity was only 200 ft/sec. Maximum range was 25 yds. Given the low pressure generated in these shells, they would not function in auto-loading shotgun.

References

1. Butler D.F. *The American Shotgun.* New York: Winchester Press, 1973.
2. Keith, E. *Shotguns by Keith.* New York: Bonanza Book, 1967.
3. Labisky, W. The ever-changing shotshell story. *Gun Digest.* Northfield, IL: Digest Books Inc., 1973.
4. Breitenecker, R., Senior, W. Shotgun patterns. An experimental study on the influence of intermediate targets. J. Forensic Sci. 12(2):193–204, 1967.
5. Breitenecker, R. Shotgun wound patterns. Am. J. Clin. Pathol. 52:258–269, 1969.

Gunshot Wounds: Miscellaneous

9

Bloody Bodies and Bloody Scenes

Violence as portrayed in the movies and television has traditionally been relatively bloodless. In real life, most gunshot scenes are quite bloody. As in many aspects of forensic pathology, this observation is not absolute. Some scenes show very little evidence of bleeding, and some show essentially none. In the latter case, hemorrhaging is internal—into the chest or abdominal cavities—or is prevented by clothing. The only observable blood may be a dime-shaped area of bleeding on the clothing overlying the entrance site.

Minimal bleeding around an entrance site usually involves small-caliber weapons and locations on the body that are clothed and elevated, i.e., not in dependent areas where bleeding or leakage of blood would occur secondary to gravity. Clothing may act as a pressure bandage. When the deceased is wearing multiple layers of clothing, blood from the wound may be absorbed by the internal layers of clothing so that there is no evidence of bleeding on the outer clothing.

Gunshot wounds of the head usually bleed freely. Again, this is not inevitable. The author has seen a case in which there was a contact gunshot wound of the back of the head from a .22-caliber rimfire weapon. The entrance was apparently sealed by the hot gases as there was no blood at the scene or visible on the body. The entrance was concealed by a bushy Afro haircut and was found only when the head was opened as part of a routine autopsy on an apparently natural death.

In scenes where the deceased has walked or run from the scene of the shooting, there is usually a trail of blood. The quantity of bleeding, however, is very variable. In some cases there may be no blood because the bleeding was internal or the victim has pressed his or her hand or a cloth against the wound, thus acting as a pressure bandage to prevent external hemorrhaging onto the floor or ground.

Physical Activity Following Gunshot Wounds

That an individual sustains a fatal gunshot wound does not mean he or she cannot engage in physical activity. Experienced forensic pathologists inevitably encounter cases in which an individual, after incurring a fatal gunshot wound of the heart, is able to walk or run hundreds of yards and engage in strenuous physical activity prior to collapse and death.

One of the most unusual cases the author has seen involving movement after a gunshot wound of the heart was that of a young man shot in the left chest at a range of 3 to 4 ft with a 12-gauge shotgun firing No. 7½ shot. The pellets literally shredded the heart, yet, this individual was able to run 65 ft prior to collapsing. Such activity is not surprising if one realizes that an individual can function without a heart for a short time. The limiting factor for consciousness is the oxygen supply to the brain. When the oxygen in the brain is consumed, unconsciousness occurs. Experiments have shown that an individual can remain conscious for at least 10 to 15 sec after complete occlusion of the carotid arteries. Thus, if no blood is pumped to the brain, an individual can function, e.g., run, for at least 10 sec before collapsing.

In another case, a 17-year-old boy was shot once in the left back with a .25 Automatic. The bullet perforated the aorta, left main pulmonary artery and left lung, embedding itself in the anterior chest wall. When the emergency medical service technicians arrived at the scene, the victim initially refused to got to the hospital with them; he had to be forced into the ambulance. This scene was actually videotaped and shown on a local television station. He arrived at the hospital approximately 30 min after having been shot. At the time, he was awake and alert with normal vital signs. Fifteen minutes after arrival at the hospital, i.e., 45 min after being shot, he was noted to be agitated and combative. Over the next half hour he gradually exhibited shock, and 1 hr and 15 min after being shot, he was brought into the operating room. At this time, he developed irreversible shock and was pronounced dead 2 hrs and 20 min after being shot.

Just as in the case of gunshot wounds of the heart or major blood vessels, individuals can perform tasks or even survive gunshot wounds of the brain—especially if they involve the frontal lobes. In documented cases of suicide, an individual has fired a bullet through the frontal lobes, to be followed by a second fatal wound into the basal ganglia. If a bullet passes through the basal ganglia, one can be certain that the individual will be incapable of any movement after the wound. Gunshot wounds of the brainstem also produce instant incapacitation, though even with this wound death may not occur immediately. One individual who had a gunshot wound of the pons survived approximately 1 wk, although in a totally vegetative state.

The fact that one can survive at least for a limited time with a wound that would ordinarily be thought to cause instant death is shown in Figure 9–1. This elderly male shot himself in the right temple with a .357 Magnum. In spite of the obvious devastating nature of the wound, he lived 1 hr and 34 min without any life support systems.

In addition to a wound not immediately causing incapacitation, in some instances individuals who have been shot do not initially realize it. This is not uncommon in combat situations, where the noise, violence, and activity so distract an individual that he may not realize that he has been wounded.

Concealed Wounds

It is quite common for a pathologist, at autopsy, to discover gunshot wounds missed by the police at the scene or physicians in an emergency room. Emergency room physicians often miss wounds of the back because they do not turn the individual over and wounds of the head because of long hair. They also often confuse entrances with exits. Therefore, one must approach medical records with a great deal of caution in trying to determine how many times a person has been shot

Figure 9–1 Contact wound of right temple with .357 Magnum. The deceased lived 1 hr and 34 min without any life support systems.

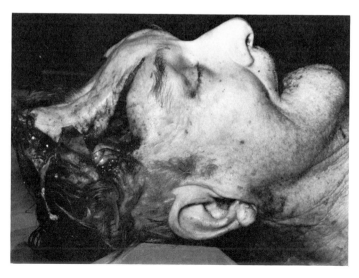

as well as whether a wound is an entrance or exit. It is also quite common for a physician to fail to note in the medical records the presence or absence of soot or powder tattooing around a wound. Occasionally, such information may be found in a nurse's notes. One also must realize that soot may have been present initially, at the entrance, but that the nurse who saw the patient before the physician may have wiped it off. These factors again point out the importance of retention of clothing, as the wounds in question may have gone through the clothing. One should instruct the ambulance crews, emergency rooms, and hospitals in one's jurisdiction never to discard clothing in cases of gunshot wounds.

Surgical intervention may make interpretation of gunshot wounds difficult as a result of the obliteration or the alteration of wounds. Thus, in gunshot wounds of the chest, the surgeon may either put his thoracotomy incision through the wound or insert a chest tube through it. In gunshot wounds of the head, it is usual for the surgeon to obliterate the entrance wound in the skin and bone when performing a craniectomy.

Some surgeons, especially those who have had military training, persist in performing wide debridement of entrance wounds in the skin from handguns and rimfire rifles even though this is unnecessary given the low wounding energy of such weapons. Often the skin removed in the debridement procedure is sent to surgical pathology and may be retrieved, but unfortunately this is not always the case.

Surgeons often recover a bullet that caused an injury. One should instruct them in the correct marking of such missiles. Unfortunately, it is not uncommon for a surgeon to inscribe his or her initials on the side of a recovered bullet rather than the nose or base, thus obliterating its rifling characteristics. In shotgun wound cases, one should also inform the surgeons that the wadding and representative pellets should be retained for evidentiary purposes.

Concealment of a wound may occur not only through the actions of a physician but also inadvertently on the basis of an unusual entrance site. At some time in his or her career, a forensic pathologist will encounter a case in which the bullet entered either the nostril or open mouth, thus, presenting the pathologist with a body with no observable entrance wound. Advanced decomposition may also conceal a gunshot wound. The use of x-rays on select decomposed bodies will prevent missing such cases.

In skeletal remains, x-ray of the bones for missiles should be done routinely. It is also wise to collect the dirt underneath the skeleton and x-ray it. The author saw a case in which a .22-caliber bullet was found embedded in a vertebrae. Up to that time no cause of death had been determined. The entrance defect had been missed on gross examination of this bone. X-ray of the dirt underneath the body revealed two other bullets.

Minimal Velocities Necessary to Perforate Skin

Before a bullet can cause a significant injury, it must be able to perforate skin. Skin differs from other tissue in that a relatively high initial velocity is necessary for a bullet to effect perforation. Knowledge of this velocity is important to the forensic pathologist in cases of assault, attempted homicide, or homicide with airguns as well as in determining the maximum range out to which a bullet is capable of penetrating the body.

The first person to attempt to determine the minimum velocity needed to perforate skin was Journee in 1907.[1] He observed that missiles of relatively low velocity 80 to 200 m/sec that rebounded from the skin of a horse could go through 20 cm of muscle after the skin had been removed. Thus, skin appeared to be more resistant to missiles than muscle. Experiments on human cadavers revealed that a lead sphere 11.25 mm in diameter and weighing 8.5 gm needed a minimum velocity of 70 m/sec (230 ft/sec), with an energy/area of presentation (E/a) of 2.13 m-kg/cm^2, to perforate the skin and enter the underlying subcutaneous tissue and muscle.

Mattoo et al. in 1974 obtained virtually the same results using human thigh muscle with intact skin.[2] A lead sphere 8.5 mm in diameter and weighing 4.5 gm required a velocity of 71.3 m/sec (234 ft/sec) to perforate skin and penetrate into subcutaneous tissue and muscle to a depth of 2.9 cm. The E/a was 2.06 m-kg/cm^2.

Both these studies involved relatively heavy large-caliber lead balls and not the lighter weight, bullet-shaped projectiles fired in modern firearms or the very lightweight projectiles used in airguns.

DiMaio et al. conducted a series of tests to determine the velocities necessary for .38-caliber lead bullets and lead airgun pellets (calibers .177 and .22) to perforate skin.[3] Human lower extremities were used in the tests. A 113-gr lead roundnose .38-caliber bullet required a minimal velocity of 58 m/sec (191 ft/sec) to perforate skin (Table 9−1). The E/a was 1.95 m-kg/cm.^{2}

Caliber .22 wasp-waist Diabolo-style airgun pellets weighing an average of 16.5 gr initially perforated skin at 75 m/sec (245 ft/sec), with perforation becoming consistent at 87 m/sec (285 ft/sec) and above (Table 9−1). The E/a at 75 m/sec is 1.30 m-kg/cm^2. At a velocity of 68 m/sec (223 ft/sec), a pellet embedded itself in but did not perforate the skin.

0.177 airgun pellets of wasp-waist Diabolo style weighing an average of 8.25 gr required a minimum velocity of 101 m/sec (331 ft/sec) to initially perforate skin (Table 9–1). At velocities of 111 m/sec (365 ft/sec) and higher, perforation always occurred. At a velocity of 88 m/sec (290 ft/sec), a pellet embedded itself in the skin. The E/a at 101 m/sec (331 ft/sec) is 1.84 m-kg/cm^2.

These studies indicate that lightweight projectiles need a higher velocity to perforate skin than large caliber heavier bullets.

Now that we know the minimum velocity necessary for bullets and airgun pellets of different weight and caliber to perforate skin, we must ask whether in perforating the skin the missiles lose this velocity. The answer is no. In an unpublished extension of the previously mentioned study, DiMaio and Copeland conducted a number of test firings using a human lower extremity to determine how much velocity was lost by a missile passing through the thigh.[4] The bullets had to pass through two layers of skin and approximately 6 in. of muscle. Two different calibers of ammunition were used—.38 Special and .22 Long Rifle. In the tests with the .38 Special ammunition, two different types of ammunition were used. The first type was loaded with a 158-gr lead round-nose bullet. Average impact velocity was 766 ft/sec. On an average these bullets lost 280 ft/sec (36.8% of impact initial velocity) in passing through the thigh (Table 9–2). The velocity lost ranged from a minimum of 214 ft/sec to a maximum of 337 ft/sec.

The second type of ammunition was loaded with 158 gr, semijacketed hollow-point bullets. The average impact velocity was 884 ft/sec. With this velocity and weight of bullet, there is no mushrooming of the projectile in the body. Therefore, mushrooming was not a factor in loss of velocity. The average velocity lost was 305 ft/sec for an average loss of 34.4% of impact velocity (Table 9–2). The velocity lost ranged from a low of 264 ft/sec to a maximum of 355 ft/sec. The increased loss of velocity by the semijacketed hollow-point bullet compared with the roundnose bullet, if significant, could be due to either one or the other of two factors if not a combination. The first factor is the greater velocity at which the semijacketed bullet was propelled and the second is the blunt

Table 9–1 Minimum Velocities Necessary to Perforate Skin

Missile	Weight (gr)	Minimum velocity (m/sec)
.177 airgun pellets	8.25	101 (331 ft/sec)
.22 airgun pellets	16.5	75 (245 ft/sec)
.38-caliber round-nose bullet	113	58 (191 ft/sec)

Table 9−2 Velocity Lost by Bullets Perforating Human Skin and Muscle[a]

Caliber	Bullet weight (gr)	Bullet style	Average velocity lost (ft/sec)	Range of velocity lost (ft/sec)	Percentage of impact velocity lost (%)
.38 Special	158	Lead roundnose	280	214−337	36.8
	158	Semijacketed hollow point[b]	305	264−355	34.4
.22 Long Rifle	40	Lead roundnose	195	187−202	18
	36	Lead hollow point	491	431−599	45.5

[a] Two layers of skin, 6 in. of muscle.   [b] This bullet did not mushroom.

shape of the tip necessitated by having a hollow point. Mushrooming of the bullet did not occur and therefore could not play a part in an increased loss of velocity. In all probability the greater impact velocity caused the greater loss of velocity. This theory tends to be confirmed by the fact that the percentage loss of impact velocity for both styles of bullets was approximately the same.

The tests with the .22 ammunition were somewhat more extensive in that the loss of velocity was determined not only for the thigh when it was enclosed by skin but also for the muscle alone. This was accomplished by the subsequent removal of the skin after test-firing with it in place. The first ammunition tested was high-velocity .22 Long Rifle cartridges loaded with 40-gr lead roundnose, bullets. The average impact velocity was 1083 ft/sec. Average loss of velocity in passing through the thigh was 195 ft/sec, with velocity lost ranging from 187 to 202 ft/sec (Table 9−2). When the skin was removed from the thigh, this same ammunition lost an average of 151 ft/sec range (85 to 229 ft/sec). Thus, in passing through two layers of skin, the bullets lost only an average of 44 ft/sec.

The second type of ammunition used was high-velocity .22 Long Rifle ammunition loaded with a 36-gr lead hollow-point bullet. The average striking velocity was 1079 ft/sec. Average velocity loss was 491 ft/sec with a range of 431 to 599 ft/sec, approximately 2½ times the velocity lost by the solid roundnose bullets (Table 9−2). When the hollow-point ammunition was tested against the thigh with the skin removed, there was an average loss of velocity of 383 ft/sec, with a range of 320 to 520 ft/sec. Thus, in passing through two layers of skin, the hollow-point bullets lost an average of only 108 ft/sec. The increased loss of velocity in passing through the skin compared with the solid lead bullets is consistent with the increased loss sustained while passing through muscle.

Bullet Emboli

Vascular embolization of a bullet is an uncommon occurrence. When it does occur, it usually involves the arterial system. Embolization should be suspected whenever there is a penetrating bullet wound with failure to discover the bullet in the expected region or to visualize the bullet on routine x-ray.[5] In the author's first autopsy on a case of bullet embolization, he spent 7 hr looking for a bullet in the chest and abdomen, when it was in the femoral artery.

The most common sites of entrance for a bullet into the arterial system are the aorta and the heart. Although embolization usually occurs immediately following entrance of the bullet into the circulation, delays as long as 26 days have been reported.[6] The site of lodgment of the bullet is predominantly the lower extremity. Whether there is predominant embolization to the right or left legs is debatable.[5]

Bullet emboli are usually associated with small caliber, low velocity missiles. Thus, in the review by DiMaio and DiMaio, in the 24 instances in which the caliber or type of weapon was known, a .22 caliber bullet accounted for 14 cases, an airgun pellet for 2 cases, and a shotgun pellet for 2 cases.[5] These missiles are all small-caliber, lightweight, low-velocity projectiles possessing low kinetic energy and usually causing penetrating rather than perforating wounds. If these missiles lose their forward velocity on penetration of a major blood vessel or the heart, they will be swept along by the blood to their final point of lodgement.

If an x-ray is not taken before autopsy, a bullet embolus secondary to a gunshot wound of the aorta may not be suspected because of the presence of both an entrance and an exit in this vessel. In such a case, the almost spent bullet, after exiting the aorta, strikes the vertebral column and rebounds back through the exit into the lumen of the aorta, where it is swept away to a lower extremity.

Bullet emboli may occur from wounds other than those in the chest and abdomen. In one of the author's cases, an individual was shot in the left eye with a .22-caliber bullet. The bullet entered the cranial cavity, traveled through the left cerebral hemisphere, and ricocheted off the inner table of the skull, penetrating into the left straight sinus. It was carried through the venous system, down the jugular vein, through the right atrium and ventricle, and into the pulmonary artery. The bullet came to rest lodged in a major branch of the left pulmonary artery.

A variant of the bullet embolus not involving vascular embolization is encountered occasionally. One such case involved an individual shot in the right back. The bullet traveled upward into the oral cavity, where it subsequently was coughed or vomited up by the victim. The bullet was found on the ground a number of feet away from the deceased in a pool of vomitus and blood. In another case, an individual incurred a gunshot wound of the chest. On admission to the hospital, the bullet was seen on x-ray apparently lodged in the parenchyma of the right lung. The individual survived a number of days in the hospital. At autopsy, the bullet was found in the bronchus of the left lung. Apparently the bullet entered the bronchial tree on the right side and subsequently was coughed up and aspirated into the left bronchial tree.

Gunshot Wounds of the Brain

Gunshot wounds of the brain constitute approximately one-third of all fatal gunshot wounds. Wounds of the brain from high-velocity rifles and shotguns are extremely devastating. Such injuries are described in chapters 7 and 8. This section will deal with gunshot wounds of the brain caused by low-velocity weapons: handguns and .22 rimfire rifles.

Bone Chips

When a bullet strikes the head, it "punches out" a circular to oval wound of entrance in the skull, driving fragments of bone into the brain. The bone chips generally follow along the main bullet track, contributing to its irregular configuration. Sometimes the bone chips create secondary tracks that deviate from the main path. These chips are detectable on digital palpation in approximately one-third of gunshot wound cases of the brain.[7] Use of high-resolution x-ray increases the percentage detected.

The presence of bone chips at one end of the bullet track through the brain provides conclusive evidence of the direction of the shot; in the author's experience, no bone chips are found in the brain parenchyma adjacent to the exit wound. This fact is of help in cases of perforating gunshot wounds where there has been surgical debridement of wounds in the skin and bone and where it is important to differentiate the entrance from the exit.

Secondary Fractures of the Skull

As the bullet perforates the brain, it produces a temporary cavity that undergoes a series of pulsations before disappearing. The pressure waves in the brain in the case of high-velocity missiles may produce massive fragmentation of the skull. In the case of handgun bullets, the pressure waves are considerably less but still may cause fractures. Linear fractures of the orbital plate are the most common because of the paper-thin nature of the bone. Fracture lines may also radiate from the entrance or exit hole or even be randomly distributed in the vault or base of the skull. These secondary fractures of the skull are seen most commonly with medium- and large-caliber handguns, though they occur even in distant .22-caliber Long Rifle wounds. No matter what the caliber, secondary fractures are more common with contact wounds, where the pressure waves from the temporary cavity are augmented by pressure from the expanding gas.

Shape of the Bullet Tracks

The shape of the permanent missile track in the brain is irregular, sometimes larger near the entry and sometimes larger near the exit or the middle.[7] The irregular shape of the cavity defies any attempt to determine the direction of travel from its configuration. The size of the permanent cavity bears no relationship to the caliber or muzzle energy of the missile. Wound tracks produced by .22 rimfire ammunition may be as large and devastating as those caused by .45 ACP bullets. The influence of gas from combustion of the propellant on the volume of the permanent cavity appears to be small or nil. In the study by Kirkpatrick and DiMaio, contact wounds accounted for both the minimum and the maximum volume of missile tracks.[7]

Point of Lodgment of the Bullet

In most handgun wounds of the head, the bullet is retained either in the cranial cavity or beneath the scalp. Most .22 rimfire, .32 revolver, and .38 Special wounds of the head are penetrating rather than perforating. Full metal-jacketed bullets have a greater tendency to perforate the head than lead or semijacketed bullets of the same or approximately the same caliber. As the caliber of the full metal-jacketed bullet increases, the likelihood of its perforating the head also increases. Thus, whereas .25 Automatic full metal jacketed bullets usually do not perforate the head, 9-mm and .45 automatic bullets usually do. The location of the entrance site and whether the wound is contact or distant in nature also influence the probability of a bullet exiting the head.

In gunshot wounds of the head caused by .22 caliber lead bullets, the bullet will exit in only about 10% of the cases. These wounds are almost invariably contact and occur in the temple, with the exit usually in the opposite temple. In another 10% of the cases, the bullet will exit the skull and be found beneath the scalp. These cases are also usually contact in nature, with the entrance in the temple.

Approximately one-third of all .38-caliber gunshot wounds of the head are perforating. The entrance wound is usually contact in nature and occurs in the temple. The statistics for .25 ACP full metal-jacketed bullet are the same. When one gets to the .380, 9-mm, and .45 full metal-jacketed rounds, the picture changes radically. As a rule, whether contact or distant, these bullets exit. Partial metal-jacketed bullets in these calibers may be retained in the cranial cavity. The author has not had enough such cases to come to any statistical conclusions.

Of the bullets that do not exit the head, the vast majority are retained in the cranial cavity. Thus, internal ricochet is fairly common, occurring in anywhere from 10 to 25% of the cases, depending on the caliber of the weapons and the diligency with which the evidence of internal ricochet is sought. As a general rule, internal ricochet is more commonly associated with lead bullets and bullets of small caliber. Thus, ricochet within the cranial cavity occurs most commonly with .22-caliber lead bullets. The type of ricochet most commonly encountered results from a bullet that passes through the brain, strikes the internal table of the skull on the other side, and is deflected in a cortical or subcortical path parallel to the internal table (Figure 9–2). This results in a shallow gutter wound track in the cortex of the brain. Less commonly, bullets ricochet back into the brain at the acute angle or along the original bullet track (Figure 9–2).

The length of the internal ricochet track may be quite long. In one case the author has seen, a .38 Special lead bullet entered the right frontal lobe and perforated the brain, exiting the left frontal lobes. The bullet then ricocheted off the bone along the lateral aspect of the left frontal, parietal, and occipital lobes; crossed the midline; and continued along the lateral aspect of the right cerebral hemisphere, coming to rest in the lateral cortex of the right frontal pole adjacent to where it had entered.

Figure 9–2 Patterns of bullet ricochet inside cranial cavity. Type B is the most common.

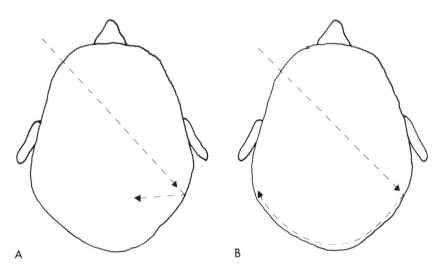

A   B

Examination of the brain in gunshot wounds reveals contusions around the entrance site in about half the cases.[7] These are probably due to inbending of the bone against the brain at the moment of perforation. Contusions are equally frequent at the exit, although they do not necessarily occur in the same cases as entry contusions. Contusions can also be seen on the inferior surface of the frontal lobe.

In virtually all gunshot wound cases involving the brain, the brain will show signs of increased intracranial pressure. These signs consist of grooves of the uncal gyri from the tentorium as well as cone-shaped molding of the cerebellar tonsils at the foramen magnum. These findings may help explain death in some cases. Examination of gunshot-wounded brains reveals many cases in which the vital centers were not directly in the path of the bullet and in which the volume of the permanent cavity was relatively small (less than many spontaneous hematomas); i.e., the volume of grossly involved brain is trivial when compared with the brain itself. In such cases, deformation of the brain toward the foramen magnum still occurs. Pressure on the brainstem secondary to this deformation may be the fatal mechanism in these cases.[7]

Intrauterine Gunshot Wounds

Gunshot wounds of the pregnant uterus are relatively uncommon.[8] Maternal death in such cases is extremely rare. The gunshot injury to the fetus or placenta usually results in intrauterine death or premature delivery with or without evidence of injury to the child.

The most significant question arising from fetal deaths due to gunshot wounds of the pregnant uterus concerns the ruling of the manner of death.[9] If the child dies in utero, no matter how advanced the stage of development, there is no criminal culpability for the child's death attached to the person who did the shooting. Legally the child is not considered an individual until it is born alive. If, however, the child is born alive and then dies, even if the time of survival is a matter of only a few minutes, the death is considered a homicide—even if the bullet did not strike the child but just induced premature labor. In the latter case, one could rule the cause of death as "prematurity secondary to gunshot wound of uterus—Homicide."

Lead Poisoning from Retained Bullets

Lead poisoning from a retained bullet or lead pellet is extremely rare in view of the large number of individuals with such retained missiles. Even rarer is death from lead poisoning resulting from the retained bullet, with only two such cases in the literature.[10,11]

There are only about 21 laboratory-documented cases of lead toxicity from a retained lead missile in the literature.[10-13] Of these cases, in 18 instances the bullet was within a joint, a bone, or an intervertebral disk. It has long been recognized that synovial fluid is capable of dissolving lead. A rich vascular supply to the tissue surrounding the bullet and prolonged bathing of the bullet with either bursal or synovial fluid makes the development of acute lead intoxication more likely.

In a fatal case of lead poisoning reported by the author, the individual was a 54-year-old woman shot in the thigh by her son with a .32-caliber revolver.[11] X-rays taken at the time the deceased was shot showed a flattened, deformed lead missile lodged in the soft tissue near the distal femur, just proximal to the condyles and anterior lateral to the bone. Small fragments of lead were present adjacent to the main mass. The location of the bullet was consistent with its being in or in communication with the suprapatellar bursa. Five months after being shot, the victim was admitted to a hospital with severe anemia. Hemoglobin was 6.9 gm/dl, hematocrit 21%, MCV 84, and platelets 388,000 mm^3, with a white blood cell count of 5600 mm^2. The reticulocyte count was 5%. A

Figure 9–3 Eosinophilic intranuclear inclusions in hepatocytes.

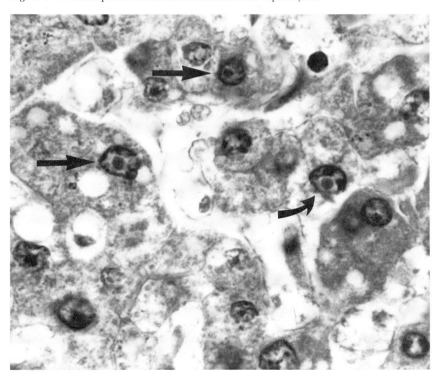

smear showed basophilic stippling. The patient had been seen 9 months previous to this admission, at which time her hematocrit was 39% and hemoglobin 13 gm/dl. One month before this last admission, she came to the hospital complaining of constipation and gnawing dull peri-umbilical and epigastric abdominal pain. She had had a 20-lb weight loss over the previous 4 mo.

During her hospitalization, a diagnosis of lead poisoning was never considered. She suffered multiple episodes of gran mal convulsions and died 14 days after admission. At autopsy, the brain was swollen with uncal herniation and necrosis. Secondary brainstem hemorrhage was present. Analysis of the blood obtained postmortem revealed a lead level of 5.3 mg/L. Fortuitously, antemortem blood obtained 5 days before death had been retained and revealed a lead level of 5.1 mg/L. Any lead level above 0.6 mg/L was considered toxic in the hospital laboratory.

Microscopic examination of autopsy tissue in this case revealed eosinophilic intranuclear inclusions in hepatocytes and cells of the proximal tubules of the kidneys (Figure 9−3). Many of the perivascular spaces in the brain contained agregates of pink-staining homogeneous material that was PAS positive. These histological lesions are described as being associated with lead intoxication. It is interesting that a neuro-logical examination conducted at the time of admission to the hospital was negative. This result most probably represents a cursory neurologic examination in a patient not expected to have neurological abnormal-ities. By coincidence, the other fatal case in the literature also involves a woman shot in the leg.[10]

Location of Fatal Gunshot Wounds

There have been no extensive civilian studies to show the location of fatal gunshot wounds in the body in nonsuicide cases. The U.S. Army has conducted a number of studies involving combat casualties.[14−16] The most recent one, and probably the most applicable in view of changes in medical therapy, was the WDMET study from the Vietnam war.[14] This study found that, although the head and neck constituted only 6.5% of the body surface, wounds of this region accounted for 37.2% of fatal gunshot wounds. The thorax, which contributes 13% of the body surface, was the source of fatal wounds in 36.4% of fatalities. The abdomen, which constitutes 10.6% of the body surface, accounted for 9.2% of the fatal wounds.

It has been the author's experience in civilian homicide cases that 40% of fatal wounds involve the brain; approximately 25%, the heart; 25%, the aorta or other main blood vessels; and 10%, solid viscera—e.g., lungs, liver, kidney, and so forth.

Behavior of Ammunition and Gunpowder in Fires

Occasionally a story appears in a newspaper describing how firefighters fought a blaze in a sporting goods store as bullets from exploding ammunition "whizzed by" and cans of gunpowder "exploded" around them. Although this type of story makes fine newspaper copy, it bears no relation to what actually happens in a fire involving ammunition and gunpowder.

Smokeless powder is used in all modern cartridges. When it is ignited in a gun, heat and gas are produced, both of which are confined initially to the chamber. As the pressure of the gas builds up, the chemical processes of combustion are speeded up so that the rate of burning becomes relatively instantaneous, and an "explosion" is then produced. This explosion, however, occurs only when smokeless powder is ignited in a confined space such as a gun. When smokeless powder is ignited outside of a gun, it will only burn with a quick hot flame.

In order to demonstrate the burning properties of smokeless powder, Hatcher conducted a series of experiments in which he burned cans of smokeless powder.[17] The amount of powder in each can varied from 1 lb to 8 oz. Each can was placed on a quantity of kindling wood, which was then ignited. After a time of from 40 sec to 1½ min, the cans burst with a mild noise, followed by a yellow-white flame 3 to 4 ft in diameter. The underlying kindling wood was practically undisturbed. There were no violent explosions.

Black powder is a different matter. It burns faster than smokeless powder and may actually produce an explosion. Black powder is not loaded in modern ammunition. Hatcher burnt a 1-lb can of black powder. After 5 min of heating, the can exploded with a heavy dull thud, producing a dense cloud of smoke but no flames. The can was hurled approximately 35 ft. It had been opened up and flattened by the explosion.

Occasionally one hears that an individual has been "wounded" when a cartridge was accidentally dropped into a fire and detonates. Investigation of such incidents usually reveals that the victim was really injured when he or another individual was playing with a gun. When small-arms ammunition is placed in a fire, the cartridge case may burst into a number of fragments and the bullet may then be propelled forward out of the case. In centerfire cartridges, the primer may blowout. None of these missiles, however, is dangerous to life. The bullet in fact is probably the most harmless of all these missiles because with its relatively great mass it will have very little velocity. Fragments of brass and the primer are the only components of an exploding round that have sufficient velocity to cause injury. These fragments can penetrate the skin or eye if the individual is very close to the exploding cartridge. With the exception of eye injury, however, no serious injury should occur, and certainly no mortal wound. As the distance between the exploding round and the individual increases, the brass particles become harmless because of their relatively small mass and irregular shape, which produce rapid loss in velocity.

Experiments have been conducted to determine at what temperature a small-arms cartridge will detonate.[18] Cartridges were placed in an oven and the furnace was heated until the round exploded. It was found that .22 Long Rifle cartridges exploded at an average of 279° F., .38 Special rounds at 290°F, .30-06 at 317°F, and 12-gauge shotgun shells at 387°F. Whereas the cartridges detonated in every case, the primers did not. In fact, in some of the detonated rounds the primers were removed, loaded into other cartridges cases, and fired.

Although unconfined cartridges are relatively innocuous in fires, ammunition in a weapon is dangerous if it is present in the chamber. Here we have the same conditions as if the cartridge had been fired in the weapon in a conventional manner. The heat of the fire may be sufficient to "cook off" the cartridge in the chamber. If the weapon is a long arm or an auto-loading pistol, only one round will be fired. If the weapon is a revolver, not only can the cartridge in line with the barrel discharge, other cartridges in the other chambers of the cylinder can discharge. In this situation, one bullet would have rifling marks whereas the other bullets would be free of such markings. The bullets not in alignment with the barrel would show shearing of one surface secondary to their striking the frame of the weapon as they exited the cylinder.

If one is in a situation in which a fired weapon is recovered from a burned-out residence or vehicle, it is usually very easy to determine whether the cartridges in the weapon have been discharged by heat rather than by firing in the conventional manner. Examination of the cartridge case in the weapon will reveal the primer to be free of the normal firing-pin impression. In weapons in which the firing pin rests on the primer, a faint mark may be present on the primer as a result of slight rearward movement of the cartridge case at the time of discharge from the heat.

Blunt Force Injuries from Firearms

Occasionally a firearm will be used not only to shoot a person but to beat that individual. Thus, individuals will be seen with evidence of "pistol whipping." This usually takes the form of triangular or less commonly semicircular lacerations of the scalp or forehead. Underlying depressed fractures may be present (Figure 9-4). The butt of a rifle may also be used to beat a victim. Figure 9-5 shows an individual who after being shot had his jaw broken with the butt of a .22 rimfire rifle.

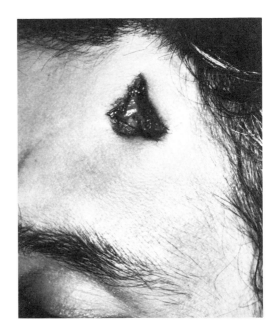

Figure 9−4 Triangular laceration with underlying depressed skull fracture caused by pistol butt.

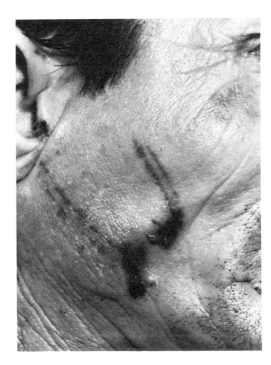

Figure 9−5 Patterned abrasion from rifle butt. Underlying fracture of mandible.

References

1. Journee, C. Rapport entre force vive des balles at la gravite des blessures qu'elles peuvent causer. Rev. d'Artilleries. 70(1):81–120, 1907.

2. Matoo, B.N., Wani, A.K., Asgekar, M.D. Casualty criteria for wounds from firearms with special reference to shot penetration. Part II. J. Forensic Sci. 19(3): 585–589, 1974.

3. DiMaio, V.J.M., Copeland, A.R., Besant-Matthews, P.E., Fletcher, L.A., Jones, A. Minimal velocities necessary for perforation of skin by air gun pellets and bullets. J. Forensic Sci. 27 (4): 894–898, 1982.

4. DiMaio V.J.M., Copeland, A.R. Unpublished study.

5. DiMaio, V.J.M., DiMaio, D.J. Bullet embolism: Six cases and a review of the literature. J. Forensic Sci. 17(3):394–398, 1972.

6. Keeley, J.H. A bullet embolus to the left femoral artery following a thoracic gunshot wound. J. Thoracic Surg. 21:608–620, 1951.

7. Kirkpatrick, J.B., DiMaio, V.J.M. Civilian gunshot wounds of the brain. J. Neurosurg. 49: 185–198, 1978.

8. Jafari, N., Jafari, K., Sheridan, J.T. Gunshot wounds of the pregnant uterus. Int. J. Gynecol. Obstet. 13:95–96, 1975.

9. Adelson, L., Hirsch, C.S., Schroeder, O. Fetal homicide victims of maternally sustained violence. An occasional paper published by the law–medicine center. Cleveland, OH: Case Western Reserve University, 1977.

10. McNally, W.D. Lead poisoning caused by a bullet embedded for twenty-seven years. Industrial Med. 18:77–78, 1949.

11. DiMaio, V.J.M., DiMaio, S.M., Garriott, J.C., Simpson, P. A fatal case of lead poisoning due to a retained bullet. Am. J Forensic Med. Pathol. 4(2):165–169, 1983.

12. Machle, W. Lead absorption from bullets lodged in tissues: Report of two cases. JAMA 115:1536–1541, 1940.

13. Dillman, R.O., Crumb, C.K., Lidsky, M.J. Lead poisoning from a gunshot wound: Report of a case and review of the literature. Am. J. Med. 66:509–514, 1979.

14. *Evaluation of Wound Data and Munitions.* Effectiveness in Vietnam, Vol. 1. Prepared by Joint Technical Coordinating Group for Munitions Effectiveness. December 1970.

15. Maughon, D.S. An inquiry into the nature of the wounds resulting in killed in action in Vietnam. Mil. Med. 135:8–13, 1970.

16. Silliphant, W.M. Beyer, J.C. Wound ballistics. Mil. Med. 113: 238–246, 1954.

17. Hatcher, J.S. Powder Fires. *NRA Illustrated Reloading Handbook.* Washington, D.C.: The National Rifle Association of America.

18. Cooking-Off Cartridges. *NRA Illustrated Reloading Handbook.* Washington, D.C.: The National Rifle Association of America.

Weapons and Ammunitions: Miscellaneous

10

Air Weapons

Air-powered guns are used throughout the world for target shooting, sport, and firearms training. These devices range from toys exemplified by the Daisy BB gun to expensive, highly sophisticated custom air rifles.

The device that most people think of when discussing an air-powered gun is the Daisy BB gun. The Daisy is in fact a toy that fires an 0.175-in. steel BB down a smooth bore at a velocity of 275 to 350 ft/sec. A BB gun can cause serious injury only if the BB strikes the eyes. In such cases, perforation of the globe may occur. BBs fired from a Daisy BB gun should not ordinarily perforate the skin.

There are, however, other air and gas-powered guns with considerably greater velocity and striking energy that the Daisy BB gun. These devices are more properly classified as weapons as they can cause significant physical injury and occasionally death. Austrian armies used air rifles against the French during the Napoleonic wars of 1799 to 1809.[1] These weapons were rifles of 12.8-mm caliber with an effective range between 100 and 150 yd. Air rifles, air shotguns, and air pistols were used for hunting and target shooting during the late eighteenth and early nineteenth centuries. Air rifles are still used extensively for target and sport shooting as well as gun training.

An air rifle is a weapon that uses the expanding force of compressed air or gas to propel a projectile down a rifled barrel.[1] The term "air rifle" is commonly but incorrectly applied to toys such as the Daisy airgun. An airgun is distinguished from an air rifle in that the airgun has a smooth-bored barrel and may be either a weapon or a toy. Air pistols may be either weapons or toys and may have either a rifled or a smooth bore.

The same projectile used in airguns and air rifles are used in air pistols.

The standard calibers for air-and gas-powered guns in the United States are the 0.177 in, the Sheridan 0.20 in., and the .22 in. The basic form of airgun ammunition is the BB. These are steel balls having an average diameter of .175 in. and an average weight of 5.5 gr. The most common form of air rifle ammunition is the waisted Diabolo pellet, a soft lead missile shaped somewhat like an hourglass (Figure 10–1A). The front edge of the pellet acts as a guide riding on the rifling lands of the bore. The bullet is waisted at the center and has a hollow base. The rear edge is flared to engage the rifling and to seal the bore. Diabolo pellets weigh an average of 8.2 gr for caliber .177 and 15 gr for caliber .22. The exact weight depends on the brand of the pellet. Because of their extremely light weight, these pellets lose velocity rapidly, becoming harmless in less than 100 yd. Air rifle pellets can be fired in smooth-bore air guns without any difficulty. The firing of BB shot in a rifled bore, however, eventually results in damage to the rifling.

Pointed conical bullets are also made for use in air rifles. The Sheridan air rifle in .20 or 5-mm caliber fires pointed conical pellets averaging 15.3 gr weight, with a hollow base and a narrow exterior flange to engage the rifling in the bore (Figure 10–1B). The forward portion of the pellet is bore diameter and rides on top of the lands.

There are three basic power systems for air-powered guns.[1] In the pneumatic type, air is pumped into a storage chamber. When the trigger is pulled, the air is released, driving the pellet down the barrel. Varying the amount of air pumped into the reservoir by varying the number of pump strokes allows control of the velocity of the projectile. Increasing the number of pumps to a maximum can produce velocities as high as 770 ft/sec in a well-made airgun or air rifle.

The spring-air compression system uses a powerful spring that is compressed by manual action. On pulling the trigger, the spring is released, driving a piston forward in the cylinder and compressing the air ahead of it. The air is driven from the cylinder through a small port behind the projectile. The air drives the missile down the barrel. Velocities of 600 to 750 ft/sec may be reached by .177 air rifles. Weapons of .22 caliber generally have slightly lower muzzle velocities. In contradistinction to pneumatic guns, spring-air compression rifles have only one power setting. Thus, the muzzle velocity is constant.

Both air rifles and toy airguns operate on the spring-air compression principle. In toy guns, however, cheap construction and low-power springs prevent the high performance achieved in quality rifles. Thus, in a Daisy airgun, the muzzle velocity varies from 275 to 350 ft/sec, depending on the model of weapon.

The third gas-compression system uses carbon dioxide from a disposable cartridge as the propellant. Carbon dioxide guns may be toys or

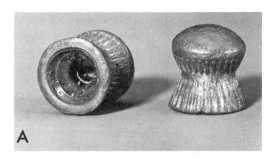

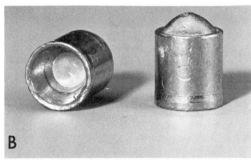

Figure 10-1 A. Diabolo air rifle pellets. **B.** Sheridan air rifle pellets.

weapons, rifles or pistols, smooth-bore or rifled. The rifles have approximately the same muzzle velocity as spring rifles of the same caliber.

Deaths from air powered guns are rare. The author has seen only two such cases.

Case 1. During a heated argument between two boys, ages 14 and 17 years, respectively, the 14-year-old grabbed an air rifle from a friend and at a range of a few feet shot the other boy in the right eye. The victim was transported to a hospital, where he was pronounced dead.

The autopsy revealed a pellet wound of entrance in the medial half of the right eyelid. The wound measured 6 mm in diameter, with a 4-mm central perforation. The pellet traveled through the soft tissue of the orbit superior to the globe, not injuring it. The missile entered the cranial cavity through the right orbital plate adjacent to the cribriform plate. The pellet moved across the ventral aspect of the right straight gyrus, across the midline, and penetrated the left straight gyrus. It traveled upward, posteriorly and laterally, along the anterior limb of the left internal capsule, and came to rest subcortically in the left posterior gyrus, 5 cm to the left of the midline. A deformed, 5-mm lead air rifle pellet with rifling marks on its surface was recovered.

The weapon was a 5-mm Sheridan air rifle with a rifled barrel. Ballistic examination of the pellet removed from the brain confirmed it to have been fired from this weapon.

Case 2. Two boys, age 7 and 8, respectively, were playing in the yard with an "empty" airgun of .177 caliber. A cousin who was baby-sitting had taken the BBs for the gun away from the boys. The 8-year-old boy pointed the gun at the 7-year-old and pulled the trigger. The weapon discharged and the 7-year-old collapsed to the ground. The boy was dead at the scene.

At autopsy, there was a single 5 × 4 mm oval pellet wound of entrance in the left forehead, just above the middle of the eyebrow. The pellet perforated the underlying frontal bone, which was 2 mm thick at this point. The pellet entered the left frontal pole and traveled medially, posteriorly and slightly upward in the left frontal lobe, exiting on the medial surface. It then entered the right cerebral hemisphere, continued left to right, posteriorly, and in a slightly upward path through the right cerebral hemisphere. The pellet was recovered from the right Sylvian fissure. The missile was a standard .175-inch, coppercoated steel BB.

Examination of the gun revealed it to be a smooth bore, pneumatic-type airgun of caliber .177. The weapon had a magazine that could hold 100 BBs. When testing the weapon, the author discovered that if a single BB is in the magazine, this BB is not delivered consistently to the firing chamber on working the action. Thus, with one BB in the magazine, it was possible to "fire" the weapon several times before the BB was actually chambered and propelled down the barrel. An individual unfamiliar with this eccentricity of the weapon might assume that the weapon was empty after discharging it a number of times and not firing a missile down the barrel. In fact, a missile might still be in the magazine and might be capable of being discharged on another firing.

The weapon used in the first case was a 5-mm Sheridan pneumatic air rifle. Average muzzle velocities for this particular rifle, as determined by tests conducted by the author for different numbers of pump stokes, is given in Table 10−1. The muzzle energy of these pellets is also listed. Fifty-eight foot-pounds of energy is considered the minimum energy neces-

Table 10−1 Performance Data of the 5 mm Sheridan Air Rifle in Case 1 (average weight of pellet, 15.3 gr)

Number of pump strokes	Average muzzle velocity (ft/sec)	Muzzle energy (ft-lbs)
1	0[a]	0[a]
2	303	3.1
3	388	5.1
4	435	6.4
5	470	7.5
6	502	8.6
7	531	9.6
8	553	10.4
9	554	10.4
10	566	10.9

[a] Pellets did not leave barrel.

sary to cause a casualty by the military.[2] The amount of energy possessed by these pellets is less than 20% of this value. Death occurred because of the site of entrance: the orbit. Test firings of the same weapon at point blank range on skull caps from cadavers resulted in the air rifle pellets being deflected off the bone without causing any damage. The only evidence that the pellets had struck the bone was 6 × 7 mm smears of lead at the point of impact.

The second death was caused by a smooth-bore pneumatic .177 air gun. By virtue of its high muzzle velocity, this gun is a weapon rather than a toy. Table 10−2 lists the average muzzle velocities for this particular air weapon as determined by the author for different numbers of pump strokes. Also listed is the muzzle kinetic energy at these velocities. All tests were conducted using BBs, as this was the form of missile that caused death.

The weapon used in Case 2 is relatively ineffective if one considers its muzzle energy. Death occurred in this case because the thin (2-mm) frontal bone of the child permitted the missile to enter the cranial cavity.

Recent reviews of the English language literature reveal only 14 reported deaths from air-weapons.[3,4] Most involved children. The portal of entry for the pellet was usually the head.

Zip Guns

The term "zip gun" as used in this book indicates either a crude homemade firearm or a conversion of a blank pistol, tear gas gun, or cap pistol to a firearm.[5] Zip guns had their peak of popularity in inner city areas during the juvenile gang wars of the 1950s. The quality of these weapons is extremely variable, with some so crude as to be a greater danger to the

Table 10−2 Performance Data of the .177 Air Gun in Case 2 (average weight of BB, 5.5 gr)

Number of pump strokes	Average muzzle velocity (ft/sec)	Muzzle energy (ft-lbs)
1	294	1.1
2	416	2.1
3	492	3.0
4	540	3.6
5	581	4.1
6	606	4.5
7	620	4.7
8	646	5.1
9	657	5.3
10	669	5.5

firer than to the intended victim. The simplest zip gun seen by the author was a metal tube in which a .22 Magnum cartridge was inserted. It was fired by striking the protruding base of the cartridge with a hammer. This weapon was used to commit suicide.

The zip guns of the 1950s in the New York area generally were constructed of a block of wood, a car antenna (the barrel), a nail (the firing pin), and rubber bands (to propel the pin). Most of these weapons were chambered for the .22 rimfire cartridge. The "chamber" was generally oversized, resulting in bulging and splitting, i.e., bursting, of the fired case. As the round was usually a low pressure .22 rimfire cartridge, injury to the firer was uncommon. The firing pin was often too long and too sharp, leading to piercing of the primer when the weapon was fired. The barrel was an unfired tube, often of greater diameter than the bullet. Thus, when the zip gun was fired, gas leaked out the ruptured case, the perforated primer, and around the bullet as it began to move down the barrel. This resulted in a very low muzzle velocity to the projectile. Because of the lack of rifling, the bullet was not stabilized and on leaving the barrel would almost immediately begin to tumble and lose velocity. The initial lower velocity combined with the inherent instability of the projectile made the zip gun an extremely short-range weapon.

Cap firing conversions are more sophisticated zip guns. Cap pistols are made of light metal castings held together by rivets. Conversion to a firearm was made by inserting a piece of car radio antenna or similar metal tubing in the barrel and providing a firing pin. The firing pin usually was made by inserting a nail or screw into the hammer or by filing the hammer to a point. If the hammer fall was too light, it was strengthened by wrapping rubber bands around the frame in back of the hammer.

Blank firing pistols were also converted to lethal weapons by reaming out the barrel and altering the cylinder chambers to accommodate live ammunition. Such a weapon at contact range may produce a characteristic soot pattern. Figure 4–5 shows such a case.

Zip guns were most commonly encountered in poverty-stricken areas where there was restrictive firearms legislation, as these weapons could be easily manufactured with inexpensive materials, few tools, and limited skills. In the 1950s in New York City, they were often manufactured in high school shop classes. The increased mobility and affluence of the population, combined with the availability of Saturday night specials, has resulted in the disappearance of the zip gun from the crime scene. The only exception appears to be conversion of tear gas pens to firearms. This still retains some popularity, perhaps because these devices do not immediately appear to be firearms and can be carried openly without eliciting suspicion.

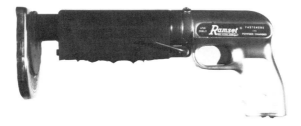

Figure 10-2 Stud gun.

Stud Guns

Stud guns are industrial tools that use special blank cartridges to fire metal nails or studs into wood, concrete, or steel (Figure 10-2). The blank cartridges range in caliber from .22 to .38. They are loaded with fast-burning propellants that develop pressures too high for a firearm to contain. Thus, they should never be used in firearms. The mouth of these blank cartridges is sealed with a cardboard disk that is color-coded to indicate the strength of the propellant.

Stud guns have a built-in safety mechanism that requires a guard at the end of the tool to be pressed firmly against a flat surface before the tool can be fired. Workers have been known to use stud guns for "plinking" at tin cans. They depress the safety guard with one hand and fire with the other.

Stud guns have caused a number of accidental deaths at industrial sites. The nails or studs have perforated walls, striking and killing other workers. There is a report of a suicide with a stud gun.[6] The deceased, a

Figure 10-3 Contact wound of forehead from stud gun.

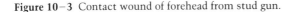

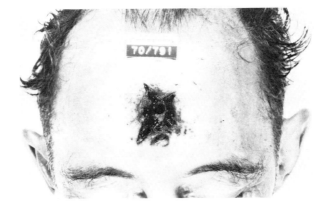

50-year-old white male, shot himself in the middle of the forehead with a gun that used a .22 industrial blank propellant cartridge. A stellate-shaped entrance wound was present (Figure 10–3). The nail perforated the head, lodging in a wall behind the deceased. Interestingly, there was no visible soot blackening in the skin, soft tissue, or skull of the deceased.

Sympathetic Discharge of Rimfire Firearms

In cheap .22 rimfire revolvers, "sympathetic" discharges may occur on firing. By "sympathetic" discharge is meant that on firing a revolver there is not only discharge of the cartridge stuck by the firing pin but also discharge of a cartridge in an adjacent chamber in the cylinder. Such multiple discharges were quite common in percussion revolvers before the introduction of metallic cartridges. In these cases, a spark from a discharging round would ignite the black powder in other cylinders.

   In the case of cheap .22 rimfire pistols, discharge of a cartridge by the firing pin may cause recoil of the cylinder with crushing of the rim of another cartridge between the cylinder and frame, producing a second discharge (Figure 10–4). As this chamber is not aligned with the barrel, no rifling will be imparted to the bullet. In addition, the inner surface of the bullet will be partially shaved away by the frame of the revolver as the bullet travels forward. In a case seen by the author a young male was shot during an argument on a bus. There was a penetrating gunshot wound of the right cheek with an apparent graze wound of the right shoulder. The bullet recovered from the head was a .22-caliber rimfire bullet with rifling marks on its sides. The bullet that caused the graze wound was found loose in the clothing. Examination of the bullet showed shortening of its length (from base to tip), absence of rifling, one side sheared off, and an expanded (flared-out) base having a granular pockmarked surface resulting from impaction of powder grains (Figure 10–5). This appearance of the bullet is classical for sympathetic discharge of a weapon. Examination of the weapon confirmed the tendency of the gun to sympathetic discharge. Sympathetic discharge can occur only in rimfire cartridges, not in centerfire cartridges, because of the centrally located primer in the latter type of cartridge.

Bullets without Rifling Marks

Occasionally a bullet recovered at autopsy will show no rifling on its surface. Lack of rifling indicates that the weapon was either a zip-gun, a smooth-bore pistol or rifle, or a revolver whose barrel has been removed. Zip guns have been previously discussed.

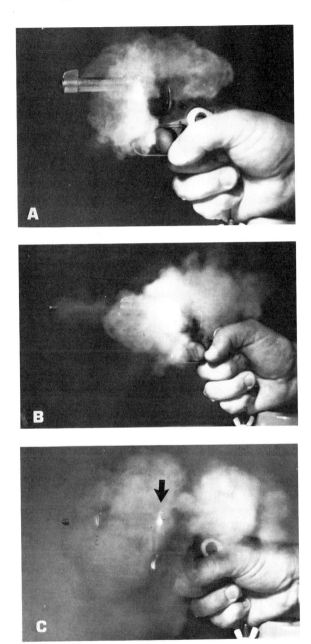

Figure 10–4 Sympathetic discharge of .22 rimfire revolver. **A.** The weapon has just been fired. **B.** A bullet has emerged from the barrel. **C.** A second bullet has come out the left side of the cylinder and is approximately 1 in. ahead of the barrel. The **arrow** indicates where the bullet emerged from.

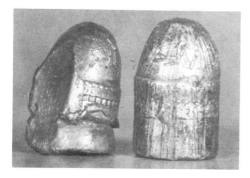

Figure 10−5 The bullet on the left is shortened, shows the absence of rifling, and has one side sheared off compared to the bullet on the right, which emerged from the barrel.

Smooth-bore weapons are almost all .22-caliber. A number of rifles in this caliber have been made for the exclusive use of .22 shot cartridges. Absence of rifling in a smooth-bore weapon does not indicate that a ballistic comparison cannot be made. The author has seen a case in which an individual was shot with a smooth-bore .22 rifle in which there was enough pitting of the bore to produce striations on the bullet, thus making possible a positive comparison with test bullets fired down the barrel.

An individual may remove the barrel of a revolver to prevent rifling marks being imparted to bullets fired from it. Such a weapon is effective only at short range, because the lack of gyroscopic spin on the bullet causes it to become unstable after leaving the revolver cylinder and to tumble end over end. Bullets fired from such barrelless revolvers often have a "flared" base. Flaring of the base of the bullet is most pronounced in ammunition that has a concave base (Figure 10−6A). Flaring out of the base can also be seen, though to a lesser degree, in bullets fired from short barrel revolvers and derringers (Figure 10−6B). In such cases, however, the bullets still have rifling marks on them.

Figure 10−6 A. .38 caliber lead hollow-base bullets fired from revolver without barrel. **B.** .38-caliber bullet fired from derringer. The base is flared.

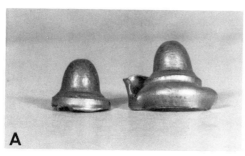
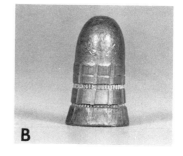

Elongated bullets

Rarely, one may recover abnormally long thin lead bullets up to 2 to 3 times normal length. They are produced by a constriction at the end of the barrel which swages or compresses the bullets as they pass through the area of constriction. The author has seen this phenomenon only in association with .22 rimfire ammunition. In all instances the end of the barrel had been compressed in a vise while part of the barrel had been sawed off.

Cast Bullets

On occasion individuals are shot with pistol ammunition reloaded with cast bullets. These bullets can usually be recognized on x-ray by the deep lubricating grooves. Upon recovery of the bullets, they usually have a dull silver-gray color. The lead is obviously harder than that used in commercial bullets, deep lubricating grooves are present, and the base of the bullet shows a circular marking caused by the sprue in the bullet casting mold (the sprue is the opening in the bullet mold through which the molten lead is poured) (Figure 10−7).

Sabot Ammunition

Sabot ammunition was introduced during World War II in an armor-piercing antitank role and is still used for this purpose. This ammunition, known as APDS (armor-piercing discarding sabot) projectiles, consists of a dense core of tungston carbide covered with a steel sheeth and a bore-and-sleeve assembly (the sabot). The sabot converts the core of the projectile to the same diameter as the gun barrel. The sabot is discarded as the projectile leaves the bore of the weapon.

The U.S. Army experimented with sabot small arms ammunition containing a flechette. It also experimented with a 5.56-mm cartridge, loaded with a 4.32-mm bullet in a 5.56-mm sabot. Smith & Wesson manufactured sabot shotgun slug ammunition that used a plastic sheath to bring the diameter of the projectile up to 12 gauge.

Figure 10−7 9-mm cast bullet showing circular mark on base resulting from sprue.

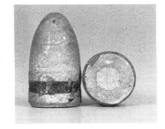

In late 1976, Remington introduced rifle ammunition loaded with a sabot round. This cartridge is sold under the trade name of Accelerator®. The round was originally introduced only in .30−06. Other calibers have appeared (.30-30 and .308) or are planned. In .30-06, a standard .30-06 cartridge case is loaded with a subcaliber .224 (5.56-mm) 55-gr, partial metal-jacketed soft-point bullet loaded in a plastic sabot weighing 5.7 gr and having four equally spaced slits down its side (Figure 10−8). The manufacturer claims a muzzle velocity of 4080 ft/sec for .30-06. This ammunition will not function in most semiautomatic rifles. A special fast-burning powder is used in this ammunition.

On firing, the rifling of the barrel engages the sabot, imparting a spin of over 200,000 rpm. On exiting, the centrifugal force and increased air resistance spread the "petals" of the sabot, causing it to drop away from the bullet (Figure 10−9). The manufacturer claims complete separation of the plastic sabot from the bullet within 14 in. of the muzzle.

Tests in which the .30-06 cartridge was fired in a Model 1903 Springfield rifle revealed muzzle velocities of 3861 to 3950 ft/sec. Test firings were carried out at 3, 5, and 10 ft. At 3 ft the sabot entered the bullet hole. At 5 ft, the sabot impacted 2 cm to the right of the bullet hole of entrance. At 10 ft it impacted 8.9 cm to the right in one test and 16.5 cm to the right in a second. In all tests the sabot impacted to the right of the bullet hole. This trait possibly has to do with the right-hand twist of the rifle. The sabot traveled approximately 50 ft.

Figure 10−8   A. .223 bullet and plastic sabot disassembled. **B.** Bullet in sabot inserted in .30-caliber cartridge case. (From DiMaio, V.J.M. Wounds caused by centerfire rifles. Clin. Lab. Med. 3:257−271, 1983. Published with permission.)

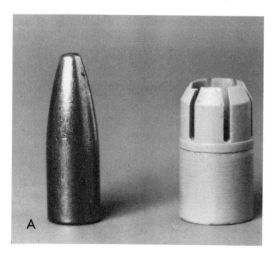
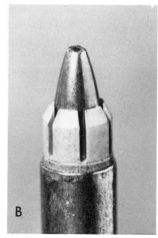

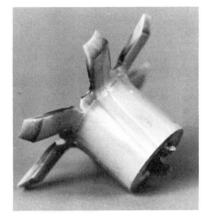

Figure 10-9 Sabot with open "petals" and rifling marks.

Animal tests by the Armed Forces Institute of Pathology using .30-06 Accelerator ammunition showed an entrance with surrounding prong marks at ranges of 3 and 6 ft.[7] At 9 ft there was an entrance with a separate abrasion from the Sabot.

The most significant facet of sabot ammunition to the forensic pathologist is that, if a bullet is recovered from an individual shot with this cartridge, the bullet will not show any rifling; rather, the rifling will be on the plastic sabot. A ballistic comparison can be made between the markings on the sabot and a test round fired through a weapon, though this is difficult.

Tandem Bullets

It is rare that, when a gun has been fired, the bullet lodges in the barrel rather than exits. This occurs because there is an insufficient quantity of propellant in the cartridge case or incomplete combustion of the propellant. The latter condition can occur if oil has leaked into the cartridge case, preventing some of the powder from being ignited or if there is a chemical breakdown of the powder because of age or prolonged exposure to high environmental temperature.

If a bullet has lodged in the barrel and the weapon is fired a second time, one of two things may happen. The increased pressure in the barrel can cause it to rupture, or both bullets can be propelled out of the barrel.[8] At close range, both these bullets can enter a body through the same entrance hole. Thus, although a single wound of entrance will be found, two bullets will be present in the body. Careful examination of the bullets, however, will generally reveal that a "piggyback" arrangement was present when they entered the body.

A very unusual variation to this was reported by Mollan and Beavis.[9]

They reported the case of an individual shot in the knee in which on surgical exploration there were found to be two bullets and a cartridge case in the knee joint. All three missiles entered through one entrance wound. The bullets were .32 ACP and .380 ACP caliber and the case was .32 ACP. It was hypothesized that a .32 ACP cartridge was inadvertently put in a .380 automatic. The cartridge slipped forward, lodging in the barrel. A .380 ACP cartridge then was chambered. On firing, the .380 bullet struck the .32 ACP primer, discharging the cartridge. The whole complex of two bullets and one case was swept down the barrel, emerged from the muzzle, and entered the victim.

New Forms of Handgun Ammunition

In order to increase the "stopping power" of handgun ammunition, a number of changes in bullet design have been introduced in the past 20 yr. The first change was introduction of lead and semijacketed hollow-point and semijacketed soft-point bullets. Up to the mid-1960s, handgun bullets were either full metal-jacketed or all lead. If one recovered a full metal-jacketed bullet, the individual had been shot with an automatic pistol; recovery of an all-lead bullet (excluding .22) indicated a revolver. The 1960s saw the introduction of semijacketed soft-point and hollow-point bullets for both automatic pistols and revolvers. In addition to the change in bullet design, the bullets tended to be lighter and were driven at higher velocities. Of the two designs, the hollow point has been the most successful. This bullet is designed to mushroom in the body, causing penetrating rather than perforating wounds, with loss of all its kinetic energy.

Hollow-Point Ammunition

The hollow-point design is successful in causing a greater loss of kinetic energy, not only because of its "mushrooming" but also because of the blunt tip necessitated by the hollow point, the lighter weight of the bullet (which causes it to be retarded more readily), the high velocity that results in its having greater kinetic energy at the time of impact. Heavier hollow-point bullets, e.g., the 158-gr semijacketed .38 Special bullet, usually do not mushroom in the body even though they lose greater kinetic energy by virtue of their increased velocity and blunter tip.

Soon after their introduction, hollow-point handgun bullets became the center of controversy. Many civil libertarian groups protested that they were "dum-dum bullets," violated the "Geneva Convention," and caused severe and more lethal wounds. All these statements are incorrect. The dum-dum bullet was in fact a .303 soft-point centerfire rifle bullet manufactured at the British Arsenal at Dum-Dum, India, in the late nineteenth century. This type of ammunition exists today as soft-point centerfire hunting rounds.

The Geneva Convention that outlawed dum-dum bullets was in fact the Hague Conferences of 1899 and 1907. The declarations issued at the conventions were applicable only to the use of expanding bullets in war. If one takes the declaration literally, even the all-lead bullets tradition-ally used by the police are outlawed.

In regard to charges that hollow-point ammunition is "more lethal" and produces "severer" wounds, in an unpublished study of over 75 fatalities from hollow-point ammunition by the author, he was unable to demonstrate any death that would not have occurred if the bullet had been an all-lead bullet. As to increased wounding, to this day the author cannot distinguish a wound by a hollow-point bullet from that by a solid lead bullet of the same caliber until recovery of the actual bullet.

As the years have passed, bullets of hollow-point design have begun to mushroom more consistently as a result of redesign of the jacket and cavity. Winchester has replaced the copper jacket in some of its hollow-point ammunition with a softer aluminum jacket that more readily permits mushrooming.

More radical bullet designs have appeared to increase the stopping power of handgun ammunition. Most have faded rapidly into oblivion. Three designs are worth mentioning, however: Glazer rounds, explod-ing ammunition, and multiple bullet loadings.

Glazer Round

The Glazer round is loaded with a bullet consisting of a copper jacket containing multiple small lead pellets rather than the traditional solid lead core (Figure 10–10). The tip of this jacket is closed with a Teflon plug. On firing, the "bullet" travels to the target just like a traditional bullet. On penetrating the target, the lead pellets force the plug and emerge from the jacket, radiating outward in a fanlike manner and producing a shotgun pellet wound effect.

Exploding Ammunition

The 1970s saw the introduction of exploding ammunition for hand-guns.[10] Exploding ammunition dates back to the early nineteenth cen-tury and was used in rifles in the American Civil War. Present-day exploding ammunition intended for handguns has been manufactured in at least three forms for centerfire cartridges and one form for rimfire cartridges. Ammunition initially manufactured for centerfire weapons used ordinary commercial semijacketed hollow-point ammunition in

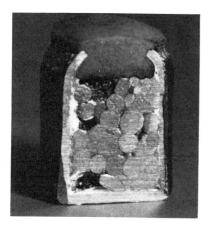

Figure 10–10 Cross-section of a Glazer round.

which the nose of the bullet had been drilled out. Into this cavity was placed black powder and a lead shot. The tip of the cavity was then sealed with a percussion cap. Because of federal regulations regarding black powder, a second form of exploding ammunition was introduced to replace the first. The black powder was replaced by Pyrodex, a smokeless powder substitute for black powder and a pistol primer replaced the percussion cap. The third form of exploding ammunition is essentially the same, but no lead shot is used.

Evaluation of a series of individuals shot with this ammunition reveals that both the entrance wound and the wound tracks are indistinguishable from wounds produced by similar nonexploding ammunition of the same caliber.[10] The fact that one is dealing with exploding ammunition may be determinable only on x-ray, as often the primer cap and primer anvil may be seen.

President Reagan was shot with .22 Long Rifle exploding ammunition. This ammunition is constructed from ordinary commercially available .22 Long Rifle hollow-point ammunition. A hole is drilled in the tip of the bullet, with insertion of an aluminum cylinder. The cylinder is filled with an explosive mixture and sealed at its open end. The cylinder is inserted with the sealed end toward the base of the bullet (Figure 10–11). Originally, RDX explosive was used in the cylinder, but this was replaced with lead azide.

Multiple Bullet Loadings

Pistol and rifle ammunition in which more than one bullet is loaded into a cartridge case has been produced by both civilians and the military. Figure 10–12 illustrates a .38 Special cartridge that has been loaded

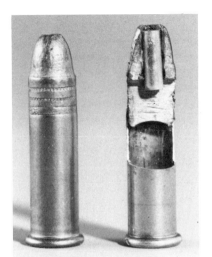

Figure 10-11 Longitudinal section through .22-caliber exploding round.

with four 50-gr lead bullets. This ammunition was produced commercially. If an individual was shot at close range with this ammunition, there would be a single wound of entrance and four bullets in the body.

The U.S. Army has used 7.62 × 51 mm Duplex round designated M-198.[11] This cartridge was loaded with two 80-gr bullets of conventional flat-based design. The base of the rear bullet, however, was canted at an angle of approximately 9 degrees (Figure 10-13). At 25 m, the velocity of the lead bullet was 2800 ft/sec (850 m/sec), with the second bullet having a velocity of 2600 ft/sec (790 m/sec). The canting of the second bullet's base was for the purpose of controlled dispersion. The M-198 cartridge had a green bullet tip for identification purposes.

Figure 10-12 .38 Special round loaded with four 50-gr bullets.

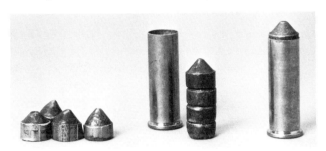

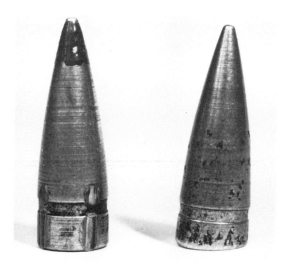

Figure 10-13 Military duplex round. Note the canted base of bullet on right.

KTW Ammunition

This is a form of armor-piercing ammunition intended for police use. It has been banned in some localities because of its potential to perforate bulletproof vests worn by police. The cartridge is loaded with a light green Teflon-coated tungsten alloy or steel bullet with a copper half jacket on its base. This jacket, rather than the bullet proper, is gripped by the lands and grooves. Thus, rifling marks will be present only on this jacket and not on the bullet. If it is fired through a body, there is the potential for this jacket to separate from the rest of the bullet and be deposited in the body.[6] The author is unaware of any homicide committed with this ammunition.

NYCLAD® Revolver Cartridges

This ammunition was originally manufactured by Smith & Wesson. When they stopped manufacturing ammunition, Federal purchased the exclusive manufacturing rights. These cartridges are loaded with nylon-coated lead bullets. This black coating significantly reduces the amount of lead particles in the air of firing ranges. Rifling is impressed on this coating and not on the lead. If these bullets go through thick bone, nylon jacketing may be shredded or stripped from the core, making bullet comparison more difficult or even impossible.

Handgun Shot Cartridges

Handgun cartridges loaded with lead shot are available in various calibers, e.g., .22 Long Rifle, .22 Magnum, and .38/357. This ammunition, often called "birdshot" or "snakeshot," is used to kill small game—usually varmints—at close range. The rimfire versions of these cartridges have been discussed in Chapter 6. The most popular centerfire shot cartridge is the .38/.357, which is primarily manufactured by Speer (Figure 10–14). This particular cartridge consists of a plastic cylinder, closed at one end and open at its base, and containing approximately 150 No. 9 shot. A cup-shaped plastic wad closes the open base. The plastic cylinder was an opaque yellow until 1975, when it was changed to a transparent blue. On firing, the plastic cylinder fragments; at close range, it can produce small cuts on the skin adjacent to the entrance (Figure 10–15). The fragments of plastic can be found embedded in the skin adjacent to the entrance and in the wound proper. The muzzle velocity of the pellets is approximately 1100 ft/sec.

Zumwalt et al carried out a series of experiments with this cartridge to determine its attributes.[12] The weapon used was a .38-caliber revolver with a 4¾-inch barrel. At a muzzle-to-target distance of 1 ft (30 cm), the pellets produced a circular defect 32 mm (1¼ in.) in diameter, having scalloped edges. At 15 in. (38.1 cm), the pellets produced a central defect 38 mm (1½ in.) in diameter surrounded by a cuff of satellite pellet holes. The whole wound complex measured 51 mm (2 in.) in diameter. At 2 ft the pellets produced individual defects.

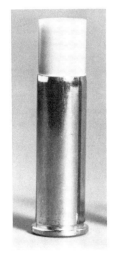

Figure 10–14 .38/.357 Speer shot cartridge.

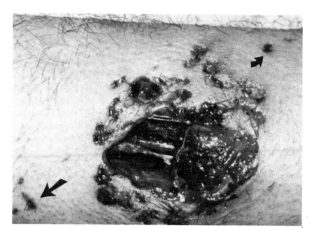

Figure 10–15 Gunshot wound of arm from .38 shot cartridge. **Arrows** indicate marks from plastic casing.

Plastic Training Ammunition

A number of European countries manufacture military blanks and training ammunition whose cartridge cases and "bullets" are made of plastic. The blanks can be identified easily by the "breaking points" or serrated lines at the nose of the cartridge (Figure 10–16). These blanks are typically color-coded as to caliber.

In the plastic military training ammunition, the plastic bullet is integral with the plastic case (Figure 10–17). On firing, the bullet breaks free of the case. The rifle projectiles have a muzzle velocity of 1280 m/sec with a maximum range of 300 m.

Although the aforementioned plastic blank and training ammunition are rarely encountered in the United States, there was a form of plastic ammunition manufactured domestically. This ammunition, manufactured by Speer, consisted of a reusable red plastic case and a black cylindrical plastic bullet that uses a large pistol primer as the sole propellant. Muzzle velocity of the plastic bullet is approximately 500 ft/sec. This ammunition is intended for indoor use at close range.

Test firings with the .38/.357 version of this plastic cartridge on cadavers at ranges varying from contact to 20 ft showed that the plastic bullets were incapable of penetrating the skin, let alone the body.[6] The wound inflicted, which was limited to the skin, consisted of a superficial, circular laceration with a diameter approximately the same as that of the bullet. Although incapable of penetrating the body, this ammunition probably can cause severe injury to the eye.

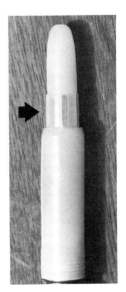

Figure 10−16 Plastic blank with breaking points on top.

Figure 10−17 Plastic training round. **Arrow** indicates where bullet breaks free from case.

Flechettes

During the Vietnam war, the United States military used ammunition loaded with steel flechettes. A flechette is a small arrow-shaped projectile with a metal tail fin. It is made in both 8- and 13-gr form. The 8-gr flechette, which is the more common type, measures 1 mm in diameter by approximately 2.7 cm in length. Flechettes were fired from 90-mm recoilless rifles, 90-mm guns, the 105-mm howitzer, and the 2.75-in.

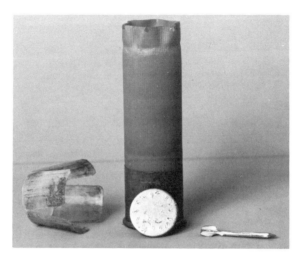

Figure 10–18 12-gauge flechette round.

air-to-ground rocket. The 90-mm gun fired from 4100 to 5600 8-gr steel flechettes per round. These flechettes were driven at sufficient velocity for them to perforate steel helmets. Entrance wounds in the skin may have an X shape due to the tail fin.

Twelve gauge shotgun shells loaded with flechettes were manufactured. These rounds have hulls of either Federal or Western manufacture. The Federal round contains 25 flechettes, the Western round 20. The tips of the flechettes are exposed in the Federal rounds but are concealed in the Western by a crimped mouth. The Winchester shells are packed in military cardboard boxes of 10 shells each. The boxes are labeled "18.5-mm Flechette Plastic Case" and state that the shells should be fired in cylinder bore guns only. The 20 flechettes in each round weigh 7.3 gr each and are packed in a plastic cup with granulated white polyethylene (Figure 10–18). A metal disk lies at the base of the cup. The shell is sealed with a pie crimp.

Blank Cartridge Injuries

A blank is a cartridge containing powder but no bullets or pellets. It is intended to produce noise. Blanks are generally loaded with ultrafast burning powder that detonates rather than burns. The case itself may appear like any other case in this caliber or may have a rosette crimped end. The wad can cause injury to a person immediately in front of the gun. If the wad is removed and a bullet is substituted, pressure generated by the ultrafast burning powder will explode the gun.

A number of European countries have manufactured blanks whose cartridge case and "bullet" are made of plastic. The blanks can be identified easily by the breaking points or serrated lines on the nose of the cartridge.

Injuries from blank cartridges are rare in civilian life. They are more commonly encountered in the military, where there is extensive use of blanks in training procedures.[13] Thus, it is not surprising that most civilian physicians are unaware of the severe wounds blanks can cause. Even fewer physicians realize that these cartridges can cause death. Gonzales et al. described the death of a 14-year-old boy shot with a pistol loaded with a .32 blank.[14] The weapon was held in contact with the skin of the left fifth intercostal space adjacent to the sternum. The blank perforated the chest wall and the right ventricle of the heart.

While serving in the military, the author had occasion to review a death from a rifle blank. A 22-year-old black male was dead on arrival at a dispensary in Germany with a blank gunshot wound of the chest. Inspection of the body revealed a circular wound of entry of the left chest in the second interspace, 5 cm from the midline. The wound measured 1.5 cm in diameter and was surrounded by a 7.5-cm area of powder blackening. Subsequent autopsy revealed a fracture of the third costal cartilage and adjacent lateral half of the sternum. There was an irregular laceration of the anterior wall of the right ventricle, the interventricular septum, and the aortic valve. A bilateral hemothorax and hemopericardium were present. The weapon involved in this incident was an M-1 rifle (caliber .30-06) loaded with a blank training round. The nature of the wound suggested either a loose or a near-contact wound.

In the civilian population, blank cartridge injuries and death are extremely rare. It is unlikely for a civilian forensic pathologist to see one in a lifetime. Injuries in the civilian population are most commonly due to blank pistol cartridges rather than rifle cartridges. Most modern blank pistol cartridges are loaded with smokeless powder. Black powder .22s and .32s are still available, however. The type of powder is important in that smokeless powder has a greater wounding capacity than black powder.

Shepard conducted a number of tests on dogs using .38 caliber blanks.[13] At a range of 1 in., he produced subdural and cortical hemorrhages in the head, penetration of the skin and pleura with laceration of the lung in the thorax, and penetration of the skin and peritoneum with lacerations of the liver in the abdomen. At 12 in., although there was injury to the skin, the pleura and peritoneum were intact. Tests with .22 Short blanks at a range of 1 in. failed to produce either skin penetration or internal injuries.

The author conducted a number of experiments on cadavers to determine the wounding capacity of blank pistol cartridges. The first test was conducted with .38 Special smokeless blanks. Test firings were conducted on human thighs, using a Smith & Wesson revolver with a 6-in. barrel and firing at ranges from 6 in. to contact. From a range of greater than 1 in. up to 6 in., focal accumulations of largely unburnt powder and shredded wad were deposited on the skin. The skin underlying the deposits was abraded. There was no powder blackening of the skin. At the 1-in. range, a faint gray halo of soot, 1 in. wide, enclosed a deposit of unburnt powder averaging ¾ in. in diameter. An underlying ¼ in. long × ½ in. deep laceration extended into the subcutaneous tissue.

Contact firings produced two different types of wounds in the thighs. In the first type, there was a ½ in.-diameter circular wound of entrance in the skin, surrounded by a faint gray sooty halo, ½ in. wide. A 3-in.-deep by 2-in.-wide cavity was present in the underlying muscle of the thigh. In the second type of wound, the entrance was irregular, measuring 1½ × ¾ in. with no detectable blackening of the wound edges. The underlying cavity in the muscle was 3½ in. deep × 2½ in. wide. Careful examination of these wound cavities revealed small shreds of wad and unburnt powder grains.

Contact test firings were conducted in the head. These tests produced stellate wounds of the scalp up to 1 × ¾ in. with no observable blackening. No fractures or injuries to the skull were produced. Deposited on the external table of the skull was a circular deposit of unburnt powder and shredded wad, averaging ½ in. in diameter.

Contact wounds of the thorax were of two types. When the muzzle of the gun was pressed firmly into the intercostal space, there was complete perforation of the anterior chest wall. Unburnt flakes of powder were deposited on the skin around the entrance wound. There was no powder blackening. When the muzzle overlaid a rib, there were no penetrating wounds, only a focal accumulation of powder with loss of the underlying superficial skin. When these areas were incised, however, there were comminuted fractures of the underlying rib with laceration of the parietal pleura. If the lungs had been expanded at the time of firing, lacerations of the parenchyma from the fractured rib wound have been produced.

Contact test firings of the anterior abdominal wall produced circular perforating wounds with laceration of the underlying small bowel. Again, there was no evidence of blackening of the skin.

Test firings with .22-caliber smokeless blanks were of a limited nature. The weapon used had a 4-in. barrel. All test firings were contact and occurred in the intercostal spaces of the chest. These blanks produced perforating wounds of the chest wall.

A final series of tests were conducted with the M-9 military .45-caliber blank. This blank is loaded with smokeless powder. Contact firings of the thigh produced irregular entrance wounds of the skin, slightly larger (1¼ × 1¼ in.) than those produced by the .38 Special.

Again, there was no observable blackening of the skin. The underlying cavity measured 4×3 in. Careful examination of this cavity revealed a small area of blackening on the surface of the femur and a few remnants of shredded wad. Both these elements were relatively inconspicuous.

Based on the experiments, we can conclude that contact wounds with pistol blanks are without doubt potentially lethal as such wounds can cause perforation of chest and abdomen. Close range noncontact wounds with pistol blanks probably would not produce significant internal injuries, though injury to the skin would be produced.

Electrical Guns

The 1970s saw the introduction of the first electrical gun—the Taser®. The Taser® is a device that uses electrical current to immobilizing victims without killing them.[15] Superficially resembling a flashlight, it has a gray plastic body in which there is a flashlight bulb, and lens. Two slots loaded with cassettes are beneath the bulb and lens. Each cassette contains two barbs connected to the case by approximately 18 ft of wire. The weapon is aimed and fired by pointing the flashlight and pressing the trigger. This procedure allows a spark to ignite the cassette, propelling the barbs out of the weapon at about a 15-degree angle of divergence. If the barbs lodge in either the skin or the clothing, continued pressure on the trigger delivers current and voltage down the wire. A current of 60 M amps is driven at 50,000 V. This current causes depolarization of the muscle cells, leading to widespread contraction and immobilization. Current can be delivered continuously for approximately 20 min. While the weapon is suppose to be nonlethal, death can result by continuous deliverance of the current with respiratory paralysis, from an arrythmia in an individual with heart disease, or from direct production of a ventricular arrythmia due to the current inadvertently affecting the polarization–depolarization cycle of the heart at a critical point. This last possibility is fairly unlikely.

Interchangeability of Ammunition in Weapons

Recovery of a bullet of a particular caliber from a body does not necessarily indicate that the weapon used to fire this missile was of the same caliber as the cartridge in which the bullet was loaded. Certain weapons will chamber and fire ammunition of a caliber different from that for which they are chambered. Some automatic pistols are capable of firing revolver ammunition, and some revolvers can fire automatic ammunition. The .32-caliber revolver is well known for its ability to chamber and fire the semirimmed .32 ACP automatic cartridge (Figure 10–19).

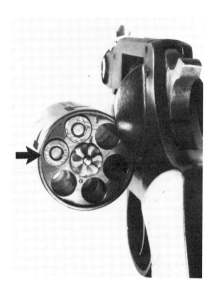

Figure 10–19 .32 revolver loaded with a .32 S&W Short revolver cartridge and a .32 ACP automatic pistol cartridge (**arrow**).

The .38-caliber Enfield revolver, chambered for the .38 Smith & Wesson cartridge, will accept and fire 9-mm Luger ammunition. Less well known is the fact that many .32 automatic pistols will chamber and fire the .32 Smith & Wesson Short revolver cartridge as well as feed the revolver ammunition from a clip and function the mechanism for at least three or four rounds without jamming. .32 cartridges have been fired in .38 revolvers by being wrapped in tape so that they completely occupy the larger chamber.

In theory, a .38 Special revolver should not be able to chamber and fire a .38 Smith & Wesson cartridge, as the latter cartridge case has a greater diameter than the former. However, a significant number of .38 Special revolvers have oversized chambers and will accept .38 Smith & Wesson cartridges.

During World War II, large numbers of revolvers were manufactured in the United States for Great Britain. These were chambered for the .38 Smith & Wesson cartridge. Since then, many of these revolvers have been brought back to the United States and rechambered for the .38 Special cartridge. These weapons will chamber and fire both cartridges.

All .357 Magnum revolvers will, of course, fire the .38 Special cartridge, as the Magnum cartridge is nothing but an elongated .38 Special. Some people believe that if one fires a .38 Special cartridge in a .357 Magnum revolver, the .38 Special travels at a greater velocity and has better ballistics; however, firing a .38 Special in a .357 Magnum does *not* improve the characteristics of this cartridge.

The Astra, Model 400, is chambered for the 9-mm Bayard cartridge, which is not available in the United States. This particular weapon will chamber and fire the .38 Super cartridge reliably and the 9-mm Luger cartridge unreliably as well as single-fire the .380 ACP cartridge. In the last case, the cartridge case usually bursts. The .32 ACP cartridge can be single-fed and fired in a .380 ACP automatic pistol. The case ruptures, however.

Mention should be made of *adapters* (Figure 10–20). These permit firing of a cartridge in a weapon not chambered for it by the use of a device that fits in the weapon's chamber and will accept a different caliber cartridge. Adapters permit the use of .22 rimfire ammunition in .22-caliber centerfire rifles as well as .32 ACP and .30 Carbine ammunition in high velocity .30-caliber centerfire rifles. At one time, one could buy adapters for shotguns so as to permit firing a handgun cartridge from a shotgun. An adapter is made that permits firing of a .410 shotgun cartridge in a 12-gauge shotgun.

Ruger manufactures a line of single-shot revolvers that have interchangeable cylinders. Thus, one weapon will fire .38 Special and .357 Magnum ammunition in one cylinder and 9-mm Luger in another interchangeable cylinder. Another weapon fires .45 ACP in one cylinder and .45 Colt in a second. A number of firearms companies manufacture .22 rimfire revolvers with two interchangeable cylinders—one for .22 Short, Long, and Long Rifle cartridges and the other for the .22 Magnum cartridge.

Pistol bullets can be loaded in rifle cartridges. Thus, in one case seen by the author an individual was fatally wounded with a 7.62-Luger bullet loaded in a .30 carbine cartridge. It is also possible to load .32 ACP bullets in any of the .30 centerfire cartridges. The .32 ACP cartridge in

Figure 10–20 Adapter for firing .22 Long Rifle ammunition in .223 rifle.

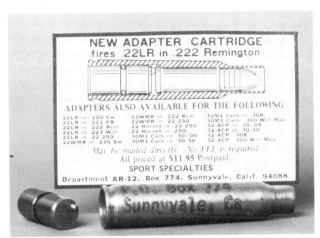

turn may be reloaded with a single 00 Buck pellet (0.33 in. diameter) rather than a bullet.

Rifles have been and still are being chambered for certain handgun cartridges. Rifles are currently available in calibers .38 Special, .357 Magnum, and .44 Magnum.

Specialized single-shot handguns chambered for rifle cartridges have been and still are manufactured. The Thompson-Contender, which features interchangeable barrels, can be obtained in calibers .223 Remington, .25-35 Winchester, .30-30 Winchester, for example.

Markings and Foreign Material on Bullets

If a bullet perforates an intermediate target before entering a body, it may carry foreign material from that target into the body. Thus, examination of a bullet recovered from a body after having passed through glass often reveals numerous fragments of glass embedded in the tip of the bullet.

A hollow point-bullet may carry fragments of the deceased's clothing in the hollow cavity into the body. In one case the author is aware of, an individual shot himself while lying next to his wife. The bullet passed through his body, entering his wife's, where it was subsequently recovered. Tissue of his blood type, which was different from that of his wife's, was recovered from the tip of the bullet.

In passing through a target prior to entering a body, a bullet may have the pattern of the target impressed on its tip. Thus, one occasionally recovers lead bullets with the weave pattern of the clothing on the tip. Bullets—lead or jacketed—can have the grid pattern of a wire screen impressed on the tip if they perforate a screen.

Sometimes in passing through a target the bullet may pick up material that is not immediately visible. Thus, a bullet suspected of having passed through a screen and recovered from a body had a slight area of discoloration of the tip. On examination by scanning electron microscopy with x-ray probe (SEM-EDX), the smear was revealed to be aluminum from the screen.

On exiting a body a bullet may carry away fragments of tissue, bone, or even clothing overlying the exit site. The case that comes to mind was a 17-year-old male shot three times by a police officer. All bullets exited. Two—one of which inflicted the fatal wound—passed through bone, with the third bullet passing through only muscle. A fourth bullet missed the deceased. Three bullets were recovered at the scene. In a civil case filed against the police, it was contended that one of the bullets recovered at the scene—let us call it A—inflicted the fatal wound. However, when the author examined the other two bullets, B and C, he found fragments of white glistening material embedded in the tips at the

Table 10–3 Effect of Temperature on Bullet Velocity (weapons used, M-16 rifles)

Temperature (F°)	Weapon 1 muzzle velocity (ft/sec)	Weapon 2 muzzle velocity (ft/sec)
−65	2983	3031
−30	3011	3078
0	3039	3144
70	3206	3253
125	3219	3281

point of junction of the lead core with the cupper jacket. Analysis by SEM-EDX and light microscopy revealed this material to be bone. Thus, bullet A was not the fatal bullet but the one that either missed the deceased or passed through muscle alone.

One other unusual mark on a bullet should be mentioned. The author has seen a case of a woman accidentally shot when the .25 automatic she was carrying fell to the ground and discharged. Etched on the jacket of the recovered full metal-jacketed bullet was the partial print of the woman. She apparently had handled the cartridge at one time, and the moisture and salt in her perspiration had corroded the jacket, with the resultant production of the partial print.

Effect of Environmental Temperature on Bullet Velocity

Environmental temperature can significantly effect the velocity of a bullet. In tests conducted by the military using M-16 rifles, two rifles having a rifling twist of 1:12 lost 167 ft/sec and 109 ft/sec, respectively, in muzzle velocity when the environmental temperature was decreased from 70°F to 0°F.[16] Table 10–3 shows the results of the experiment with the two rifles at different temperatures.

References

1. Smith, W.H.B *Gas, Air and Spring Guns of the World.* Harrisburg, PA: Military Service Publishing Company, 1957.
2. Beyer, J.C. (ed.). *Wound Ballistics.* Washington, D.C.: Office of the Surgeon General, Department of the Army, 1962.
3. DiMaio, V.J. Homicidal death by air rifle. J. Trauma 15:1034–1037, 1975.
4. Green, G.S., Good, R. Homicide by use of a pellet gun. Am. J. Forensic Med. Pathol. 3(4): 361–365, 1982.
5. Koffler, B.B. Zip guns and crude conversions—identifying characteristics and problems. J. Crim. Law, Criminol. Police Sci. 60(4): 520–531, 1969. Part II, 61: 115–125, 1970.
6. DiMaio, V.J.M., Spitz, W.U. Variations in wounding due to unusual firearms and recently available ammunition. J. Forensic Sci. 17:377–386, 1972.

7. Thompson, R.L., Gluba, M., Johnson, A.C. Forensic problems associated with the acceleration (sabot) cartridge. Paper presented at the American Academy of Forensic Sciences, 34th Annual Meeting, February 8–11, 1982, Orlando, FL.

8. Timperman, J., Cnops, L. Tandem bullet in the head in a case of suicide. Med. Sci. 15(4): 280–283, 1975.

9. Mollan, R.A.B., Beavis, V. A curious gunshot injury. Br. J. Accident Surg. 9(4): 327–328, 1978.

10. Tate, L.G., DiMaio, V.J.M., Davis, J.H. Rebirth of exploding ammunition—a report of six human fatalities. J. Forensic Sci. 26(4) 636–644, 1981.

11. Archer, D.H.R. (ed.). Jane's Infantry Weapons—1977. Jane's Yearbooks. London: Paulton House, 1977.

12. Zumwalt, R.E., Campbell, B., Balraj, E., Adelson, L., Fransioli, M. Wounding characteristics of "shotshell ammunitions: A report of three cases. J. Forensic Sci. 26(1): 198–205, 1981.

13. Shepard, G.H. Blank cartridge wounds. Clinical and experimental studies. J. Trauma 9(2): 157–166, 1969.

14. Gonzales, T.A., Vance, M., Helpern, M., Umberger, C.J. "Legal Medicine," in Pathology and Toxicology, 2nd ed. New York: Appleton-Century-Crofts, 1954.

15. Wright, R.K.: Injuries caused by electrical guns. News and Views in Forensic Pathology. 6:2–3, 1978.

16. Piddington, M.J.: Comparison of the exterior ballistics of the M-193 projectile when launched from 1:12 in. and 1:14 in. twist M16A1 rifles. Ballistic Research Lab. Report 1943, October 1968.

X-Rays

11

The use of X-ray is invaluable in the evaluation of gunshot wounds. As a general rule, x-rays should be taken in all gunshot wound cases, especially those in which there appears to be an exit wound.

X-rays are useful for a variety of reasons:

1. To see whether the bullet or any part of it is still in the body
2. To locate the bullet
3. To locate for retrieval small fragments deposited in the body by a bullet that has exited
4. To identify the type of ammunition or weapon used prior to autopsy or to make such an identification if it cannot be made at autopsy
5. To document the path of the bullet

Use of x-ray equipment to locate a bullet will save valuable time at autopsy whether one is dealing with a routine or a special situation. In instances of bullet emboli, x-rays are invaluable in locating the bullet. Hours of tedious dissection can be saved. X-rays are also helpful in instances where a bullet track abruptly ends in muscle and no missile is present at the end of the track. Theoretically, one should have a hemorrhagic track from the entrance to the site where the bullet finally lodges. However, in some instances—especially with small-caliber bullets such as the .22 rimfire—the last 3 to 4 in. of the track, if it is in skeletal muscle, may be free from hemorrhage and virtually unidentifiable because the bullet has slipped in between and along fascial planes. Such an occurrence is seen most commonly in the arm.

X-rays should be performed in all cases where a bullet exits, because an "exit wound" does not necessarily indicate that the bullet did indeed exit. Occasionally an exiting bullet will have enough energy to create a defect in the skin but will rebound back into the body. This may be due either to the elastic nature of the skin or to resistance from overlying clothing. The "exit" also can be due to a fragment of bone being propelled through the skin ahead of the missile, with the bullet itself remaining in the body.

A special situation can arise with partial metal-jacketed bullets. Here separation of the jacket and the core can occur as the missile moves through the body. The lead core may exit while the jacket remains (Figure 11–1). The core is of no use for purposes of bullet comparison. Only the jacket is useful as the rifling is present on the jacket. At autopsy, if one is unaware that the jacket is present in the body, it can readily be missed. This is especially true if the jacket lodges in the muscle adjacent to the exit. To compound the problem, the core may be recovered at the scene by the police and then be mistaken for the complete bullet. The medical examiner may be informed that the "bullet" was recovered. Facilitating the misidentification of a lead core as a bullet is the fact that the lead may have very faint "rifling" marks impressed on it through the jacket. These marks, however, are class characteristics, not individual characteristics; thus, ballistic comparison is not possible.

Figure 11–1 Copper jacket retained in jaw. Lead core exited.

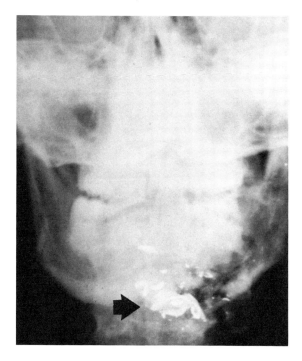

An artifact seen on the lead core of Remington .38 and .357 partial metal-jacketed bullets of older manufacture can be mistaken for rifling marks. As these bullets were assembled, they underwent a mechanical process by which the lead core was inserted into the jacket, resulting in six land- and groovelike marks being impressed on the core. These marks differ from lands and grooves in that they are vertical rather than canted as one would expect in rifling marks.

Although in most instances the lead core exits and the jacket remains, sometimes the opposite situation occurs, with the jacket exiting the body.

Sometimes, the jacket and core will separate in the body, but neither will exit. The forensic pathologist may recover the core with "rifling" on it and assume it to be the complete bullet. He or she will then inadvertently leave the jacket in the body or discard it with the viscera. Such mistakes can be prevented by an x-ray of the body, which will reveal whether separation of the core and jacket has occurred. With an x-ray, it is very easy to distinguish between the core and jacket by the different densities.

Introduction of Silvertip® pistol ammunition by Winchester has complicated the whole process of detecting bullet jackets on x-ray. In Silvertip® ammunition the jacket is in most calibers aluminum instead of copper alloy. If separation of the jacket and lead core occurs in the body, the jacket is not seen on routine x-rays because it is aluminum (Figure 11−2). The recovered bullet core will show the impressed marks of the lands and grooves. Ballistic comparison cannot be made, however, as these are only class characteristics.

In through-and-through gunshot wounds, small fragments of lead from the missile may be deposited along the wound track or in bone perforated by the bullet. These fragments, 1 to 2 mm or less in size, are

Figure 11−2 9-mm Silvertip® bullet.

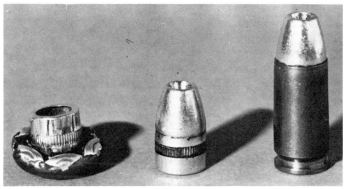

readily missed at autopsy, especially if only two or three are present. It may be important, however, to recover such fragments. They can be analyzed by EDX and spectrograph to determine the metals present. A comparison can then be made with a bullet recovered at the scene and suspected to be the lethal missile. The trace metal content of these fragments may also be compared with bullets in a box of cartridges that is thought to have been the source of the fatal cartridge. Although no one can testify absolutely that a fragment came from a specific bullet or lot of ammunition, one can testify that the fragment and the other ammunition are identical in all measurable properties. If these properties are very unusual and the combination of trace metals is very rare, one can say that the probability of the bullet coming from another source is extremely small.

X-rays may give a pathologist an idea of what type of weapon or ammunition he or she is dealing with before autopsy. Thus, the pathologist can recognize partial metal-jacketed pistol bullets or pistol shot cartridges. X-rays of close-range shotgun wounds may reveal a slug or buckshot rather than birdshot. Complete absence of a missile on total body x-ray (thus excluding embolization) and lack of an exit wound would suggest a blank cartridge.

In through and through gunshot wounds, the presence of small fragments of metal along the wound track virtually rules out full metal-jacketed ammunition, such as may be used in an automatic pistol. The reverse is not true, however; absence of lead on x-ray does not necessarily rule out a lead bullet.

One of the most characteristic x-rays and one that will indicate the type of weapon and ammunition used is that seen from high-velocity rifles firing hunting ammunition. In such a case, one will see a "lead snowstorm" (Figure 11–3). Such a picture rules out a full metal jacketed rifle ammunition or a gunshot slug. The autopsy examination of the organs themselves cannot rule out these other forms of ammunition, as both produce internal injuries similar to if not identical to those from high-velocity hunting ammunition.

Routine x-rays in deaths from gunshot wound may reveal old bullets, pellets or bullets fragments unrelated to the patient's death. There is usually no problem distinguishing them from new bullets when they are recovered, as the old bullets are encapsulated in fibrous scar tissue. These bullets usually have a black color as a result of oxidation. Black coloration can occur in a new bullet, however, if the bullet is exposed to the contents of the gastrointestinal tract. One case that initially puzzled the author was an individual shot in the left upper arm with a single 00 buckshot pellet. The pellet passed through the soft tissue of the upper arm, entering the left chest cavity between the fifth and sixth ribs. The pellet perforated the left lung, coming to rest in the musculature of the

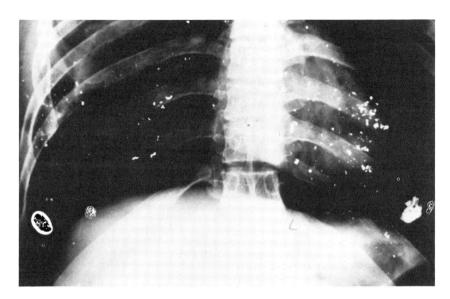

Figure 11−3 "Lead snowstorm."

back adjacent to the spinal column. A routine chest x-ray, however, revealed two "pellets," the second of which was embedded in the fifth rib, adjacent to the wound tract (Figure 11−4A). On recovery of the "pellet," it was found to be a deformed .22 Long Rifle bullet. Reexamination of the x-ray and rib showed a bony callus, indicating that the bullet had been lodged in the bone for a considerable amount of time (Figure 11−4B). In fact, the deceased had been shot almost exactly 1 yr earlier by the same perpetrator.

In gunshot wounds of the skull, a large fragment of lead may be deposited between the scalp and the outer table of the skull at the entrance site. This piece of lead is sheared off the bullet as it enters. With lead .32 revolver bullets and less commonly with .38 bullets, this fragment usually has a C or comma-shaped configuration (Figure 11−5).

X-rays may also show evidence of internal ricochet. This is manifested by a trail of small lead fragments which doubles back on itself.

Less information can be learned by x-ray in the case of shotgun wounds. Fiber shotgun wads may on rare occasions be seen on x-ray. These fiber wads appear as faint opaque circles, resulting from lead deposits on the edge of the wad picked up from the barrel as the wad moved down it (Figure 11−6).

In shotgun wounds in charred bodies, the range at which the individual was shot is often an important question. Determination of range cannot be made from the spread of the pellets on x-rays, however. A contact wound of the chest can produce an x-ray picture identical to that

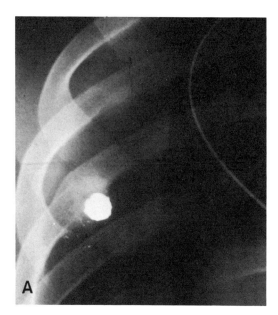
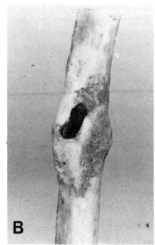

Figure 11-4 A. Old .22-caliber bullet embedded in rib. Note callus formation on x-ray. **B.** Rib with callous. The defect was from where the bullet was recovered.

in an individual shot at 10 ft. This is due to the "billiard ball" effect.[1] Pellets entering the body in a mass strike one another, dispersing at random angles throughout the tissue.

In "explosive" contact shotgun wounds of head with birdshot, virtually all pellets may exit. This situation has caused confusion when no x-rays were taken of the head and the pathologist was unable to recover any pellets at autopsy. The pathologist then doubted the hypothesis that the individual had died of a shotgun wound. An x-ray in such cases will reveal at least a few pellets.

Winchester recently introduced a .25-caliber cartridge loaded with a 42.6-gr lead bullet having a hollow-point filled with a No. 4 steel birdshot pellet.[2] On striking bone, the lead bullet usually is deformed and is easily mistaken for a .22 Long Rifle bullet. The steel ball usually pops out and can be seen next to the bullet thus presenting a very characteristic x-ray picture.

X-rays have some limitations. The exact caliber of a bullet cannot be determined with certainty by use of an x-ray. This is due to magnification of the bullet image depending on its distance from the source of x-ray. Bullets close to the origin of x-rays will appear larger and have fuzzier margins than those close to the film. Approximate caliber estimations can, of course, be made, and certain calibers can be ruled out.

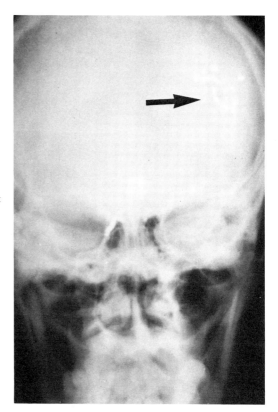

Figure 11-5 C-shaped fragment of lead under the scalp at entrance site.

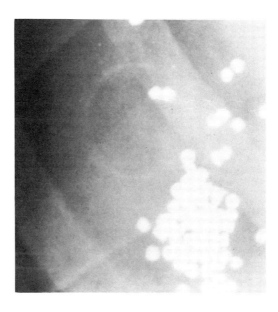

Figure 11-6 Shotgun wad outlined by thin coat of lead.

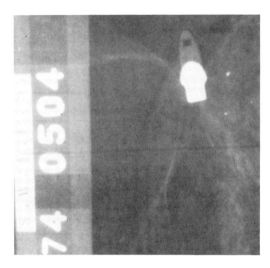

Figure 11–7 Zipper

X-rays in gunshot wound cases may show artifacts that can be mis-construed as bullets. The "stem" of a zipper often has the appearance of a slightly mushroomed bullet (Figure 11–7). The dislodged crown from a tooth may appear as a flattened bullet (Figure 11–8).

X-rays should always be taken while the deceased is fully clothed. This practice will reveal bullets that exited the body and are retained in

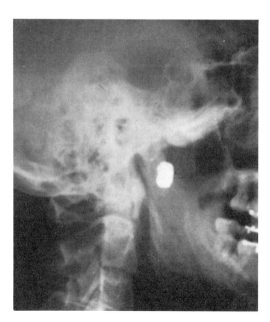

Figure 11–8 Aspirated gold cap of tooth.

the clothing. In a case seen by the author, the bullet exited the right chest, impacting the inner surface of the front of a suit jacket the deceased was wearing, and then, having lost all its velocity, fell into the inside coat pocket. There was a hole in the bottom of this pocket, however, and the bullet fell through into the lining.

References

1. Breitenecker, R. Shotgun wound patterns. Am. J. Clin. Pathol. 52:269–285, 1969.
2. Rao V.J., May C.L., DiMaio V.J.M. The behavior of the expanding point .25 ACP ammunition in the human body. Am. J. Forensic Med. Pathol. 5(1):37–39, 1984.

Detection of Gunshot Residues

12

The ability to determine whether an individual has fired a firearm is of great significance in the investigation of both homicides and suicides. Thus, over the years a number of tests have been developed in an attempt to fill this need. The first such test was the "paraffin test" also known as the "Dermal Nitrate" or "diphenylamine test."[1] It was introduced in the United States in 1933 by Teodoro Gonzalez of the criminal identification laboratory, Mexico City police headquarters. In this test, the hands were coated with a layer of paraffin. After cooling, the casts were removed and treated with an acid solution of diphenylamine, a reagent used to detect nitrates and nitrites that originate from gunpowder and may be deposited on the skin after firing a weapon. A positive test was indicated by the presence of blue flecks in the paraffin. Although this test often but not invariably gave positive results on the hands of individuals who fired weapons, it also gave positive results on the hands of individuals who had not fired weapons because of the widespread distribution of nitrates and nitrites in our environment. The paraffin test is in fact nonspecific and is of no use scientifically.

In 1959, Harrison and Gilroy introduced a qualitative colormetric chemical test to detect the presence of barium, antimony, and lead on the hands of individuals who fired firearms.[2] These metals, which originate from the primer of a cartridge on discharge of a weapon, are deposited on the back of the firing hand as discrete particulate matter (Figure 12-1). In revolvers these metallic particles come primarily from the cylinder-barrel gap, and in automatic pistols from the ejection port. The technique developed by Harrison and Gilroy was intended as a relatively simple inexpensive test for detection of these residues. In the test a square of white cotton cloth was moistened with hydrochloric

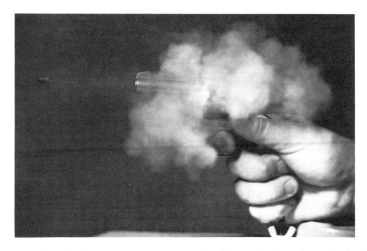

Figure 12−1 Gas cloud containing primer residue flowing backward onto back of firing hand.

acid and then used to swab the hand. The swab was treated with triphenylmethylarsonium iodide for the detection of antimony and sodium rhodizonate for the detection of barium and lead. The limited sensitivity of this test prevented its widespread adoption.

At present, there are three generally accepted methods of analyzing for gunshot residues: neutron activation analysis, FAAS, and analysis using the scanning electron microscope.[3−6] All three tests are based on the detection of barium, antimony, and lead originating in primers and deposited on the back of the hand firing the weapon. Although all three compounds are found in the primers of virtually all centerfire cartridges, this is not necessarily the case in rimfire primers. Thus, Remington rimfire cartridges contain only lead in their primers; CCI and Winchester lead and barium; and Federal, lead, barium, and antimony. Geco (Dynamit Nobel) produces a 9-mm Parabellum cartridge developed for use in indoor firing ranges, the Geco Sintor. This cartridge has a primer that does not contain either lead or barium. The bullet is full metal-jacketed with a sealed base, thus preventing vaporization of lead from the lead core.

The metallic components of the primer are removed from the hands employing cottom tip swabs moistened with either hydrochloric or nitric acid. An adhesive material may be used to remove these metallic elements in the case of the scanning electron microscope. The cotton-tipped swabs should have a plastic swab as wool shafts may contain barium.

Neutron activation techniques detect only antimony and barium and not lead. Therefore, neutron activation is usually employed in conjunction with FAAS to detect the lead. Neutron activation analysis would be useless in the case of an individual firing .22 Remington ammunition the primer of which contains only lead. Because of the limitation of analysis and especially because of the need for access to a nuclear reactor, the use of neutron activation is not suitable for most crime labs.

Use of FAAS techniques is increasing in crime laboratories in this country. The method combines relatively cheap cost, ease of analysis, and adequate sensitivity. FAAS will detect antimony, barium, and lead from the primer as well as copper vaporized from either the cartridge case or the bullet jacketing.

In this method of analysis, four cotton swabs moistened with 5% nitric acid, are used to swab the palms and backs of the hands (Figure 12–2). (See Appendix C for more detailed instructions.) A fifth swab is moistened with the acid and acts as a control. Based on the amount of antimony, barium, and lead detected on the four surfaces of the hands, one then concludes that the quantity and distribution of these metals is or is not consistent with gunshot residue and thus with firing a weapon. Detection of primer residue on the palms of the hands instead of on the back of the suspected firing hand is suggestive of a defensive gesture rather than of discharge of a weapon. However, it does not rule out that the suspect handled a gun coated with firearms residue from its having been fired in the past. In suicides with handguns, primer residue on the palm or back of the nonfiring hand may be due to cradling the gun at either the muzzle or, in the case of the revolver, at the cylinder at the time of firing. With rifles and shotguns, residue is virtually never detected on the firing hand. Residue is often detected, however, on the nonfiring hand that has been used to steady the muzzle against the body. The residue is detected more commonly on the back rather than on the palm of the hand.

In the author's laboratory, levels of antimony, barium, and lead are considered significant only when they are at or above 35 ng for antimony, 150 ng for barium, and 800 ng for lead. For a hand washing to be positive for a centerfire weapon, all three elements must be present and at least the lead must be elevated. Marked elevation of barium alone may be due to the presence of soil rich in barium on the hand.

For a positive hand washing in an individual who fired a handgun, antimony, barium, and lead must be present and at least lead elevated on the back of the firing hand. If the individual instead of firing the weapon put the hand up, palm out, in a defensive gesture toward the weapon at the time of discharge, elevated levels of primer residue will be present on the palm and sometimes on the back of the hand. In such cases, primer residue on the back of the hand occurs when the whole hand is engulfed in a cloud of vaporized primer residue. The levels of metal on the back of the hand will be lower than those on the palm.

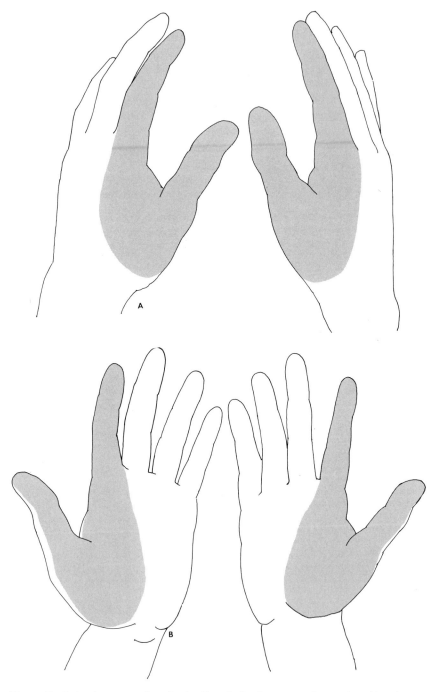

Figure 12-2 A. Area to swab on back of hands. **B.** Area to swab on palm of hands.

The following are actual cases worked on by the author's laboratory. They represent a fair cross section of the type of cases that are encountered.

Case 1. Handwashings in this case showed no evidence of gunshot residue. This is as it should be, as the individual was a young male dying during an episode of diabetic ketoacidosis.

Hand area	Antimony(ng)	Barium (ng)	Lead (ng)
Right back	2.0	86	8
Left back	1.2	4	25
Right palm	0.4	0	16
Left palm	1.6	33	50

Case 2. This case was also negative for firearm residues. The individual died of stab wounds. The markedly elevated levels of barium present on the back and palms of the hands were due to contamination, probably by soil, which is very rich in barium in some areas of the country. The levels of lead and antimony were in background concentrations not consistent with the gunshot residue.

Hand area	Antimony (ng)	Barium (ng)	Lead (ng)
Right back	2.4	390	58
Left back	0.8	1387	159
Right palm	0	826	168
Left palm	0	1409	478

Case 3. This test was interpreted as positive for gunshot residue on the back of the deceased's right hand. The deceased shot himself in the head with a .38 Special revolver, using the right hand.

Hand area	Antimony (ng)	Barium (ng)	Lead (ng)
Right back	78	212	1537
Left back	12	75	345
Right palm	5	90	210
Left palm	21	79	320

Case 4. This was a case of suicide with a .357 Magnum revolver. The deceased shot himself in the right temple. Hand washings were negative for gunshot residue. This has in fact been our experience with the .357 revolver.

Hand area	Antimony (ng)	Barium (ng)	Lead (ng)
Right back	3	12	110
Left back	7	71	73
Right palm	21	23	210
Left palm	5	5	80

Case 5. This individual shot himself in the mouth with a .38 Special revolver. At the scene, the deceased's left hand was around the barrel. Hand washings were positive for primer residue on the back of the right hand and thus were consistent with the individual having used this hand to fire the weapon. Markedly elevated levels of primer residue were also present on the back and palm of the left hand. This hand was used to hold the muzzle in the mouth.

Hand areas	Antimony (ng)	Barium (ng)	Lead (ng)
Right back	81	232	975
Left back	250	635	67,292
Right palm	5	21	190
Left palm	193	804	45,360

Case 6. This is a case of an individual who shot himself in the right temple with a .410 shotgun. The deceased used his left hand to hold the muzzle of the weapon against his head. The right hand, which was used to fire the weapon, not unexpectedly with this type of weapon, is negative. The back of the left hand shows elevated levels of primer residue.

Hand area	Antimony (ng)	Barium (ng)	Lead (ng)
Right back	1.6	202	210
Left back	98.8	233	3738
Right palm	6.8	112	840
Left palm	12.0	152	344

Case 7. This is an example of an individual trying to ward off his attacker. There were significant levels of antimony, barium, and lead on the palm of the right hand.

Hand areas	Antimony (ng)	Barium (ng)	Lead (ng)
Right back	10.4	102	344
Left back	22.8	92	705
Right palm	54.8	301	1999
Left palm	12.4	58	722

Case 8. This is a variation on Case 7. Significantly elevated levels of primer residue were present on the palms of the hands. The backs of the hands show-elevated levels of lead and, in the case of the right hand, antimony. In this case the hands were probably outstretched toward the weapon and were enveloped by a cloud of residue, thus accounting for the elevated levels of lead on the back of the hands.

Hand area	Antimony (ng)	Barium (ng)	Lead (ng)
Right back	81.2	30	3166
Left back	18.2	5	1646
Right palm	262.8	416	9273
Left palm	148	349	2931

Case 9. This is an example of a lead cloud from a high-velocity missile that has passed through an object with resultant pulverization of the lead core, production of a lead cloud, and coating of the individual who was in the vicinity of the lead cloud. The deceased was shot through a car door with a high-velocity hunting bullet. Lead levels are markedly elevated. Barium levels are negative, with antimony levels elevated. The elevated antimony may have resulted because antimony is used to harden lead.

Hand area	Antimony (ng)	Barium (ng)	Lead (ng)
Right back	149.2	92	10054
Left back	57.2	0	2646
Right palm	52.4	0	3561
Left palm	75.2	52	4880

The difficulty with both these methods of analysis, i.e., FAAS and neutron activation analyses, is that one can never be assured absolutely that one is dealing with firearms' residues. Both methods of analysis are bulk, elemental analytic methods involving measurement of the total quantity of metallic residues removed. One cannot distinguish the source of the metals. In addition, both techniques have a high percentage of false negatives. If one asks 100 individuals to fire 100 different centerfire handguns, in only 40 to 50% of the individuals will the hand-washings will be positive. This percentage is even lower for rimfire weapons. In living individuals, as the time interval between firing and the taking of samples increases, there is a rapid loss of the residue from the hands. This can be produced not only by washing the hands but just by rubbing them against materials.

The third method of analysis employs a scanning electron microscope (SEM) with an x-ray analysis capability.[5,6] Gunshot residue particles are removed from the hand using an adhesive lift. The material removed is scanned with the SEM for gunshot residue particles. These consist of discrete micrometer-sized particles, often of a characteristic shape. The x-ray analysis capability is used to identify the chemical element in each of the particles.

The appearance of the particles is fairly specific, making them easily identifiable from other debris on the hands. X-ray analysis then identifies them as gunshot residue. Some particles can be absolutely identified as gunshot residue, from the x-ray analysis of the particles; others, when the x-ray analysis is combined with the physical appearance of the particles. Some particles, however, cannot be identified with certainty. They may be typical but not unique. Based on testing, it has been found that in individuals who have fired handguns, 90% of the time residue will be detectable; for rifles and shotguns, the figure is 50%.[5] In long arms, rifles accounted for the majority of negative results.

Because particles can be identified absolutely as gunshot residue, analysis by SEM is not as time-dependent as flameless atomic absorption and neutron activation analysis. These latter tests depend on quantitation and distribution of metal levels to make determination of firearms residues. SEM involves qualitative analysis. Thus, large quantities of metallic residues are not necessary for a positive determination. Analysis on the hands of firers by SEM has been positive as long as 12 hr after they fired the weapon.

Some police agencies in an attempt to link a gun with an individual use a trace metal detection technique (TMDT). These tests depend on the detection of trace metals left on the hand as a result of handling a gun. The metal forms characteristic color complexes with a reagent sprayed on the hand. Different metals produce different colors. The pattern and color produced depend on the shape and metal content of the weapon. Whether the pattern and color are present depends on how long the weapon was held and whether the individual was sweating. As sweating increases, the pattern and color increase in prominence. The initial TMDT involved the use of 0.2% 8-hydroxyquinoline solution with viewing the hand for color patterns under ultraviolet light. Positive results were obtained for 36 to 48 hr after handling metal. A new reagent— 2-nitroso-1-naphthol—does not require viewing under ultraviolet light.[7] Metallic patterns using this reagent last only 4 hr or less. The problems inherent with TMDT are its lack of specificity and in the case of the original reagent the long time period during which trace metal can be detected. Only rarely in actual practice is the characteristic pattern of a weapon produced on the hand, e.g., emblems or designs. More often, one has only a poorly defined area of color change. The trace metal that produced this color change could have come not only from a gun but an iron railing, a tire tool, and so forth. If the original reagent is used, the individual could have handled a metal object other than the weapon as long as 1 to 2 days previously. Thus, in actual practice this test is more subjective than objective.

Gunshot Wounds Through Clothing

In gunshot wound cases, examination of the clothing is often as important as examination of the body. The interposing of clothing between the muzzle of the gun and the skin can alter the appearance of close-range gunshot wounds on the body. Clothing can prevent soot or powder, either completely or in part, from reaching the skin as well as produce a redistribution of this powder and soot. In hard contact wounds of the body, where soot and powder ordinary would be driven completely into the wound track, clothing can cause dispersion of soot and powder among the layers of clothing or onto the skin surrounding the entrance, thus altering the appearance of the wound from that of a hard contact wound to that of a loose contact wound (Figure 12–3). With near-contact wounds the clothing may absorb soot that would ordinarily be deposited on the skin as well as preventing or decreasing searing of the skin by hot gasses.

Complete absorption of the soot and powder by clothing can occur in what ordinarily would be called an intermediate range wound. The resultant absence of powder tattooing on the skin results in an intermediate-range wound having the appearance of a distant wound.

Whether powder perforates clothing to mark the skin depends on the nature of the material, the number of layers of cloth, and the physical form of the powder. Ball powder can readily perforate one and even two layers of cloth to produce tattooing of the underlying skin. Under unusual circumstances it will perforate three layers. It cannot penetrate

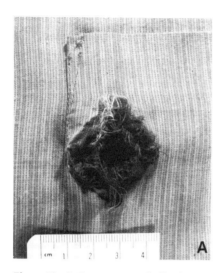 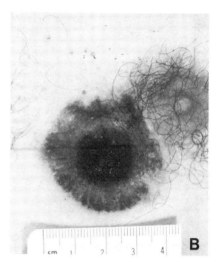

Figure 12−3 Contact wound of body through two layers of cloth. Note the appearance of the wound in chest, which simulates a loose contact.

four layers, however. Flake powder, on the other hand, usually does not perforate even one layer of cloth. This is not absolute, and the author has seen a number of cases involving weapons ranging in caliber from .22 to .38 where flake powder perforated a layer of cloth to produce tattooing of the underlying skin. In these instances, the flake powder usually consisted of small thick disks.

In intermediate-range wounds involving clothed areas, apparent absence of powder on the outside of the clothing can be associated with dense powder tattooing of the underlying skin (Figure 12−4). The type of powder in such cases is spherical ball powder. The ball powder, because of its shape, readily perforates the weave of the cloth, producing powder tattooing of the skin. Although powder may seem to be absent on the outside of the shirt with the naked eye, use of the dissecting microscope will reveal occasional balls of powder caught in the weave of the material. If for some reason the clothing has been separated from the body and the clothing is examined by one source and the body by another, different conclusions may be reached as to the range from which the individual was shot. This is especially true if only a cursory examination of the shirt is made and no dissecting microscope is employed. Thus, the individual who examined the clothing may say that one is dealing with a distant wound, whereas the individual who examined the body may say that one is dealing with an intermediate-range wound.

In view of these facts, one can see why examination of the clothing is part of the autopsy. This examination should be conducted not only

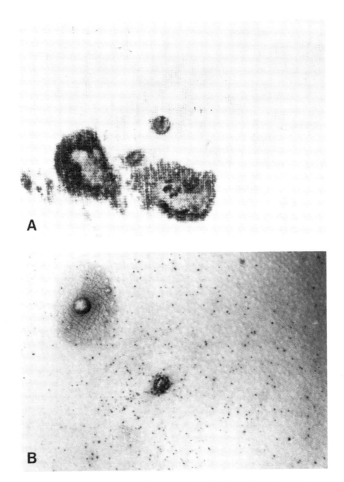

Figure 12–4 Intermediate-range gunshot wound of chest form .22 Magnum revolver. Note the absence of powder on the outside of the clothing with powder tattooing of the underlying skin.

with the naked eye but with the dissecting microscope. The presence of one or two grains of powder on clothing does not necessarily mean that the deceased was shot at close range. Powder grains can travel as far as 20 ft from muzzle to clothing. This topic was discussed in detail in Chapter 5.

In addition to aiding in range determination, clothing may give an idea as to what the position of the deceased was at the time he or she was shot by correlating the holes in the clothing with the entrance and exit wounds in the body.

Just as the bullet and powder gases produce alterations on the body, so they will alter clothing. In contact wounds through clothing, depending on the type of fabric and the amount of gas produced, tearing of the material can occur. This is true whether the garment is hanging loose or pulled tightly against the skin. Contact wounds in cotton cloth and cloth composed of a cotton mixture with medium and large-caliber weapons (.38 Special and above), usually result in tears with a cruciform appearance (Figure 12−5). Contact wounds in 100% synthetic material (nylon, triacetate, and so forth) result not in tears but in "burn holes." The heat of the gases causes the material to melt producing large circular holes, usually with scalloped margins (Figure 12−5).

A contact shot in cotton material using a 4-in. barrel .38 Special revolver firing a semijacketed hollow point bullet resulted in a 9 × 8 cm (maximum dimensions) cruciform tear in the material. Similar shots with 100% synthetic materials resulted in roughly circular holes 4 to 5.5 cm in diameter whose edges were scalloped.

With large- and medium-caliber weapons, tears in material may occur not only at contact range but at near-contact range. Thus, tests with the aforementioned weapon using 158-gr roundnose ammunition resulted in tears of the cloth occurring with shots up to 0.5 cm from muzzle to target.

Ammunition that produces a small amount of gas, such as the .22 rimfire cartridge, tends to produce either a single tear or an incomplete cruciform tear in cotton material. In synthetics .22 Long Rifle ammunition produces burn holes averaging 1 cm in diameter.

Some of the older forensic literature mentions that clothing can be ignited by close-range firing. This refers to black powder cartridges, however. Black powder emerging from the barrel is often still burning. It

Figure 12−5 (a) Contact wound through 100% synthetic. (b) Stellate-shaped defect through cotton material.

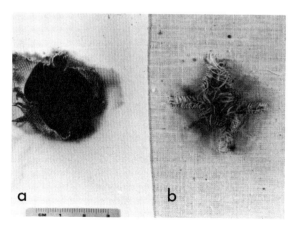

can land on clothing, continue to burn, and ignite the clothing. This does not occur with smokeless powder.

Occasionally, a pillow is used to muffle a gunshot. If the weapon is a revolver, in addition to a blackened seared entrance hole, one can see a linear or more commonly an L-shaped blacked zone of seared material on the pillow where it was wrapped around the cylinder of the gun (Figure 4–10). This mark is due to soot and hot gases that have escaped from the cylinder gap of the gun. Measurement of the distance between this mark and the entrance hole will give one an idea of the barrel length of the weapon (Figure 4–11). If 100% synthetic material overlaps the cylinder gap, the gases may burn completely through the material.

"Bullet wipe" is a gray to black rim round an entrance hole in clothing. It is seen around holes made by both lead and full metal-jacketed bullets. It is not, as some people contend, lead wiped off the bullet but is in fact principally soot. Lubricant and small amounts of metallic elements from the primer, cartridge case, and bullet may also be present in the bullet wipe. As the bullet moves down the barrel it is coated with soot, lubricant, and the previously mentioned metallic elements. In addition, the bullet may pick up debris left in the barrel by prior discharge of the weapon. The bullet carries this material on itself to the target. As it passes through the clothing, it "wipes off" this material, producing the bullet wipe. If one takes a barrel and cleans it repeatedly until there is no material left in it and then fires a bullet down the barrel, this bullet on striking cloth will produce a light gray bullet wipe. As more and more rounds of ammunition are discharged down the barrel, the bullet wipes produced will become increasingly darker in color until finally the color will stabilize as a dark black. This is true for both lead and full metal-jacketed ammunition. Bullet wipe is not seen around all entrance defects. If a bullet goes through multiple layers of cloth, bullet wipe may be present only around the defect in the cloth that was perforated first.

Careful examination of both sides of a bullet hole in clothing, using a dissecting microscope, may suggest the direction in which the bullet was moving by which way the fibers are bent. It should be realized that not all fibers are bent in the direction of the path of the bullet, and in fact some fibers may point in the opposite direction. Therefore, differentiation of entrance versus exit holes in cloth is of dubious reliability if one uses only the direction in which the fibers are bent. Deposition of small fragments of tissue on the inner surface of clothing around a defect strongly suggests that it is an exit. One has to realize that—at least with centerfire rifles—blow-out of tissue can occur at the entrance as a result of positive pressure waves generated in the temporary cavity formed by the bullet.

Analytic Examination of Clothing for Range Determination

Although in many cases soot and powder grains are readily seen on the clothing, thus indicating a close-range shot, on occasion examination with the naked eye and the dissection microscope is insufficient. Thus, in heavy bloodstained garments, one may have to resort to infrared photography to demonstrate the soot pattern. In addition, in some instances more exact determination of the range may be necessary rather than just saying it is close-range. To make such determinations, crime labs traditionally have used the Walker test or some modification of it.

The Walker test was developed to detect the nitrites of gunpowder residue on clothing.[8] This test documents the presence of nitrites as well as showing the size and configuration of the pattern on the clothing. A firearms examiner can attempt to duplicate this pattern by firing the same weapon and type of ammunition at known distances at the same type of material. This procedure will give the examiner the range at which the individual was shot. The test involves desensitizing glossy, photographic paper in a hypobath, washing and drying it, immersing it in a 5% solution of sulfanilic acid; drying it, dipping the paper in a 0.5% solution of α-naphthylamine in methyl alcohol drying the paper, placing the clothing to be examined on the paper, placing a layer of cloth moistened with 20% acetic acid over the clothing to be examined, and pressing down on this cloth with a warm iron for 5 to 10 min. The paper is removed and washed in hot water and methyl alcohol. When nitrites are present, they will appear as orange-red spots on the paper.

Because α-naphthylamine has been identified as a carcinogen, Watson introduced a variation on this test using α-napthol or naphthoresorcinol.[9] The former chemical will cause the nitrites to appear orange; the latter will make them appear yellow. Neither one of these chemicals will interfere with subsequent lead tests using sodium rhodizonate.

The sodium rhodizonate test, long used as a spot test for lead and barium, constituted one portion of the Harrison and Gilroy test for the detection of gunshot residue on the hands. Many laboratories now use it for the detection of metallic primer residues around an entrance hole in clothing. In a modification proposed by Bashinski et al., the material to be tested is pretreated with 10% acetic acid.[10] This step improves the sensitivity of the test. The material is then sprayed with sodium rhodizonate followed by pH 2.8 tartaric acid buffer. Lead becomes visible as a bright pink reaction. Barium has an orange color.

A less commonly used method of examining clothing in order to make range determination involves the use of EDX. The edges of the entrance hole are analyzed for the presence of antimony, barium, lead, and copper. Multiple readings are taken at varying distances from this hole. Thus, a reading will be taken 1 in. from the 12 o'clock position of the hole, followed by additional readings at 2 in., 3 in., 4 in., 5 in., and so forth. Readings will then be taken in a similar manner from the 3, 6, and 9 o'clock positions. The distribution of the metallic residue around the entrance hole can thus be mapped out in a semiquantitative manner. This pattern can be duplicated on identical cloth, with the same weapon and type of ammunition. This procedure gives one the range at which the wound was inflicted. Identical cloth must be used as differences in cloth can produce marked differences in the deposition of the metals.

Use of the EDX has the advantage that it is nondestructive and extremely rapid. There is no preparation of the garment. A 100-sec count is taken for each reading. Thus, a garment can be analyzed in a matter of minutes. If desired, after analysis with EDX, the garment can be submitted for analysis by the Walker test or the sodium rhodizonate test. The metallic primer residues are detected out to ranges of 2 to 3 ft.

It has been observed that, on firing Remington .22 rimfire ammunition at cloth, one may detect antimony, barium, and lead on the cloth even though only lead is present in the primer of this ammunition. The source of the antimony and barium are deposits of antimony and barium in the bore of the weapon caused by previous firing of other rimfire ammunition that had these metals in their primers.

Range Determination in Decomposed Bodies

Determination as to whether a gunshot wound in a decomposing body is either close-range or distant can be difficult for a number of reasons. First are the changes of decomposition itself. Decomposition results in a blackish discoloration of the skin and subcutaneous tissue, which can either simulate or conceal soot. There is slippage of the epidermis, which can produce complete loss of powder tattooing and soot. Blood around the wound clots and dries out. Fragments of this desiccated blood can simulate partly burnt powder fragments.

In addition to the changes of decomposition, insect activity can obliterate as well as simulate wounds. Maggots and beetles are attracted to injury sites where blood is present. They can completely obliterate the entrance in the skin and thus any evidence of soot or powder. Insects can burrow into the skin, producing circular defects resembling gunshot entrance wounds. If there is subsequent drying of the edges, this may simulate the blackening and searing of a contact wound from a small caliber weapon (Figure 12−6).

Although nothing can be done if insects have obliterated a wound, it is possible to differentiate close-range versus distant wounds, provided

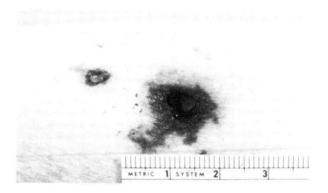

Figure 12-6 Hole in skin from insect. Note drying of edges which simulates contact wound.

that one has adequate instrumentation. In all decomposing bodies, the suspected wound should be examined in situ with the dissecting microscope for the presence of soot and powder. It should then be excised and the underlying subcutaneous tissue examined for soot and powder as well. In many instances, one cannot say with certainty whether soot is or is not present. If one sees unburned powder grains, one will know that one is dealing with a close-range wound. As mentioned, fragmented, dried-out, desiccated blood can simulate partly burnt grains of powder. The suspected material can be tested with a hot probe to see if it burns, or it can be retained and submitted for thin-layer chromatography. This latter method can differentiate single- from double-base powder as well.[11]

After examination with the dissecting microscope, the wound can then be examined by EDX. Here one is looking for vaporized metal from the primer, cartridge case, and bullet deposited on the skin. Low levels of lead at an entrance are not significant in range determination, as the lead may have "wiped off" the bullet as it punched its way through the skin. This lead is either from the bullet itself or the primer residue that coats the fired bullet as it moves down the barrel.

Extremely high counts of lead found by EDX indicate close-range firing. The significance of specific levels or counts of lead depends on the time of counting and the machine used and have to be worked out for each machine. Detection of either antimony or barium in significant levels by EDX indicates a close-range wound, as they are from the primer compounds. In addition, zinc and copper may be vaporized from the cartridge case; if this occurs in high enough concentrations, it will indicate close-range wounds. One has to have a control sample from the adjacent skin to see what is the normal background for the previously mentioned metals detected. If one does not have access to EDX, a swab of the skin around an entrance can be made and analysis performed by FAAS for the primer residues.

In contact wounds from shotguns and rifles, only lead may be detected by EDX at the wound entrance. The other metallic elements of the primer may not reach the entrance site in high enough concentrations to be detected by this method of analysis.

After initial examination by EDX, saline swabs can be taken from the interior of the wound for analysis by FAAS for antimony, barium, lead, and copper. The wound itself can be split down the center and the interior reexamined with a dissecting microscope for powder and soot. Examination of the wound track by EDX should be carried out as the original EDX analysis detected trace metals deposited on the skin rather than in the wound track. Again, the presence of extremely high levels of lead or the presence of antimony and barium by EDX indicates that a wound is close-range.

Interpretation of the results of the analysis of the swabs of the wound by FAAS is more difficult than analysis with EDX, as the former method is very sensitive and detects very small amounts of trace metal. One has to run controls to determine the normal background level. Since copper is very common, it usually is of no help. Very high levels of lead and significantly elevated levels of barium or antimony indicate that the wound to be close range.

Determination that a defect in a body is a pseudogunshot wound caused by an insect, is usually made by examining the wound and attempting to follow its bullet track. Usually, the insect burrows down only to the subcutaneous tissue and it is obvious that one is dealing with an insect defect. These alleged gunshot wounds can also be examined by EDX and FAAS. They will, of course, be negative. However, this finding does not rule out that they are gunshot wounds, as it is possible to have a negative analysis by both methods (EDX and FAAS) with known gunshot wounds.

References

1. Cowan, M.E., Purdon, P.L. A study of the "paraffin test." J. Forensic Sci. 12(1): 19–35, 1967.
2. Harrison, H.C., Gilroy, R. Firearms discharge residues. J. Forensic Sci. 4(2): 184–199, 1959.
3. Krishnan, S.S. Detection of gunshot residue on the hands by neutron activation and atomic absorption analysis. J. Forensic Sci. 19(4): 789–797, 1974.
4. Stone, I.C. Petty, C.S. Examination of gunshot residues. J. Forensic Sci. 19(4): 784–788, 1974.
5. Wolten, G.M., Nesbitt, R.S., Calloway, A.R., Loper, G.L., Jones, P.F. *Final Report on Particle Analysis for Gunshot Residue Detection.* El Segundo, CA: The Aerospace Corporation, 1977.

6. Wolten, G.M., Nesbitt, R.S., Calloway, A.R., Loper, G.L., Jones, P.F. Particle analysis for the detection of gunshot residue (I–III). J. Forensic Sci. 24(2): 409–422, 423–430, 1979; 24(4):864–869, 1979.

7. Kokocinski, C.W., Brundage, D.J., Nicol, J.D. A study of the use of 2-nitro-1-naphthol as a trace metal detection reagent. J. Forensic Sci. 25(4): 810–814, 1980.

8. Walker, J.T. Bullet holes and chemical residues in shooting cases. J. Crim. Law Criminol. 31:497, 1940.

9. Watson, D.J. Nitrites examination in propellant powder residue. AFTE 2(1): 32, 1979.

10. Bashinski, J.S., Davis, J.E., Young, C. Detection of lead in gunshot residues on targets using the sodium rhodizonate test. AFTE J. 6(4): 5–6, 1974.

11. Peak, S.A. A thin-layer chromatographic procedure for confirming the presence and identity of smokeless powder flakes. J. Forensic Sci. 25(3): 679–681, 1980.

Correct Handling
of Deaths from Firearms 13

The correct handling of deaths from gunshot wound begins at the scene. Here valuable evidence on the body can be lost or altered and bogus evidence may be inadvertently introduced through mishandling of the body.

The most important rule at the scene is to handle the body as little as possible so as not to dislodge trace evidence that may be clinging to garments or to the body surface. Hands should never be pried open, and fingerprints should never be taken at the scene. Prying the fingers apart may dislodge material such as fibers, hair, or powder. Black fingerprint ink can either mimic or obscure powder soot as well as introducing contaminating materials that may render subsequent examination of the hands for primer residues of questionable validity. Manipulation of the hands is of even greater potential danger if it is done by a police officer, who theoretically can transfer primer residues from his hands to that of the deceased. After all, as part of the job, the officer handles and fires weapons, thus putting him or her in an environment where the hands may be contaminated with primer residues.

Before transportation of the body to the morgue, paper bags should be placed over the hands to prevent loss of trace evidence. Paper bags should be used rather than plastic, because if plastic bags are placed on the body and the body is refrigerated there will be subsequent condensation of moisture in the bags. This can wash away primer residues and make fingerprinting more difficult. Some authorities have claimed that it is possible for the hands to be contaminated by barium in the paper of the bags. In the author's experience, this has never happened.

After the paper bags are placed securely around the hands, the body should be wrapped in a white sheet or placed in a clean crash bag. This is done to prevent loss of trace evidence from the body. It also avoids the acquiring of bogus evidence from the vehicle used in transporting the body to the morgue, as this vehicle has probably transported numerous other bodies previously.

On arrival at the morgue, the body should be logged in as to name, date, and time of arrival; who transported it; and who received it. A case number should be assigned. At this time or some time before the autopsy, an identification photo should be taken of the deceased with the case number prominently displayed in the identification photo.

If the deceased did not die immediately after being shot and was transported to a hospital, a number of surgical and medical procedures may have been carried out. Because of this, complete medical records of the deceased from the time of admission to death should be obtained before autopsy. All hospitals in the area served by the medical examiner system should be informed that in all medical examiner cases, no tubing should ever be removed from the body after death, e.g., endotracheal tubes, intravenous lines, and Foley catheters. Injection sites should be circled in ink by the hospital staff to indicate that they are of therapeutic origin and did not antedate hospitalization. Thoracotomy, laparotomy, and surgical stab wounds should be labeled or described in the medical records. If death occurs within a few hours after hospitalization, paper bags should be placed on the hands, just as if the death had occurred at the scene. The body and any clothing worn by the deceased should be transferred to the medical examiner's office. All medical records detailing the procedures performed should accompany the body. Any blood obtained on admission to the hospital should be obtained for toxicology. Admission blood obtained for transfusion purposes often is saved for 1 to 2 wk in the hospital blood bank.

Before examination by the forensic pathologist, the body should not be undressed or embalmed. Examination of the clothing is as much a part of the forensic autopsy as examination of the body. Embalming can induce artifacts, change the character of wounds, and make toxicological analyses impossible or extremely difficult. The best example of an artifact created by embalming is shown in Figure 13–1. The deceased was a young child who allegedly was accidentally shot by the father at a distance of 10 ft. The justice of the peace who handled the case saw no reason for an autopsy and had the body embalmed. When it initially was viewed, there appeared to be a muzzle imprint in the left upper chest. This was in fact the outline of an embalming button that was used to "seal" the distant wound of entrance. During embalming, the tissue swelled around the button, producing the mark.

After receipt of a body, the pathologist immediately should have x-rays taken. X-rays should be taken in all gunshot wound cases whether the missile is believed to be in the body or to have exited. The clothing

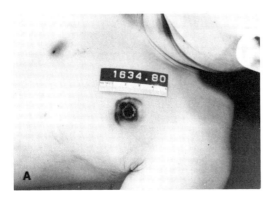

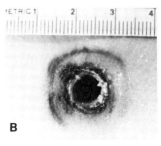

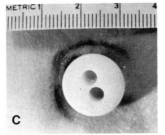

Figure 13–1 **A.** Gunshot wound of left upper lateral chest. **B.** Circular mark around defect, suggestive of muzzle imprint. **C.** Embalming button in place, acting as causative factor for "imprint."

should not be removed before x-ray. On occasion bullets have exited the body and become lodged in or among the clothing. In a number of cases seen by the author, the bullet would not have been found unless it was known to be in the clothing. In one case the bullet exited the right chest and fell into the inside pocket of a jacket. A hole was present in the bottom of the pocket, and the bullet then fell into the lining. It would not have been found had x-ray not shown it to be in the clothing.

The next step is to recover any primer residues from the hands. This can be done by the use of swabs moistened in acid or by adhesive materials. At the same time the hands should be examined for the presence of trace evidence, powder, and soot. Powder and soot may be found on the hand if the deceased had tried to reach for the weapon or had his or her hand around the weapon at the time of discharge. Fingernails may be clipped and retained at this time if indicated.

After this procedure, fingerprints may be taken. It is suggested that at least two sets of prints be made, one for the police and the other for the autopsy file. In homicides, palm prints may also be of use.

Next the body is examined with the clothing on the body. Attention is paid to see whether the defects in the clothing correspond in location to wounds in the body. The clothing should be examined for the presence of powder or soot. Following this, the clothing is removed and laid out on a clean, dry surface. The clothing should not be cut from the body except under very unusual circumstances.

The body is then examined without the clothing and without clean-ing. One should search for powder grains and soot. One may want to take photographs of the uncleaned wounds at this time if this material is present. The body is then cleaned and reexamined for any other wounds that may have been concealed by dried blood. The prosector should go back to the clothing and again correlate the observed entrances and exits with defects in the clothing. He or she should reexamine defects in the clothing for the presence of powder or soot. The use of a dissecting microscope is strongly recommended.

Photography of the wounds on the body is suggested. At least two photographs of each entrance wound should be taken. One should be a placement shot showing where the wound is in relationship to other body landmarks. The second should be a close-up showing the appear-ance of the wound. Most individuals take a third shot between the two extremes. In all photographs it is helpful if there is a scale and the number of the case.

Each wound should be examined, and notes should be taken as to its exact location and appearance. Pertinent negatives should be noted. It is strongly recommended, almost mandatory, that the wounds be exam-ined with a dissecting microscope. If there is any question as to range which cannot be settled at this time, the wound should be excised and retained for analysis by either EDX or FAAS. In routine gunshot wounds it is not necessary to retain entrances and exit sites. Microscopic sec-tions of the entrance and exit do not ordinarily contribute any informa-tion that cannot be gained by examination with the naked eye or with a dissecting microscope. In difficult cases, EDX and FAAS analysis are more useful in terms of their findings than is a microscopic section.

In homicide cases, a complete autopsy involving the head, chest, and abdominal cavities should be performed. All viscera should be removed and examined. The track of the bullet should be followed. Measure-ments as to its final point of lodgement or point of exit in relationship to the entrance should be made. If it is still present in the body, the bullet, should be recovered. In shotgun cases, it is not necessary to recover all pellets but only a representative sample. Wadding should always be recovered. Wounds ordinarily should not be probed. Use of probes can create false wound tracts, distort a wound, or dislodge a missile.

If powder, polyethylene filler, or fragments of the bullet are on the surface of the body, these should be retained and submitted with the bullet or pellets to the crime laboratory.

The Autopsy Report

In preparing an autopsy report in a death caused by gunshot wounds, it is always best to group the description of wounds in one area labeled "Evidence of Injury," rather than scattering this information throughout the protocol. Thus, when a bullet entering the left chest perforates the left lung, the heart, and the right lung; and exits the right back, one should have all this information in one area of the autopsy report rather than scattering it among the external examination and the description of the individual internal organs. Once the description of the injury to the organ has been made in this section, there is no need to redescribe the injury in the area of the report devoted to the organ.

Each gunshot wound should be described individually and fully as to location, appearance, path, and site of lodgement or exit before description of any other bullet wound is given. The first information to be noted in the autopsy report is the location of the entrance wound. The wound should be located in terms of its general geographic area, e.g., the left upper chest, followed by its distance from either the top of the head or the soles of the feet; the distance from the right or left of the midline; and most importantly its relationship and distance from a local landmark such as the nipple.

Measurements may be in either the English or the metric system. Describing a gunshot wound in relation to a local landmark is usually of greater value than locating the wound from the top of the head or so many centimeters or inches to the right or left of the midline. Thus, it is easier to visualize the location of a gunshot wound of a left chest as being "1 in. above the level of the nipples" and "1 in. medial to a vertical plane through the left nipple," rather than "20 in. below the top of the head" and "3 in. to the left of the midline." This does not, however, remove one's responsibility from locating the entrance from the top of the head and to the right or left of the midline.

After the entrance wound is located, the size, shape, and characteristics of this wound should be given. Measurements should be in the metric system for greater accuracy. The presence or absence of an abrasion ring, its symmetry, and its width should be described. The presence or absence of soot and powder should be noted in all cases. When soot is present, the configuration of the deposit along with its size and density should be described. Searing of the edges of the wound or adjacent skin should be noted and described in detail. When powder tattoo patterns are present, the maximum dimensions of the pattern and its density should be described. In measuring the pattern, occasional stray tattoo marks from the main powder tattoo pattern should be ignored. Unburned or partially burned grains of powder should be recovered, and an attempt should be made to identify them as flake, ball, or cylindrical powder. Grains should be retained for identification by a firearms examiner if the prosector is unsure of the type of powder present or wishes independent confirmation. The relationship of the bullet entrance hole to the distribution of the tattooing around it should be noted.

In contact wounds, if a muzzle imprint is present, the imprint should be described fully. If the weapon that is alleged to have produced the wound is available, comparison should be made of the muzzle end of the weapon with the imprint.

Description of the abrasion ring or zone of searing around the entrance can be done by relating the appearance of these wound characteristics to a clockface whose center is the center of the bullet hole. Thus, an eccentric abrasion ring may be said to average 1 mm wide, except from the 3 to 6 o'clock positions, where it averages 3 mm wide.

After the external appearance of the wound is described, the path of the missile through the body should be given. The organs injured and the amount of blood present in the body cavities should be noted. The point where the bullet either lodges or exits the body should be described. It is helpful to describe the point of lodgement or the point of exit in relation to the wound of entrance, e.g., "3 in. below the level of the wound of entrance, 1 in. to the left of the posterior midline." This description often aids one in visualizing the trajectory of the bullet through the body. A brief sentence about the overall direction of the bullet as it passed through the body is often helpful to an individual who has to read the autopsy protocol. Thus, the bullet may be said to have traveled from "front to back, downward and from right to left." The prosector should try to avoid terms, such as "medial," "dorsal," "ventral," "superior," or "inferior" in describing the bullet trajectory, since most lay people are unfamiliar with this terminology and forensic autopsies are more often read by lay persons than by physicians.

Exact calculation of the angle that the bullet traveled through the body is not possible. The results of such calculations are often misleading. At the time of autopsy, the body, is in an unnatural position, e.g., flat on its back and not upright. Calculations of the angle fail to take into account movement of the thorax, diaphragm, and internal viscera during the normal processes of breathing; distention of viscera by fluid, air, or food; the effects of gravity on the position of the internal viscera; and bending and twisting of the body at the time of bullet impact.

When a bullet is recovered from a body, removal should be done with the fingers, not with an instrument. Using instruments to recover a bullet can result in scratching of the surface and interference with ballistic comparison. If a bullet is recovered, it should be described briefly in the autopsy protocol. The general appearance of the bullet—i.e., deformed or not deformed; whether it is a lead bullet, jacketed, or partial metal-jacketed; and the approximate caliber, if known—should be stated. The prosector should then mark the bullet with initials or numbers so that he or she can identify it later. This marking should never be inscribed on the side of the bullet, as it would obliterate rifling marks. Any inscription should be put on either the tip or the base of the bullet. After the bullet is inscribed, it should be placed in an envelope.

The envelope should be labeled with the name of the deceased, the autopsy number, the date of autopsy, what was recovered, where it was recovered, and the inscription put on the bullet. The prosector should then sign his or her name under this information. The envelope should be kept in a secure place. At the appropriate time, it should be turned over to a representative of the criminal investigation laboratory. At this time, a receipt for the bullet should be obtained as proof of maintenance of the chain of evidence. Occasionally, a cartridge case will be recovered from the clothing of the deceased; in such as case, the casing should be retained. It may be marked with a number or initials with these marks placed either in the mouth or near the mouth of the casing.

In the case of shotgun wounds, a representative number of pellets and all wadding (if any) should be recovered. The size of the shotgun pellet pattern or the hole (if the pellets have not "opened up") should be described in the autopsy report. With shotgun pellet patterns of the skin, just as in tattooing, one should ignore stray pellets and measure only the primary pattern.

After the first gunshot wound is described, the process should then be repeated for any other gunshot wounds. Each description should be complete in itself from entrance to either recovery of the bullet or exit. There is no need to redescribe the injuries in areas of the report devoted to the individual organs.

After description of the gunshot wounds, there should be a description of the clothing in regard to defects produced by entering and exiting bullets. These defects should be located at least in a general way. It should be noted whether powder or soot is present around these defects. Examination of the clothing with a dissecting microscope is strongly recommended. One should note whether the defects correspond to the wounds. The clothing should be air-dried, packaged in paper (not plastic), and either retained or sent on to the crime laboratory for further examination.

In all gunshot wound cases, blood should be retained for typing and toxicologic analysis. Unless there has been prolonged hospitalization, a complete toxicological analysis of blood should be performed. This should include analysis for alcohol, acid, basic, and neutral drugs; morphine when narcotics are felt to be involved; and volatiles when "sniffing" of solvents is suspected. Vitreous should also be retained for alcohol determination and selective analysis. The blood should also be typed.

Appendix B may be consulted for a more general approach to the forensic autopsy as well as how it may be constructed.

Suicide by Firearms 14

The most common method of suicide in the United States is by firearm. The great majority of male suicide victims shoot themselves. For women, while drugs are still more popular as a method of suicide, they are gradually being surplanted by firearms. Handguns are used more often than rifles or shotguns. In rural areas, however, the reverse is often true.

Most people who commit suicide with a firearm, like suicide victims as a whole, do not leave a note. Notes are left in only 25% of all suicides. Therefore, absence of a note does not indicate that a death is not a suicide.

In firearm deaths it is not uncommon for the individual to attempt to make the suicide appear to be an accident. This may take two forms. The first of these is the "gun cleaning accident." The individual is found dead of a gunshot wound with gun cleaning equipment neatly laid out beside him or her. The proof that one is dealing with a suicide and not an accident usually is the nature of the wound: contact. An individual does not place a gun against the head or chest and then pull the trigger in an attempt to clean the weapon. The author has never seen a death caused by a self-inflicted wound incurred while the deceased was "cleaning" a weapon that he believes was truly an accident.

Self-inflicted wounds to the chest and abdomen from rifles and shotguns often have characteristic trajectory that acts as confirmatory evidence that one is dealing with a suicide. The individual intending suicide usually braces the butt of the gun against the ground. He or she then leans over the weapon, placing the muzzle of the gun against the chest or abdomen, holding the muzzle in place with the left hand and reaching with the right hand (if he or she is right-handed) for the trigger.

In order to reach the trigger, the individual has to rotate the body counter clockwise. Thus, the bullet or pellets will follow a right-to-left path through the body because of this rotation. Because the victim is "hunched" over the gun, the trajectory of the bullet or pellets is downward and not the upward path one would expect. Thus, the trajectory of the bullet or pellets through the body will be downward and right to left. If the individual uses the left hand to fire the weapon, he or she will rotate the body clockwise, and the path of the bullet or pellets, while still downward, will be from left to right.

The second way an individual may attempt to make a suicide appear as an accident is the "hunting accident." Here the individual goes out hunting and is subsequently found dead of a gunshot wound. Again, the nature of the wound (contact) will indicate that one is dealing with a suicide. As virtually all hunting is done with long arms, the previous discussion of the trajectory of the bullet and pellets through the body is also applicable in this situation.

The location of the self-inflicted wound varies depending on the type of the weapon, the sex of the victim, and whether the victim is right- or left-handed. In individuals who shoot themselves with handguns, the most common sites for the entrance wound are the head, chest, and abdomen, in that order. Thus, in a study by Cohle,[1] 79% of all wounds were in the head, 18% in the chest, and 3% in the abdomen. A study by Eisele et al[2] showed similar findings (Table 14–1).

In the head, the most common site for a handgun entrance wound is the temple. Although most right-handed individuals shoot themselves in the right temple and left-handed individuals in the left temple, this pattern is not absolute. Some right-handed individuals hold the muzzle of the gun against the left temple with the right hand, using the thumb of the left hand to depress the trigger. For left-handed individuals, the reverse may occur (Figure 14–1). In both instances, one may see deposition of soot on the hand holding the muzzle end of the gun. The soot is found either on the palm of the hand or on a strip of skin running along

Table 14–1 Sites of Suicidal Handgun Wounds

Site	Cohle[a]		Eisele et al.[b]	
	Number	Percent	Number	Percent
Head (including neck)	95	79	117	83
Chest	22	18	23	16
Abdomen	4	3	2	1
Total	121	100	142	100

[a] Reference 1.
[b] Reference 2.

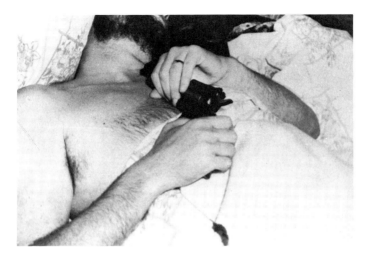

Figure 14–1 Note deceased's left hand around barrel of gun and use of thumb to fire a weapon.

the radial surface of the index finger and palm and the ulnar and palmar surface of the thumb (Figure 14–2A). Deposition of soot in this zone as well as on the radial half of the palm is usually due to muzzle blast. Soot on the ulnar half of the palm is usually due to cylinder blast (Figure 14–2B). The distribution of soot also is influenced by barrel length and where the gun is held. Even if there is no visible powder or soot deposit on the hand, analysis for primer residues is often positive.

After the temple, the most common sites in the head, in decreasing order of occurrence, are the mouth, the undersurface of the chin, and the forehead. There are people, however, who will be different and shoot themselves on the top of the head, in the eye, in the back or even in the back of the head. The fact that a wound is in an unusual location does not necessarily mean that it cannot be self-inflicted, but one must always start with the assumption that such a wound is a homicide. In rare unquestioned instances, individuals have committed suicide by shooting themselves in the back of the head. These have occurred not only with handguns but also—in one case involving an individual with whom the author was personally acquainted—with a .22 caliber rifle.

Some individuals have constructed devices to shoot themselves at a distance or in unusual locations of the body. These devices may be as simple as clamping a gun to a chair and running a string through a pulley to the trigger up to electric motors and timers. A high school student shot himself in the back with a 12-gauge shotgun by wedging the gun partly under a mattress and inserting a baton in the trigger guard. While lying on his stomach, he used his feet to push the baton against the trigger, thus firing the weapon.

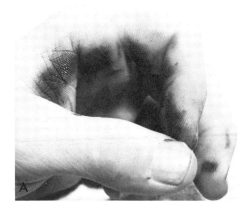

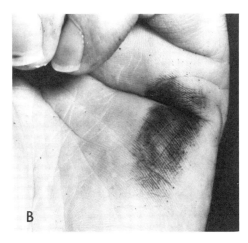

Figure 14−2 A. Soot deposited on radial aspect and edge of palm of hand. **B.** Soot deposited on ulnar aspect of palm of hand.

The sex of the victim appears to play a part in determining where individuals shoot themselves with handguns. In the study by Cohle, whereas 88.9% of the men shot themselves in the head, only 48.4% of the women did.[1]

In suicides with rifles and shotguns, just as with handguns, the preferred sites are the head, chest, and abdomen, in that order.[2,3] If one considers rimfire and high-velocity rifles in the same category (rifles), there is very little difference in the percentage distribution of wound sites in these locations compared with handguns (Table 14−2). With shotguns, however, the distribution of wound sites between the head, chest, and abdomen is not as dramatic. Thus, in the published studies concerning shotguns, the head was chosen as the entrance site in 50.5% and 51% of the time compared with the chest in 36.2% and 35% of the time, respectively (Table 14−2).

Table 14-2 Sites of Suicidal Long Arm Wounds

Site	Rifles[a]		Shotguns[a,b]			
	Number	Percent	Number[a]	Percent	Number[b]	Percent
Head (including neck)	46	81	12	51	53	50.5
Chest	8	14	8	35	38	36.2
Abdomen	3	5	3	13	14	13.3
Total	57	100	23	99	105	100

[a] Eisel et al., reference 2.
[b] Mitchell and Milvenan, reference 3.

In deaths, involving rifles, the forehead is chosen with greater frequency than it is with handguns. Still, most wounds are in the temple region.

For shotguns, although most of the entrance wounds are in the temple, entrance wounds of the mouth are almost as common.[3] Interestingly, the number of individuals shooting themselves in the right temple verses the left temple is not as marked as with handguns,[3] perhaps because it takes two hands to shoot oneself with a shotgun: one hand to steady the end of the barrel and the other to depress the trigger. Some right-handed individuals might prefer to steady the muzzle of gun with the right hand rather than using it to depress the trigger. In such a case, the individual may use the left temple rather than the right.

Just as with handguns, women tend to avoid shooting themselves in the head with shotguns.[3] However, irrespective of sex, the percentage of people shooting themselves in the head with shotguns is not as great as with handguns. This preference may be due to the fearsome reputation of the shotgun. People do not mind shooting themselves in the head but do not want to "blow their head off." In deaths due to long arms, just as in those with handguns, one should examine the hands for the presence of soot as well as do swabs for primer residues.

Suicides in which multiple gunshot wounds are present are uncommon, but not rare. These wounds may involve only one area, e.g., the head, or multiple areas, such as the head and chest. A lack of knowledge of anatomy, flinching at the time the trigger is pulled, defective or wrong ammunition, or just sheer chance in missing a vital organ account for such multiple wounds. Occasionally individuals have shot themselves simultaneously with two different weapons.

Multiple gunshot wounds confined exclusively to the head are the least common, whereas those of the chest are the most common. Multiple gunshot wounds in the head may be due to defective ammunition, use of the wrong caliber ammunition, or poor placement of the weapon. The first two may result in insufficient velocity being imparted to the bullet to penetrate the skull. More commonly, the bullet entering the cranial cavity does not strike a vital area of the brain. The victim then continues to fire until a bullet strikes a vital incapacitating area.

Wounds that on external examination may appear to be fatal may not be so on autopsy. Thus, an individual shot himself four times in the chest and once in the head with a .22-caliber pistol. One would assume that the head wound was the fatal shot, but the autopsy revealed that although the bullet did penetrate the skin, it flattened out against the frontal bone. Death was due to one of the four gunshot wounds of the chest, with the bullet going through the heart.

The largest number of gunshot wounds in a suicide that this author is aware of is nine.[4] The weapon used was a 9-shot .22-caliber revolver. All nine shots were in the left anterior chest. One bullet perforated the left lung, causing massive hemorrhage, hemothorax, and death.

Occasionally an individual will use two totally different methods in an attempt to commit suicide. Thus, one finds individuals dead of a gunshot wound with potentially lethal levels of drugs. Apparently the drugs do not work fast enough and the individual decides to shoot himself. Another individual shot herself twice in the chest with a .22 rifle. Only one bullet went into the chest cavity and this pierced the left lung, producing internal hemorrhage. This apparently was not quick enough for the woman, who then cut her wrists with a broken bottle.

Another individual, wishing to make absolutely sure he would die, placed a noose around his neck, tied one end to a support, and then shot himself in the head. The bullet itself would have been fatal, but as he collapsed, he suspended himself by the neck. If he had survived any length of time from the gunshot wound, he would have hanged himself.

The most unusual case the author has seen in this vein was a young woman who while standing on the end of a pier shot herself in the chest with a revolver. She was seen to collapse immediately after the discharge of the weapon, with the gun falling onto the pier and the woman tumbling backward into the harbor. The body was recovered a few hours later. At autopsy, she was found to have a through-and-through gunshot wound of the left breast. The bullet did not enter the chest cavity and did not injure any major blood vessel. The cause of death was drowning.

Most people who shoot themselves do so in private. Exceptions are numerous, however. Individuals have shot themselves in front of friends, spouses, relatives, and even crowds. The place chosen for the suicide may be quite bizarre. Individuals have shot themselves while driving, in police cars, and on television. One individual climbed into the trunk of his car, closed it, and then shot himself with a shotgun.

Sometimes the fatal bullet will exit the victim and either reenter another area of the body or strike another individual. Thus, an individual shot himself in the head while at the same time holding his other arm across his head, almost as if covering his ear. The bullet entered one temple, exited the other, and then lodged in the upraised arm. Another individual shot himself while lying in bed with the bullet exiting and striking his wife.

Suicide is not acceptable in American society, and thus there is often strenuous objection to the ruling of a death as suicide. The objections can vary from the naive "he wouldn't do such a thing" to a sophisticated and complicated explanation for why a weapon "accidentally" discharged. These objections can be motivated by guilt, religious belief, social pressures, or avarice.

Individuals may contest the ruling of suicide by stating that the deceased, though previously depressed, had recently been happy. In fact, it is not uncommon for individuals who have decided to commit suicide to show an elevation in mood before the suicide. After all, they have solved the problem - they are going to kill themselves.

Occasionally, someone will object to the ruling that a death is a suicide because the alleged suicide weapon had been fired several times. In fact, it is not uncommon to find that the suicide weapon has been fired at least once before the fatal shot. Why this occurs one cannot say with absolute certainty. Perhaps the individual is trying out the weapon. The other possibility is that he is building up courage to kill himself.

In all suspected suicidal gunshot wound cases, one should examine the hands for the presence of soot or powder. This is seen typically not on the firing hand but on the hand used to steady the weapon. The distribution of this soot has been discussed previously in this chapter. Even if nothing is seen grossly, one should take swabs for primer residues even if one does not have the equipment to do such analysis, as the swabs can be preserved indefinitely. If any question arises concerning the case, one can arrange to have the analysis done. It must be remembered, however, that in only 30 to 50 percent of the cases of suicide by a handgun will the handwashings be positive if one uses neutron activation or FAAS. When the weapon is a long arm, a positive correlation between firing and deposition of residue on the hand used to fire the weapon is virtually nil. More commonly, one will get a positive test for the hand that cradles the end of the long arm.

The weapon will be found clutched in the hand of the deceased in approximately 20 percent of all suicides. On rare occasions one will find an orange-brown discoloration of the skin of the palm as a result of deposition of iron in the epidermis (Figure 14−3). In such cases, the deceased will have been found with a firearm clutched in the hand. It is hypothesized that the iron of the barrel or frame, aided by water and salt in perspiration, produced rust stains. This stain will not wipe away. The fact that this material is iron has been confirmed by EDX and special

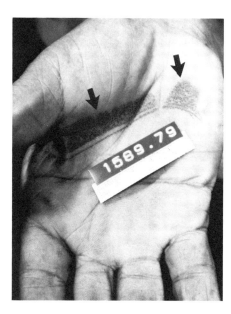

Figure 14-3 Discoloration of palm from deposits of iron.

stains for iron.[5] Of the four cases the author has seen personally, a long arm was the weapon involved in three, with the barrel of the weapon clutched in the hand. The fourth case involved an automatic pistol. Stains were present on the palms of both hands. The weapon was found clutched in the right hand, with the gun's magazine in the other.

Textbooks, articles, and lecturers commonly make mention of deposition of high-velocity blood droplets on the back of the hand used to fire a handgun in suicides, implying that this is a fairly common finding. In fact, deposition of high-velocity blood droplets on the firing hand is relatively uncommon (fewer than 5% of cases). Such a spray may in fact be present not only on the back of the hand firing the gun but also on the back of the hand used to steady the muzzle (Figure 14-4). This is also a rare finding. In one case the author has seen, the blood spray was present on the backs of both hands.

In addition to examining the hands, if possible one should examine the gun for the presence of blood or tissue. The author examined handguns used in 20 consecutive suicides in which death was due to a contact gunshot wound of the head. Each weapon was examined for the presence of visible blood and tissue at the muzzle, in the bore, and on the barrel. In only one case was tissue found. This was brain tissue at the muzzle end of the weapon in a contact wound of the head with a .38 Special. Interestingly, no blood was visible. In addition to examining the guns for the visible presence of blood, a chemical test for the identification of occult blood was performed. This was carried out by swabbing

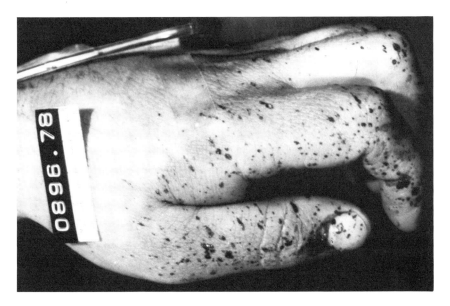

Figure 14—4 Spray of blood on hand used to steady muzzle of weapon.

the muzzle end and the bore of each gun with a moistened cotton swab and analyzing for occult blood using p,p-benzylidine. Of the 20 cases, in 8 instances (40%) blood was neither visible grossly nor demonstrated on chemical testing. In three cases, although no blood was present visibly, the chemical test revealed the presence of blood.

Five cases of contact wounds of the chest with a handgun were examined by the author. In three of the five, no blood or tissue was seen grossly and the chemical tests for the presence of blood were negative.

A less extensive study was done for shotguns. There were three contact wounds of the head. Not unexpectedly, blood was present at the muzzle end as well as inside the bore in all three instances. All three weapons were 12-gauge shotguns. In three contact wounds of the chest, blood was found on the outside of the barrel and in the bore in two of them and was absent both grossly and chemically from the muzzle end and bore in the third case. The weapons involved were a 12-gauge, a .410, and a 20-gauge shotgun, respectively.

Before ending our discussion on suicides we should consider deaths resulting from "Russian roulette". In the author's opinion, the majority of such deaths are suicides. When an individual puts a weapon to his head that he knows to be loaded and pulls the trigger the ensuing death is a suicide. The only time the author would rule such a death an accident is when it occurs in a situation in which there are multiple participants in the "game" and when the weapon is being passed around among the participants. Usually in such cases a high blood alcohol level will be found in the deceased.

Accidental Deaths from Firearms

In order to decide whether a death from gunshot wound is an accident, one must know the circumstances leading up to and surrounding the death, who was present, the type of weapon, the result of the examination of the weapon by a firearms examiner, the findings at autopsy, and the results of the toxicology study.

The exact number of accidental firearm deaths that occur each year is difficult to determine, as suicides are not uncommonly labeled as accidents. This decision may result for a multitude of reasons: lack of knowledge concerning weapons or the circumstances surround the death, naiveté, or an attempt to "make things easier" for a surviving spouse or family. In large urban areas, where the police must investigate numerous homicides, certain firearm deaths may be "classified" by the police agencies as accidents in direct contradiction to how the medical examiner rules the manner of death. This decision by the police reduces not only the work load of the homicide squad but the homicide rate, both of which are desirable goals in urban areas. The concept of what constitutes an accident as viewed by the police department is often not the same as it is for the medical examiner. Thus, if an individual is fatally shot while "struggling" over a weapon with another individual, the death may be called homicide by the medical examiner but an accident by some police departments. Another common situation involves the death of a child from a gunshot wound. The author has seen a number of such cases in which other children were present at the time of the death and which the police "ruled" as accident because it was a self-inflicted wound. The medical examiner ruled the cases homicides on the basis of the range determinations, with the children having been shot by the other individuals. Since the perpetrator was most likely another child and no criminal action would be taken, the police paid no attention to the medical examiner's ruling and wrote off the case as "self-inflicted gunshot wound—accident."

It is the opinion of the author that, if an individual is holding a weapon and this weapon discharges, killing another individual, this death is a homicide. This is true even if the individual who was holding the weapon did not intend to kill the other individual. The decision as to intent is not for the medical examiner to make but is up to the courts. Guns do not discharge by themselves while being held. Someone has to pull the trigger. The gun does not "magically" go off. The only exception to such a ruling might be if the individual holding the weapon was a very young child who does not realize the consequences of pulling the trigger.

A firearms death should be labeled as an accident if the weapon falls to the ground and discharges. Such an accidental discharge is due to the design of the weapon or a defect in it.

Handguns that will discharge on dropping fall into five general categories:

1. Single action revolvers
2. Old or cheaply made double-action revolvers
3. Derringers
4. Striker-operated automatics
5. Certain external hammer automatics

Single-action revolvers are involved in most instances of discharge of a dropped weapon.[6] Unlike double-action revolvers, the hammer of a single-action revolver must be cocked manually before pressure on the trigger will release the hammer. The firing pin in this weapon may be either intergral with the hammer or in the frame separate from the hammer. Whatever the case, single-action revolvers have traditionally been dangerous in that, when the hammer is down , the firing pin projects through the breech face, resting on the primer of the cartridge aligned with the barrel. If the weapon is accidentally dropped and lands on the hammer, the force transmitted through the hammer to the firing pin and then to the primer may be sufficient to discharge the weapon. Because of this characteristic, single-action revolvers traditionally have been carried with the hammer down on an empty chamber.

Ruger is the major manufacturer of single-action revolvers. In 1973, because of the large numbers of accidents reported from the dropping of single-action weapons, the design of their weapons was changed so that a safety lever permits discharge only when the trigger is held all the way back. The operation of a safety lever will be discussed later in this chapter.

Most revolvers now manufactured are double-action. Modern, well-made double-action revolvers are equipped with safety devices that prevent contact between the firing pin and the trigger if the weapon is dropped. Modern Smith & Wesson revolvers are equipped with two safety systems: the rebound slide and the hammer block (Figure 14–5). The older of these systems, the rebound slide, was introduced in 1896 and modified in 1908. It prevents forward rotation of the hammer unless the trigger is held to the rear. In 1915, Smith & Wesson added a second safety system to this revolver, the hammer block. This is an L-shaped metal rod whose foot is automatically interposed between the hammer and the frame except when the trigger is held to the rear.

Colt double-action revolvers are equipped with a rebound lever and a hammer block (Figure 14–6). The hammer of a Colt revolver lies in a cut in the rebound lever. The hammer cannot rotate forward because of the metal of the lever. Only when the trigger is pulled and the rebound lever

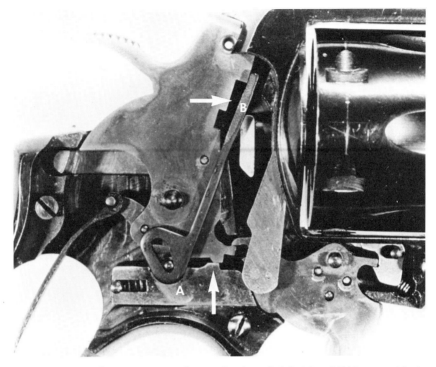

Figure 14–5 Smith & Wesson revolver with rebound slide (a) and (b) hammer block. (Reprinted with permission from the J. Forensic Sci. 19(4), 1974. Copyright © ASTM, 1916 Race Street, Philadelphia, Pennsylvania.)

elevated out of the way can the hammer rotate forward to fire the weapon. The Colt hammer block system was introduced in 1905 and has been standard with all double-action Colt revolvers since 1910. Its action is identical to that of the hammer block in the Smith & Wesson revolver.

Charter Arms revolvers, the new version of the Ruger single-action revolvers, and all Ruger double-action revolvers are equipped with a device called a "safety lever" (Figure 14–7). In these weapons, the hammer rests against the steel frame above the firing pin. When the trigger is pulled, the safety lever rises, interposing itself between the firing pin and the hammer. When the hammer falls, it strikes the safety lever, which transmits the force to the firing pin, which in turn strikes the primer, firing the cartridge. When the trigger is released, the safety lever drops below the firing pin and the hammer again comes to rest against the frame. The safety lever is also present in Colt Mark III revolvers.

These safety systems are often not present in cheap double-action revolvers known as Saturday night specials. In these weapons, safety

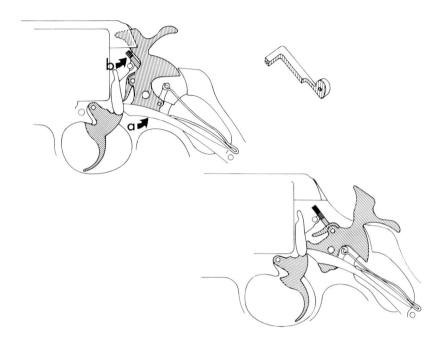

Figure 14−6 Colt revolver with (a) rebound lever and (b) hammer block.

Figure 14−7 Revolver with safety lever.

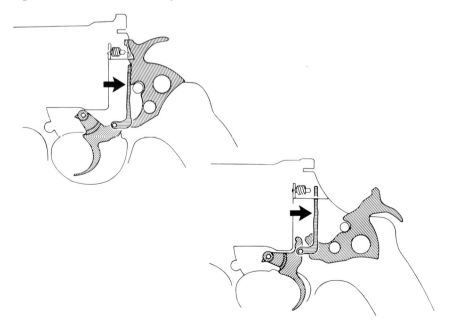

devices may vary from non-existent to excellent in concept but poor in execution. Some Saturday night special revolvers use a hammer block consisting of a thin steel wire. The metal of the hammer, however, may be so soft that a number of sharp blows to the hammer causes the wire to indent the soft metal of the frame of the weapon, thus permitting the hammer to strike the firing pin, discharging the weapon.

In derringers with external hammers, just as in single-action re-volvers, the firing pin rests on the primer of the chambered round. Dropping a derringer on the hammer will cause it to discharge. This does not happen with the hammerless derringer manufactured by High-Standard.

With automatic pistols, the firing mechanism is of two possible designs: striker-operated or hammer-operated. The cheaper automatic pistols are usually striker-operated. Here a rodlike firing pin travels inside the breech block propelled by a coiled spring. When the weapon is cocked, the slide is pulled back and the striker is engaged by the sear and held in a rearward position. On pulling the trigger, the sear disengages the striker, and the spring drives it forward, firing the cartridge. With poorly made, cheap weapons, the internal tolerances of the parts may be such that if the weapon is dropped, the striker may jar loose from the sear, go forward, and fire the weapon.

Hammer-operated automatic pistols may have either an internal or an external hammer. For all practical purposes, accidental discharge of a dropped automatic pistol involves only external hammer weapons. Whether an automatic with an external hammer is safe or dangerous depends on the presence or absence of safety devices as well as the position of the hammer at the time of fall. Thus, both the Colt Model 1911A1 and the Browning Hi-Power are completely safe if dropped on their hammer when it is down. These weapons are equipped with a "flying firing pin." The pin is shorter than the length it has to travel in the breech block. To propel the pin forward far enough to strike the primer, the hammer has to fall a great enough distance to impart suffi-cient inertia to the firing pin. If the hammer is down, a blow to it cannot be transmitted to the primer. If the weapon is at half cock when dropped, discharge can occur. The blow to the hammer, however, has to be sufficient to break off the half-cock notch or the tip of the sear engaging the notch. The forward travel of the hammer then may be sufficient to fire the weapon. If the weapon is at full cock and is dropped, it theo-retically can discharge. Discharge is unlikely, however, because the force would have to be sufficient to break not only the full-cock notch but the half-cock notch. If only the full-cock notch was broken off, the half-cock notch would catch the hammer and the weapon would not discharge. The author is unaware of any Colt Model 1911A1 having discharged when dropped on a fully cocked hammer as long as the weapon had not been tampered with. Thus, weapons such as the Colt M1911A1 or Browning should be carried only with the hammer all the way down or at full cock.

There is one way a weapon such as the Colt M1911A1 theoretically can be discharged if dropped even if the hammer is down. This occurs if the gun falls on its muzzle from a distance of 6 ft. or more. The inertia given to the firing pin by a fall of this height may be sufficient to discharge a primer. Since the gun would have fallen on its muzzle, the bullet would go into the floor or ground.

In addition to automatic pistols such as the Colt and Browning, numerous double-action automatic pistols, such as the Walther PPK/S, are made. These are equipped with a hammer block that performs the same function as in a double-action revolver.

Not all external-hammer automatics are equipped with flying firing pins or hammer blocks. In these weapons the hammer should never be down when there is a round in the chamber because the firing pin rests on the primer as in a single action revolver.

Just as for handguns, it is possible under certain circumstances for a rifle or shotgun to discharge when dropped. This can be due to design defects, poor workmanship, or broken parts. Such accidental discharges are rare compared with discharge of handguns. In all alleged cases of accidental discharge of a long arm, as for a handgun, the weapon should be examined by an experienced firearms examiner for defects in design or construction, broken parts, or wear.

Occasionally an individual will put a loaded rifle or shotgun in the back of a vehicle. When he attempts to take it out, he will grab it by the muzzle and pull it toward him. A projection in the vehicle may catch the trigger, discharging the weapon. This would be a true accidental death. One must be sure, however, that this is not a staged suicide.

Another category of death that may be considered accidental are "hunting accidents." Here one has to make a decision as to what constitutes an accident. One has to be careful that the death is not either a homicide or a suicide. Each case has to be examined individually and decided on its own merits.

References

1. Cohle, S. Handgun suicides. Forensic Sci. Gaz. 8(2): 2, 1977.
2. Eisele, J.W., Reay, D.T., Cook, A. Sites of suicidal gunshot wounds. J. Forensic Sci. 26(3): 480–485, 1981.
3. Mitchell, J.S., Milvenan, J. Shotgun suicides. Forensic Sci. Gaz. 8(2):3, 1977.
4. Coe J. Personal communication.
5. Norton, L.E., DiMaio, V.J.M., Gilchrist, T.F. Iron staining of the hands in suicides with firearms. J. Forensic Sci. 24(3): 608–609, 1979.
6. DiMaio, V.J.M., Jones, J.A. Deaths due to accidental discharge of a dropped handgun. J. Forensic Sci. 19(4): 759–767, 1974.

Appendix A
Hollow-Point Pistol Ammunition
Myths and Facts

A major controversy over the use of hollow-point pistol ammunition has appeared recently in the public press. The arguments against the use of the ammunition generally have been emotional, with claims of "mutilating wounds" and organs reduced to "unidentifiable chopped meat." Most of the arguments heard for and against the use of hollow-point ammunition are based on myths, tall tales, false assumptions, and secondhand stories spread by both opponents and proponents of this type of ammunition.

In the early 1960s, many police organizations began to complain about the .38 Special cartridge. Handguns chambered for the .38 Special cartridge are used by the majority of police forces in this county. The traditional round for a .38 Special revolver has been an all-lead, 158-gr, roundnose bullet, traveling at velocities from 700 to 850 ft/sec. This round has remained basically unchanged since its introduction in the early part of the twentieth century. Police departments have complained that this round did not have any stopping power. They cited numerous instances in which officers firing this cartridge in self-defense were unable to stop their attacker before he injured either them or an innocent bystander. What police agencies desire is a pistol cartridge that will stop a person "dead in his tracks." There is no such cartridge and there never will be. "Stopping" an individual depends not only on the stopping power of the bullet but also on the organs injured and the physiologic makeup of the person who is shot.

In scientific terms, the stopping power of a bullet is the amount of

Reprinted from "Opinion and Commentary," The Forensic Sci. Gaz. 5(4):1–2, 1974.

kinetic energy the impacting bullet transfers to the target. It is desirable that the bullet give up all its energy in the tissue, coming to rest within the target. It is more desirable that the kinetic energy given up be lost in vital organs rather than the soft tissue, muscle and skin, behind the organs.

When a bullet strikes tissue, it produces two types of injuries: visible anatomic injuries, and physiologic injuries that impair the function of the organ. As a bullet moves through tissue, it creates not only a permanent wound track but also a temporary cavity. The size of this temporary cavity is directly related to the amount of kinetic energy lost in the tissue. A hollow-point bullet may lose in vital organs up to four times the kinetic energy lost by the traditional roundnose, lead bullet. Therefore, the temporary cavity produced by the hollow-point bullet will be greater in size than that from a solid bullet. The key word in discussing cavity formation is "temporary." This cavity lasts only 5 to 10 msec before the tissue springs back into position as a result of the tissue's inherent elasticity and resiliency. This latter phenomenon explains the finding that in .38 Special hollow-point bullet wounds, the physical appearance and extent of the wounds are basically the same as those produced by the roundnose lead bullet.

As a hollow-point bullet travels through the tissue, it theoretically expands, creating greater resistance to its course, decelerating more rapidly, and losing more kinetic energy. It is not, however, only the mushrooming action of the hollow-point bullet that causes the greater loss of kinetic energy. The amount of kinetic energy possessed by a bullet is directly proportional to its weight and to the square of its velocity. Hollow-point bullets, though generally lighter than solid lead bullets, are loaded to considerably higher velocities. Because of this, hollow-point bullets possess greater kinetic energy. In turn, when they travel through tissue, they lose more kinetic energy. Thus, hollow-point bullets are more effective not only because they expand but also because of their increased velocity. This fact is important because a number of the common hollow-point bullets do not expand in the body. Testing of these rounds, however, reveals them to be more effective than the conventionally designed bullet. What makes these nonexpanding hollow-point bullets so effective if they do not expand? The answer is the increased velocity.

Whether using either a hollow-point or a solid lead bullet, to inflict a mortal injury, one must strike a vital organ. Although hollow-point bullets, in comparison to traditional solid lead bullets, theoretically have a greater ability to kill by virtue of greater physiologic injury to an organ, such differences are probably only theoretical. An individual struck through the heart with a solid, roundnose bullet is just as likely to die as an individual shot through the heart with a hollow-point bullet.

In a case of a gunshot wound of the lung, theoretically the hollow-point would be more likely to cause death. In reality, the speed at which a wounded individual is transported to the hospital is a greater determining factor as to whether the individual will live or die than the type of ammunition used.

In addition to greater stopping power, hollow-point ammunition possesses two other virtues. The first is that such bullets tend to stay in the body. Therefore, it is unlikely that they will exit and injure innocent bystanders. Second, hollow-point bullets tend to break up rather than ricochet if they strike hard objects. Again, this trait works to prevent injury to innocent bystanders.

There are a number of myths about hollow-point pistol ammunition which tend to impart a bad reputation to this type of ammunition. First, it should be said that .38 Special hollow-point bullets do not mutilate organs or destroy them any more than their solid-nose, all-lead counterparts. The wounds in the skin as well as those in the internal organs are the same in appearance for both types of ammunition. One cannot examine the wounds in a body and say that the individual was shot with a hollow-point rather than a solid lead bullet. No organs are reduced to "chopped meat" by a pistol bullet. The second often quoted myth is that hollow-point bullets fragment or "blow up" in the body. This is false. Fragments may break off a hollow-point bullet if it strikes a bone, but this is also true of solid lead bullets.

What has caused the origin of these myths? Part of the explanation is the normal exaggeration and distortion that occurs in stories when they are passed from person to person. Second is the fact that many people inexperienced with hollow-point pistol ammunition do not let this inexperience stand in the way of their offering "expert" testimony on the topic. Third is the fact that some people confuse high-velocity missile wounds caused by rifle projectiles with those caused by pistol bullets. Individuals shot with high-velocity rifle bullets, whether full metal-jacketed military rounds or soft-point hunting rounds, show more severe wounds than people wounded by pistol bullets. This is especially true of hunting ammunition. It is also true that hunting ammunition, because it is soft-point or hollow-point, does fragment in the body. Confusion between pistol and rifle bullets or statements based on experience only in the military, where high-velocity rifle bullets are the rule, may have caused the origin of some of these myths about hollow-point pistol bullets.

Appendix B
The Forensic Autopsy

The forensic autopsy differs from the hospital autopsy in its objectives and relevance. Besides determining the cause of death, the forensic pathologist has to establish the manner of death (natural, accidental, suicidal, or homicidal), the identity of the deceased if unknown, and the time of death or injury. The forensic autopsy may also involve collection of evidence from the body, which can be used subsequently to prove or disapprove an individual's guilt and to confirm or deny his or her account of how the death occurred.

Because of the possible medicolegal implications of forensic cases, not only do these determinations have to be made, but the findings or lack of findings must be documented. In many cases the cause and manner of death may be obvious. It is the documentation of the injuries or lack of them as well as the interpretation of how they occurred and the determination or exclusion of other contributory or causative factors that is important.

The forensic autopsy involves not only the actual examination of the body at the autopsy table but consideration of other aspects that the general pathologist does not consider part of the autopsy—the scene, clothing, and toxicology. The forensic autopsy begins at the scene. No pathologist should perform a forensic autopsy unless he or she knows the circumstances leading up to and surrounding the death. This is a very basic principle that is often violated. What would one think of a physician who examined a patient without asking what the patient's symptoms or complaints were? As in all examinations of patients, one must have a medical history. In the case of the forensic pathologist, the "patient" is unable to render this history. Therefore, the history has to be obtained by either medical examiner or police investigators. This history should be known before the autopsy.

The scene should be documented with diagrams or photographs, preferably both. People should be interviewed, and a written report should be given to the pathologist before the autopsy. At the scene, the body should be handled as little as possible. It makes good television dramatics to poke and prod a body at the scene, but it does not make sense scientifically. At a homicide scene, often there is pressure to move the body; people are milling around, and there are inadequate lighting, no instruments, and no running water. You cannot examine a body adequately at such a scene. What you can do, however, is destroy evidence or introduce fallacious evidence. One can dislodge powder from the clothing, wipe away primer residue from the hands, contaminate the body with one's own hair or with the hair of the police officer who helps one turn, poke, and prod the body, and so forth.

In cases of violent death, paper bags should be secured about the hands so that no trace evidence will be lost. If one uses plastic bags and then puts the body in a cooler, there will be condensation of water vapor on the hands (with possible loss of trace evidence) when it is moved back into a warm environment. Before transportation, the body should be wrapped in a clean, white sheet or placed in a clean body bag. One does not put a body directly onto a cart in the back of an ambulance. Who knows what or who was lying on the cart prior to the body transport? Trace evidence from a prior body may be deposited on this body, or trace evidence from this body may be lost and subsequently transferred to another body.

At the morgue, the body should never be undressed before the medical examiner sees it. This includes removing shoes and socks to place toe tags on the body. Examination of the clothing is as much a part of the autopsy as examination of the wounds. One has to examine the clothing for bloodstains and trace evidence as well as determine whether the wounds in the body correlate with the defects in the clothing. How does one know that the individual was not shot and dressed?

The body should never be embalmed before autopsy. Embalming ruins toxicologic analysis, changes the appearance of the wounds, and can induce artifacts. The body should never be fingerprinted before examination of the hands. In fingerprinting you pry the hands open and ink the fingers. In the process, you can lose trace evidence or deposit false evidence. One can render tests for firearms residue invalid in prying apart fingers and fingerprinting a body.

In all gunshot deaths and severely burned bodies, x-rays should be taken. X-rays are especially important in gunshot wound cases in which the bullet appears to have exited. This is due to the fact that the bullet may not have exited but rather only a piece of the bullet or a piece of bone. With the semijacketed ammunition now in widespread use, it is common for the lead core to exit the body and for the jacket to remain. The core is of no interest ballistically; it is the jacket that is important. The jacket may be retained beneath the skin adjacent to the exit site. It is very easy to miss the jacket at autopsy unless one knows that it is there by x-ray.

The Autopsy Report

The first part of the forensic autopsy is the external description. This should include age, sex, race, physique, height, weight, and nourishment. Congenital malformations, if present, should be noted. Next, one should give a description of the clothing. This description initially does not have to be very detailed. A simple listing of the articles found or accompanying the body should be given, e.g., a short-sleeve white shirt or a long-sleeve white shirt unbuttoned down the front, a blood-stained white T-shirt, and so on. If the case is a traumatic death with significant alterations of the garments as a result of trauma, the clothing will be described in further detail in another section of the autopsy.

Following the description of the clothing, one should then describe as a minimum:

Degree and distribution of rigor and livor mortis

Hair and eye color

Appearance of the eyes

Any unusual appearance to the ears, nose, or face, e.g., congenital malformations, scarring, and severe acne (excluded should be evidence of trauma, which will have its separate section)

Presence of teeth and or dental plates.

Presence of vomitus in the nostrils or mouth

Significant scars, tattoos, or moles

External evidence of disease

Old injuries

Evidence of recent medical or surgical intervention (Note: You may want to put this in a separate section entitled "Evidence of Medical and/or Surgical Intervention.")

At this time, if fingerprints have not been taken, they should be. In addition, it is strongly recommended that identification photos, with the number of the case, should be taken.

If there is injury to the body, it should now be described in the next section, entitled "Evidence of Injury." All recent injuries, whether minor or major, external or internal, should be described in this section. There is no need to repeat the description of these injuries in the subsequent "Internal Examination" section or to describe them in the "External Description." The age of the lesions should be described, if possible at least in a general way.

There are many ways to handle this section ("Evidence of Injury"). Excluding gunshot and stab wounds, it is easiest to divide it into two broad areas: external evidence of injury and internal evidence. Some people intermingle the two. They will describe the external evidence of injury to the head and then say, "Subsequent autopsy reveals. . . " and go on to describe the internal injuries of the head. They will then describe the external injuries of the trunk, followed by the internal injuries of the trunk.

Gunshot wounds and to a degree stab wounds represent a different situation. In gunshot wound cases, if at all possible each individual wound should be described in its entirety before going on to a second wound. The gunshot wound should be located on the body (in inches or centimeters) in relation to the top of the head or the sole of the foot and to the right or left of the midline. It should be described (in inches or centimeters) in regard to a local landmark such as the nipple or the umbilicus. The features of the wound that make it an entrance and that determine at what range it was fired should be described, i.e., abrasion ring, soot, tattooing, and so forth. Pertinent negatives should be noted. Then the course of the bullet through the body should be described. All organs perforated or penetrated by the missile should be noted.

It is useful to give an overall description of the missile path through the body in relation to the planes of the body. Thus, one will say, "The bullet traveled from back to front, left to right, and sharply downward." If the bullet exits, the exit wound should be described in relation to the entrance.

If the bullet is found, one should state where it was found; whether it is intact, deformed, or fragmented; whether the bullet is lead or jacketed; and the approximate caliber. A letter or number should be inscribed on the bullet. The bullet then should be placed in an envelope with the name of the victim, the date, the case number, the location from which the bullet was recovered, the letter or number inscribed on it, and the name of the prosector.

In the case of stab wounds, if at all possible the same general procedures should be used. One should indicate if possible whether the weapon was single- or double-edged, which edge of the wound was produced by the cutting edge of the knife, the exact dimensions of the stab wound, and an estimation of the depth of the wound track. In instances where there are dozens of knife wounds, it may not be possible to handle each wound separately, and they may have to be handled in groups.

The last part of the "Evidence of Injury" section should concern the clothing.

The location of defects, whether they correspond to the injuries and the presence of trace evidence, e.g., powder, soot, and car paint, should be described.

Following the section devoted to "Evidence of Injury," one comes to the "Internal Examination." In this section one systematically describes the major organ systems as well as the organ cavities. The usual subdivisions of this section are:

Head

Body cavities

Neck

Respiratory tract

Cardiovascular system

Gastrointestinal tract

Biliary tract

Pancreas

Spleen

Adrenals

Urinary tract

Reproductive tract

Musculoskeletal system

In these sections, one would give organ weights (not necessarily for adrenals and pancreas) as well as a brief description of the organs with pertinent negatives. With the pancreas, adrenals, and spleen, if there are no positive findings, use of the term "unremarkable" as the sole description is acceptable. Do not use the term "normal" as organs are rarely "normal," whatever that may mean.

The next section is the "Microscopic Examination." Microscopic slides should be made when indicated. Samples of tissue from all major organs should be saved, but microscopic slides often are not needed in forensic cases, especially in trauma cases.

After the "Microscopic Section" comes the "Toxicology Section," where one lists the results of the toxicologic analyses.

The next section is "Findings." This and the last section, the "Opinion," should be on separate pages. List the major findings in order of importance. One does not have to list every minute or extraneous finding as is done in some hospital autopsies. This autopsy will most likely be seen by nonphysicians. Having spent a half hour trying to explain acute passive congestion of the liver to a jury in a gunshot death case, the author believes that inconsequential observations should not be listed in the "Findings."

The last section is the "Opinion." This should briefly describe the cause of death in as simple language as possible as well as stating the manner of death. This section is intended for the public and not for physicians. Thus, for example, one can say that " . . . died of a heart attack due to coronary atherosclerosis ("hardening" of the blood vessels that supply blood and oxygen to the heart muscle)." Or ". . . . died of massive internal bleeding due to a gunshot wound of the aorta (the major blood vessel of the body)."

Speculation about circumstances surrounding the death should be absent or kept to a minimum.

Appendix C
Gunshot Residue Procedures

Handwashings of persons for gunshot residue analysis should be performed as soon as possible. These residues are easily lost or removed from living individuals.

1. If no plastic gloves are available, the technician performing the handwashing must wash his or her hands carefully before proceeding.
2. Moisten one of the cotton swabs provided with only two or three drops of dilute acid solution from the plastic bottle.
3. Swab the area of the back of the left index finger, thumb, and web as shown in Figure 12−2. About 20 sec. of swabbing is recommended per swab. Place the swab in the plastic envelope provided. Label and initial the envelope as being from the left hand back.
4. Repeat the procedure for the back of the right hand. Each hand area requires separate swabbing with separate cotton swabs.
5. Moisten a cotton swab from another envelope with two or three drops of dilute acid solution from the bottle. Swab the area of the palm side of the left index finger and thumb for about 20 sec. The area to be swabbed is shown in Figure 12−2. Place the swab in the plastic envelope. Label and initial the envelope.
6. Repeat step 5 for the right palm.
7. The fifth specimen is in an envelope labeled "control." Moisten this swab with two or three drops of dilute acid and replace in the plastic envelope.

Index

A

Abrasion rings
   absence of in entrance wounds, 70–71,
      78,121
   concentric vs eccentric, 68
   in entrance wounds, 67–72
   unusual configuration, 69–70
Accidental deaths from firearms, 302–307
   accident-prone weapons, 303
   "accidents" involving children, 302
   auto-loading pistols, 306–307
   Derringers, 306
   gun cleaning "accidents," 293
   handgun accidents, 303–307
   hunting "accidents," 294, 307
   medical examiner's viewpoint, 302–303
   police "rulings," 302
   rifle and shotgun accidents, 307
   Russian roulette, 5, 301–302
   safety systems in auto-loaders, 306–307
   safety systems in revolvers, 303–306
   suicides disguised as accidents, 293, 294
   weapons dangerous if dropped, 303
Adapters, 253
Air-powered guns, 227–231
   air rifles, 227
   calibers, 228
   Daisy BB gun, 227
   deaths from, 229–231
   Diabolo pellet, 228
   power systems, 228
   steel BB, 228
   used in war, 227

velocity necessary for pellet to perforate
   skin, 213–214
Aluminum jacketed ammunition, 259
Ammunition, 11
   automatic ammunition fired in
      revolvers, 251–252
   blanks, 11, 246, 248–251
   caliber, 10–11
   cartridges cases, 12–13
   common centerfire rifle calibers,
      159–162
   common handgun calibers, 121–125
   dummy cartridges, 11
   flechettes, 247–248
   handgun shot cartridges (centerfire), 245
   handgun shot cartridges (rimfire), 132
   head stamps, 13–14, 130–131
   interchangeability in weapons, 251–254
   lots, 131
   plastic blanks, 246
   plastic training ammunition, 246
   primers, 14–17
   propellants (gunpowder), 17–19
   revolver ammunition fired in auto-
      loaders, 251–252
   rimfire, 16–17, 127–134
   Wildcat, 11
Auto-loading pistols, 5–8
   clip, 5–6
   definition, 5
   double-action, 8
   magazine, 5
   methods of operation, 6–7

Auto-loading pistols [*cont.*]
  preparing to fire, 8
  safeties, 7–8
Automatics. *See* Auto-loading pistols
Autopsy. *See* Forensic autopsy
Autopsy report, 288–291

B

Ball powder
  development, 18
  distance can travel, 116–117
  in centerfire rifles, 153–155
  in handguns, 112, 113–114
  in shotguns, 188, 191, 204
  marks on base of bullets due to powder,
    33
  perforation of epidermis, 72
Ballistics, 41. *See* Bullet and cartridge case
  comparisons, Wound ballistics
BB gun, 227
Black powder, 17, 223, 278–279
  marks on base of bullets due to powder,
    34
Black powder weapons, 22–24, 35–37
  flintlocks, 22
  in shootings, 35–37
  lock, stock, and barrel, 22
  mark due to loading rammer, 35–37
  percussion locks, 22–23
  percussion revolvers, 23
  replicas, 23
  synchronous discharge, 35–37
Blank firing pistols,
  conversion to zip gun, 65, 232
  unusual soot pattern, 65
Blanks, 11
  construction, 248
  deaths from, 249
  plastic blanks, 246
  wounds from, 249–251
Blood, at scene, 209–210
Blunt trauma injuries from firearms,
  224–225
Body
  collection of primer residue, 287, 321
  preservation of primer residue, 285
  transportation to morgue, 285–286, 316
  x-rays, 286–287, 316–317
Bone, 92–97
  beveling, 93
  bone chips at entrance in head wounds,
    217
  differentiation of extrance vs exit, 93
  gutter wounds, 94
  internal ricochet due to, 91
  irregular entrance wounds over bone,
    104

keyhole wound of bone, 95
secondary fractures of skull, 95–96, 135,
  137, 217–218
soot deposited on bone, 106
temporary cavity in, 93
velocity needed to penetrate, 92
Bullet and cartridge case comparisons,
  31–33
  alterations in individual characteristics,
    31–32
  cartridge case comparison, 33
  class characteristics, 30–31
  individual characteristics, 31, 32
  recovery of bullets, 31
  shaving of bullet, 33
  skid marks, 32
Bullet emboli, 216–217
Bullet wipe, 97, 279
Bullets, 19–22
  appearance due to ricochet, 90
  base markings due to powder, 33–34
  breakup in body, 47–48, 146
  cast lead pistol bullets, 237
  cast lead rifle bullets, 20–21, 143
  centerfire rifle, 143–146
  disintegration due to ricochet, 90
  disintegration on striking glass, 82
  dum-dum, 240–241
  elongated, 237
  exploding ammunition, 241–242
  flared base, 236
  foreign material carried by bullet, 80,
    254–255
  Glazer round, 241
  gyroscopic spin, 46–47, 80–81
  hollow-point, 20, 240–241, 311–313
  hunting, 22, 143–145
  hunting vs military rifle bullets, 145–
    146
  jacketed, 21–22
  jacket-core separation after passing
    through intermediary target, 81–84
  KTW, 244
  lead, 20–21, 240
  M16 cartridge, 146
  marking the recovered bullet, 212,
    290–291
  marks on, from intermediary targets, 80,
    254
  military, 21, 143, 145–146
  Minie, 19–20
  multiple bullet loadings, 242–243
  Nyclad®, 244
  old, 260
  partial metal-jacketed, 22
  propelling intermediate target into body,
    83–84
  recovery, 290–291
  sabot, 237–239

semiwadcutter, 20
stability of military bullets, 46–47,
    48, 146
unstable in body, 46–47
veolcities necessary for deformation,
    47
wadcutter, 20
wire marks on, 80, 254
Bullets without rifling marks, 234–236
due to sympathetic discharge, 234
in revolver with barrel removed, 236
in sabot ammunition, 239
in smooth-bore weapons, 236
in zip guns, 65, 232

C
Caliber, 10–11
.30 Carbine, 141–142
common centerfire rifle calibers,
    159–162
common handgun calibers, 121–125
European nomenclature, 11
"Magnum," 11
rifled weapons, 10–11
.38 Special vs .357 Magnum, 11
U.S. nomenclature, 10–11
Wildcat cartridges, 11
Carbon monoxide in muscle,
of entrance wounds, 102, 150, 191
of exit wounds, 102, 150, 191
Cartridge cases, 12–13
Cartridges, 14–17
centerfire, 14–16
components, 11
rimfire, 16–17
susceptibility to detonation from heat,
    224
Cast bullets
centerfire rifle, 20–21, 143
handgun, 237
Centerfire rifle bullets, 143–146
breakup in body, 47–48, 146, 155
cast lead bullets, 20–21, 143
evolution of modern rifle cartridges,
    139–141
hunting, 22, 143–145
intermediary targets, 82–83, 157–158
jacket-core separation due to
    intermediate target, 81–82
M16, 146
military, 21, 143, 145–146
sabot ammunition, 237–239
Centerfire rifle wounds, 146–158
carbon monoxide in muscle, 150
comparison of wounds between Minie
    bullets and modern military bullets,
    141

contact wounds of chest and abdomen,
    148–150
contact wounds of head, 146–148
distant wounds of trunk, 150–152
exits, 152
"explosive" wounds, 140, 141
intermediate range and distant wounds
    of head, 150
intermediary targets, effects on
    appearance and extent of wound, 158
lead snowstorm, 155
micro-tears of entrance wounds, 152
Minie bullets and their wounds, 140
muzzle imprints, 148–150
of empty skull, 45
of head, 45
of mouth, 148
patterned abrasions due to temporary
    cavity, 152
perforating tendency of bullets, 157
powder tattooing, 152–155
severity and extent of wounds, 142–143
smooth-bore weapons and their wounds,
    139–140
stellate distant wounds, 150
unusually large distant wounds of
    thorax, 152
x-rays, 155
Centerfire rifles, 139, 141–142
common calibers, 159–162
Clothing
absorption of soot and powder by
    clothing, 121, 275
analytic examination for range
    determination, 280–281
"bullet wipe," 97, 279
"burn holes" due to hot gases, 278
direction of firing, 279
EDX and range determination, 280–281
emergency rooms, 286
examination on body, 287
gunshot wounds through, 275–281
ignition of clothing by close-
    range firing, 278–279
importance of, 286
markings on cloth due to cylinder blast,
    61, 279
melting of synthetics by hot gas, 61, 278
perforation of clothing by powder grains,
    275–276
position of deceased, 277
powder grains on clothing, 116–117, 277
tears due to gas, 61, 277–278
Walker test, 280
Concealed gunshot wounds, 211–212
Contact wounds, 51–53
angled, 52–56
angled contact vs angled near contact,
    54–57

Contact wounds [cont.]
  Hard, 51
  incomplete, 53
  loose, 51–52
  over bone with soot deposition, 106
  showing absence of soot and/or powder,
    106–107
  simulated by insect activity, 281
Cylinder gap
  emergence of soot, gas, powder, 39–40,
    120, 279
  lead fragments, 33, 40, 120
  melting of synthetics by hot gas, 61
  soot pattern used to determine barrel
    length, 61
  soot patterns, 61, 279
  tattooing and lead stippling, 120
  velocity lost, 99
Cylinder rotation, direction of, 5
Cylindrical powder,
  appearance of tattoo marks, 117, 154
  in centerfire rifle cartridges, 153
  in handgun cartridges, 113
  maximum range out to which tattooing
    occurs with centerfire rifles,
    153–155

D

Decomposed bodies, 212
  range determination in, 281–283
  usefulness of x-rays, 212–213
Dermal nitrate test, 267
Derringers, 1, 306
Discharge of weapon, 37–40, 183
Distant gunshot wounds, 66–73
Dum-dum ammunition, 240–241

E

Electrical guns, 251
Embalming, artifacts due to, 286
Emboli, bullet, 216–217
Entrance wounds,
  abrasion ring, 67–72
  absence of abrasion ring, 70–71, 78, 121
  angled contact, 52–56
  angled contact vs angled near contact,
    54–57
  angled near contact, 54–56
  atypical due to intermediary target,
    80–84
  atypical entrance wounds, 77–79, 81, 90
  bullet wipe, 97, 279
  caliber determination from, 97
  changes in dermis, 72–73
  contact, 51–53
  distant, 66–73

  due to ricochet bullets, 90
  excision of, for examination by EDX
    and FAAS, 288
  from high velocity rifles, 70
  graze wound, 77
  hard contact, 51
  "hot bullets," 72–73
  in bone, 93
  in palm and sole, 70
  incomplete contact, 53
  intermediate targets, altering entrance
    wounds, 80–84
  intermediate-range, 57–59, 72
  loose contact, 51–52
  microscopic appearance, 72
  micro-tears, 70, 152
  missed, 211–212
  near contact, 53–57
  of open mouth, 212
  pseudo-powder tattooing, 80, 84–88
  pseudo-soot, 88
  re-entry wounds, 78
  shored entrance wounds, 78
  superficial perforating wounds, 77–78
  tangential wound, 77
Exit wounds, 73–77
  cause of irregular appearance, 73
  due to bone, 258
  general appearance, 73
  incomplete and partial exits, 76
  of bone, 93
  path of bullet after exiting body, 76–77
  pseudo-exit wounds, 257–258
  shored exits, 73–75, 78
  size and shape affected by location, 75
  size and shape does not correlate with
    type of bullet, 75
  stellate, 73, 75
Exploding ammunition, 241–242

F

Fingerprints,
  on bullet, 255
  on cartridge cases, 34
  on weapon, 34
Fire
  behavior of ammunition and gunpowder
    in, 223–224
  discharge of weapons from, 224
Firearms. See Small arms
Flake powder
  distance can travel, 116–117
  in handguns, 112, 113
  in shotguns, 191, 204
  perforation of epidermis, 72, 117
Flame, 39

Flash suppressors, 61–64, 146–148
  soot patterns from, 64
Flechettes, 247–248
Flintlock weapons. *See* Black powder
  weapons
Foreign material carried or embedded in
  bullet, 80, 254–255
Forensic autopsy in general
  autopsy report, 317–320
  clothing, 316
  concept of, 315–317
  embalming, 316
  fingerprinting, 316, 317
  identification photographs, 317
  scene investigation, 315–316
  securing the body, 285–286, 316
  x-rays, 316–317
Forensic autopsy (in gunshot cases)
  admission blood, 286
  angle of bullet path in body, 290
  clothing, 286, 287, 291
  collection of gunshot residue, 287
  description of clothing, 287, 291
  description of wounds, 288, 290
  dissecting microscope, 288
  EDX and FAAS, 288
  embalming, 286
  fingerprinting, 287
  marking of bullet, 290–291
  medical records and intervention, 286
  photography, 288
  recovery of bullet, 290
  recovery of pellets and wads, 291
  recovery of powder grains, 288, 289
  scene, 285
  securing the body, 285–286, 316
  toxicology, 286, 291
  x-rays, 286–287, 316–317
Frangible ammunition, 134
Full metal-jacketed bullets, 21–22
  carrying of powder grains, 34
  centerfire rifles, 141, 143, 145–146
  handguns, 240

G

Gas-port, 65
Glazer round, 241
Gonzalez, T., 267
Graze wound, 77
"Gun-cleaning accidents," 293–294
Gunpowder, 17–19
  ball powder, 18, 112, 113–114, 153–154,
    191, 204
  black powder, 17, 223, 278–279
  creators of smokeless powder, 17
  cylindrical powder, 113, 153
  distance powder can travel, 116–117

double-base, 17–18
filtered out by clothing, 121, 275
flake powder, 112, 113, 191, 204
identification of powder grains, 72, 282
marks on base of bullet due to powder,
  33–34
on clothing, 277, 116–117
perforating clothing, 275–276
powder grains carried by bullet, 34
Pyrodex®, 18–19
simulated by blood, 281–282
single-base, 17–18
smokeless powder, 17–19
special stains for, 72
Gunshot residue
  centerfire cartridges, 267, 268
  collection of, 268, 269, 274, 321
  constituents of primers, 268
  criteria for positive test, 269
  detection by FAAS, 117, 283
  detection on clothing, 117, 280–281
  EDX testing of tissue, 117, 282–283
  EDX tests on clothing, 117, 280–281
  flameless atomic absorption analysis,
    117, 268–269
  Gonzalez, T., 267
  Harrison and Gilroy test, 267–268
  history of, 267–268
  in suicides, 295, 299
  lead free primer, 268
  levels, 269
  metals analyzed for, 268
  methods of analysis, 268
  neutron activation analysis, 268–269
  paraffin test, 267
  patterns of deposition, 267, 269–273,
  preservation on hands, 285
  reliability and accuracy of tests, 267,
    274
  rimfire ammunition, 268, 281
  scanning electron microscope, 268, 274
  soft x-ray, 117
  trace metal detection techniques,
    274–275
  Walker test, 280
Gunshot wounds,
  atypical entrances, 77–79
  categories based on range from muzzle
    to target, 51
  concept of wounding, 41
  contact, 51–53
  describing clothing, 291
  description and location of, 289–290
  distant, 66–73
  exit, 73–77
  in bone, 92–97
  intermediate-range, 57–59
  marking the bullet, 290–291

Gunshot wounds [cont.]
  obliteration and alteration by medical
    therapy, 212
  near contact, 53–57
  penetrating vs perforating, 51
  "powder burns," 58–59
  recovery of bullet, technique, 290
  reliability of medical records, 211–212
  theory of wounding, 41–48
  wound track without blood, 257
Gunshot wounds of the head
  bone chips at entrance, 217
  internal richochet, 219–220
  probability of exiting, 218–219
  secondary fractures, 95–96, 217–218
  shape of bullet tracks, 218
  signs of increased intracranial pressure,
    220
Gutter wounds of bone, 94

                  H
Hair, charred or seared, 110
Handgun ammunition,
  .25 ACP, 121–123
  .32 ACP, 123
  .32 S&W and .32 S&W Long, 123
  .380 ACP, 124
  .38 Colt Super Auto, 124
  .38 S&W, 123
  .38 Special, 123–124
  9-mm Luger (Parabellum), 124–125
  .357 Magnum, 124
  .44 S&W Magnum, 125
  .45 ACP, 125
Handgun wounds,
  absent abrasion ring, 121
  carboxyhemoglobin in entrance and exit
    wounds, 102
  contact and near-contact wounds in
    hairy regions, 110
  contact wounds, 100–109
  contact wounds of head, 101, 103–104,
    106–107
  contact wounds of trunk, 107
  contact wounds over bone, 103–104, 107
  dissecting microscope and hard contact
    wounds, 101
  distant range, 120–121
  EDX and FAAS and hard contact
    wounds, 101–102
  effects of clothing on range
    determination, 121
  gas injuries, 110–111
  hard contact wounds from .22 Short or
    .32 Smith & Wesson Short
    cartridges, 101
  intermediate range, 111–119

  irregular contact wounds of chest, 107
  loose contact wounds, 108–109
  muzzle imprints, 107–108
  near contact wounds, 109–110
  postmortem powder tattoo marks,
    111–112
  powder blackening, 111
  powder grains at exit, 102–103
  stellate or cruciform entrance wounds,
    103–105
Handguns
  advertised velocities, 99
  auto-loading pistols (automatics), 5–8
  common calibers, 121–125
  Derringers, 1
  muzzle velocity of Saturday Night
    specials, 100
  revolvers, 1–5
  single-shot pistols, 1
  types, 1
  vented test barrel, 99
Harrison and Gilroy test, 267–268
Head stamps, 13–14
  absence of, 14
  rimfire, 130
High-velocity rifle. See Centerfire rifles
High-velocity rifle wounds. See Centerfire
    rifle wounds
Hollow-point ammunition, 20, 240–241,
    311–313
  appearance of wounds due to, 312, 313
  break up on ricocheting, 313
  confusion with high velocity rifle
    wounds, 313
  controversy over, 311
  mortal wounds due to, 312–313
  myths, 313
  severity of wounds, 241
  tendency to stay in body, 313
  theory of effectiveness, 312
"Hot bullets," 72–73
  bacterial culture, 73
Hunting "accidents," 294, 307

                  I
Insect activity
  destruction of wounds, 281
  simulating powder tattooing, 86
  simulating wounds, 281, 283
Intermediary targets, 80–84
  alteration in entrance wounds, due to,
    80, 81, 158
  causing atypical entrance wound, 80–81
  causing separation of jacket and core,
    81–84
  fragments of, embedded in bullet, 80–84
  fragments of, propelled into target, 80

wire screen pattern on tip of bullet, 80
Intermediate-range wounds, 57−59
  "powder burns," 58−59
  powder tattooing, 57−59
Intrauterine gunshot wounds, 220

K

Keyhole wound of bone, 95
Kinetic energy
  concept of wounding, 41
  factors determining loss of, 46−48
  formula, 41
  in relationship to severity of wound,
     45−46
  minimum energy necessary to cause a
     casualty, 230−231
Kinetic energy loss
  along wound track, 43
  effect of tissues, 48
  major determinants of, 142
KTW ammunition, 244

L

Lead bullets
  cannelures, 20
  gas checks, 20, 21
  gilding, 20
  in centerfire rifles, 20−21, 143
  made out of, 20
  roundnose wadcutter, semiwadcutter,
     hollow point, 20
Lead fragments
  analysis by EDX and spectograph, 260
  in wound track on x-ray, 259, 260
Lead poisoning from retained bullets,
     221−222
Lead snowstorm, 155, 260
Location of fatal gunshot wounds,
     222−223

M

Machine guns, 10
Medical intervention prior to death
  alteration of wounds, 86−88, 212
  inaccurate medical records, 211−212
  misinterpretation of wounds, 211−212
  missed (concealed) wounds, 211
Micro-Groove® rifling, 27, 30, 129
Micro-tears, 70
  in centerfire rifle entrance wounds, 152
Minie bullet, 19−20, 140
Missed (concealed) gunshot wounds, 211,
     212
Multiple bullet loadings, 242−243
Muzzle flash, 39
Muzzle-break, 61

N

Near contact wounds, 53−57
  angled, 54−56
  angled near contact vs angled contact,
     54−57
Nonhemorrhagic wound tracks, 257
Nyclad®, 244

O

Old bullets. See Retained bullets

P

Paraffin test, 267
Partial metal jacketed bullets, 22, 143−145
  disintegration on striking glass, 82
  jacket-core separation in body, 258, 259
  separation of core and jacket due to
     intermediary target, 81−82, 84
Percussion weapons. See Black powder
     weapons
Photography of wounds, 288
Physical activity following gunshot
     wounds, 210−211
Pistol whipping, 224−225
Powder. See Gunpowder
Powder burns, 58−59
Powder soot, 60−66
  blank conversion, 65
  factors determining pattern of soot, 60,
     111
  flash suppressors, 61−64
  gas-ports of semiautomatic rifles, 65
  maximum distance out to which
     deposition occurs, 60, 111
  muzzle-breaks, 61
  on the hand in suicides, 294−295, 299
  pseudo-soot, 88
  silencers, 61, 115−116
  soot pattern from cylinder-barrel gap, 61
Powder tattooing, 57−59
  antemortem vs postmortem phenomena,
     58, 111−112
  appearance, 111
  appearance depends on form of powder,
     117−118
  ball powder (centerfire rifles), 154
  ball powder (handguns), 111−119
  ball powder (shotguns), 191
  centerfire rifles, 152−155
  cylindrical powder tattooing, 154
  dependent on range and barrel length, 115
  description, 58
  eccentric pattern of tattooing, 58, 119
  flake powder (shotguns), 191
  from cylinder gap, 120

Powder tattooing   [*cont.*]
  healing, 59
  lack of tattooing on palms and soles, 59,
      118
  maximum distance out to which it
      occurs for handguns, 113–114
  maximum range (centerfire rifles),
      153–155
  maximum range (shotguns), 191
  penetration into dermis, 59, 72, 117, 118
  perforation of hair and clothes by
      powder, 116, 121
  postmortem "tattooing," 58
  powder grains at exit, 102–103
  pseudo-powder tattooing, 80, 84–88
  shotguns, 191–193
  silencers, 115–116
  types of powders in handgun cartridges,
      112
  used to determine range, 118–119, 119
Primer, 14–17
  Berdan, 15
  Boxer, 14–15
  centerfire, 14–16
  construction, 14–17
  ingredients, 16–17
  lead free, 268
  operation, 15–16
  rimfire, 16–17
  sizes, 15
  types, 14–15
Progressive burning, 39
  theory, 39
  varying barrel length, 39
Pseudo-exit wounds, 257–258
Pseudo-powder tattooing, 80, 84–88
  causes of, 84–88, 92
  due to intermediary targets, 80
  due to ricochet, 92
  due to silencers, 86
Pseudo-soot, 88

R

Range determination, in decomposed
      bodies, 281–283
Re-entry wounds, 78
Retained bullets
  appearance, 260–261
  lead poisoning from, 221–222
Revolvers, 1–5
  break-top, 3–4
  direction of rotation of cylinder, 5
  double-action, 4–5
  "half-cock" notch, 5
  principle of operation, 1–2
  safeties, 8
  single-action, 4

  solid-frame, 4
  "swingout," 2–3
  types, 2–4
Revolvers built to fire automatic
      ammunition, 33
Ricochet
  affect on appearance of bullet, 90
  bullets, 88–92
  causing pseudo-powder tattooing, 86, 92
  inside cranial cavity, 219–220
  internal, 91
  internal track on x-ray, 261
Rifles, 9   *See* Centerfire rifles, Rimfire
      weapons
Rifling, 10
  artifacts due to manufacturing of
      bullets, 259
  gyroscopic effect, 25
  direction of, 25–27, 28–30
  lack of, 65, 232, 234–236, 239
  lands and grooves, 10, 25
  Micro-Groove® rifling, 27, 30, 129
  number of lands and grooves, 27–30
  polygonal rifling, 25
  rifling marks on bullet cores, 258, 259
  twist, 25
Rimfire ammunition, 16–17, 127–134
  BB and CB caps, 134
  construction, 16
  copper plating of bullets, 131
  estimated production, 127
  frangible ammunition, 134
  full metal-jacketed bullets, 130
  headstamps, 130–131
  history and development, 127–129
  interchangeability in rifles and
      handguns, 129
  loading, 130
  .22 Long, 127, 131
  .22 Long Rifle, 127, 129, 131–132
  lot, 131
  .22 Magnum, 127, 128
  manufacturers, 130
  mushrooming of bullets, 137
  new high velocity loadings, 132, 134
  noninterchangeability of the .22
      Magnum, 128
  primer ingredients, 16–17
  5-mm Remington magnum, 128–129
  .22 Short, 127, 131
  shot cartridges, 132
  standard velocity vs. high velocity
      loadings, 130
  tracer, 130
Rimfire weapons
  bore diameter, 129
  interchangeability of ammunition in
      rifles and handguns, 129

.22 Magnum, groove diameter of barrel, 128
micro-groove rifling, 129
nature of wounds, 139, 143
noninterchangeability of the .22 Magnum, 128
Rimfire wounds
absence of lead on x-rays of head, 136
analytical examination of, 135
apparent absence of soot and powder in .22 Short contact wounds, 135
ball powder at exit, 136
contact wounds—.22 Long Rifle, 136
contact wounds—.22 Magnum, 136
contact wounds—.22 Short, 135
distant wounds, 137
frangible ammunition, 134
intermediate range wounds, 136–137
internal ricochet in head, 135
maximum range of ball powder tatooing, 136–137
maximum range of flake powder tattooing, 137
penetration of flakes of powder into dermis, 137
powder tattooing, 136–137
secondary fractures of skull, 135, 137
shot cartridges, 132
use of dissecting microscope, 135, 136
Russian roulette, 5, 301–302

S

Sabot ammunition, 237–239
absence of rifling on bullet, 239
Accelerator® ammunition, 238–239
military, 237
prong marks, 239
rifles, 238–239
shotguns, 237
Safeties
on auto-loading pistols, 7
on revolvers, 8
Safety devices in handguns, 303–307
flying firing pin, 306
half-cock notch, 5, 306
hammer block, 303, 304, 307
rebound lever, 303
rebound slide, 303
safety lever, 303, 304
Saturday Night Specials, 4
muzzle velocity, 100
Sawed-off shotguns,
marks on wads, 200, 203
size of patterns, 203
Semijacketed bullets. See Partial metal-jacketed bullets
Semiwadcutter, 20

Shored entrance wounds, 78
Shored exit wounds, 73–75, 78
Shotgun ammunition,
birdshot, 175–176
brass shotgun shells, 207
Brenneke slug, 179
buckshot, 176–178
"cup" wad, 170
color coding of shells, 168
defects of traditional shot shells, 169
dram equivalent, 174
Federal, 206
Federal Triple-plus® wad, 172
flechette rounds, 248
Foster slug, 179, 180
jury-rigged slugs, 181–182
Magnum shotgun shells, 168
"pie" crimp, 170
plastic shot shells, 166
polyethylene filler, 172–174, 176–178
polypropylene filler, 172–174, 177
Power Piston®, 170
Remington Modi-Pac, 207–208
Remington-Peters, 204
sabot slug, 180
shot, 175–178
shot collar, 170
slugs, 179–182
stipple marks due to polyethylene and polypropylene granules, 177–178
tracer rounds, 207
wads, 166
Winchester-Western, 204–206
Shotgun wads and pellets,
recovery of, 288, 291
Shotgun wounds
buckshot wounds, 201
carbon monoxide in muscle, 191
close range wounds of head, 188
contact wounds of head, 183–188
contact wounds showing absence of soot, 188
due to slugs, 180–182
exit wounds, 200, 201
gunshot residue on hands, 185
intermediary targets, 197–199, 200
internal injuries, 199–200
intraoral shotgun wounds, 186
measurement of patterns, 194–195, 200
muzzle imprint, 189
pellet patterns, 193–194
petal marks from Power Piston®, 195–196
powder tattooing, 191–193, 201
range determination, 193–195, 200
recovery of wads, 200
soot, 186, 188, 189–191
soot on hands, 185

Shotgun wounds [cont.]
  stipple marks due to polyethylene and
      polypropylene filler, 177−178
  wad marks, 195, 197
  wound ballistics, 182−183
  wounds of face, 186
  x-rays, 199, 261−262
Shotguns, 9
  automatic ejection of fired hulls in
      pump shotguns, 204
  barrel, 163
  choke, 164−165
  description, 9, 163
  diverters, 203
  gauge, 163−164
  sawed-off, 203
Silencers, 61, 86
Single shot pistol, 1
Skeletal remains, 212−213
Skin
  velocity lost perforating skin, 214−215
  velocity necessary to perforate, 213−214
Small arms
  categories, 1
  handguns, 1−8
  machine guns, 10
  rifles, 9
  shotguns, 9
  submachine guns, 9−10
Soot. See Powder soot
"Stopping power"
  hollow-point ammunition, 312−313
  police concept, 311
  theory, 311−312
Stud guns, 233
Submachine guns, 9−10
Suicide
  automatic ejection of fired hulls from
      pump shotguns, 204
  elevation in mood, 299
  examination of the hands, 299
  examination of the weapon for blood
      and tissue, 300−301
  exiting bullet striking another
      individual, 299
  gun cleaning "accidents," 293
  gunshot residue, 299, 295
  high-velocity blood spray on hands, 300
  hunting "accidents," 294
  iron deposit on hands, 299−300
  location of self-inflicted handgun
      wounds, 294−296
  location of self-inflicted rifle and
      shotgun wounds, 296−297
  multiple gunshot wounds, 297−298
  multiple methods, 298
  multiple weapons, 297
  objection to ruling of, 299

  public suicide, 298
  right vs left handedness, 294
  Russian roulette, 301−302
  sex differences, 293, 294, 296, 297
  scene, 298−299
  soot on the hand, 294−295
  suicide notes, 293
  "the extra shot (s)," 299
  trajectory of bullet or pellets when using
      a rifle or shotgun, 293−294
  triggering devices, 295
  unusual location of self-inflicted
      wounds, 295
  weapons clutched in hand, 299−300
  wounds of the back of the head, 295
  wounds of the eye, 295
Surgical and medical alteration of
    wounds, 212
Survival following gunshot wounds,
    210−211
Superficial perforating wounds, 77−78
Sympathetic discharge, 233−234

T
Tandem bullets, 239−240
Tangential gunshot wound, 77
  simulating contact wound, 106
Tattooing. See Powder tattooing
Tear gas pens, conversion to gun, 232
Temperature, effect of environmental
    temperature on bullet velocity, 255
Temporary cavity, 41
  duration of, 41−42
  from rifle bullets, 42
  from pistol bullets, 42
  in different tissues, 42, 43
  maximum volume, 42
  pressure waves, 42−43
  production of skull fractures, 217−218
  shape determined by, 42, 43
  size determined by, 42, 43
  "tail splash," 42
Toxicology, 291
  obtaining admission or pretransfusion
      blood, 286
Trace evidence, preservation of, 285−286,
    287
Trace metal detection technique, 274−275

U
Uterus, gunshot wounds of pregnant
    uterus, 220

V
Vieille, 17

W

Wadcutter, 20
Walker test, 280
Wildcat cartridges, 11
Wound ballistics, 41–49
    critical level of kinetic energy lost, 45
    critical velocity, 43–45
    definition, 41
    kinetic energy of projectile, 41
    loss of kinetic energy, 45–48
    temporary cavity, 41–45
Wounds
    artifacts due to medical treatment, 286
    critical energy loss, 45
    critical velocity, 43–45
    description of, 289, 290
    examination by EDX and FAAS, 288
    microscopic examination of, 288
    photography of, 288

X

X-rays, 257–265
    absence of lead in wound tracks, 260
    absence of pellets in contact shotgun
        wounds of head, 262
    artifacts simulating bullets, 265
    bullets in clothing, 287

"C"-shaped fragments of lead, 261
cannot determine caliber on x-ray, 262
exiting bullets, 257–258
hollow point .25 ACP bullets, 262
identification of type of ammunition or
    weapon, 260
internal ricochet, 261
lead snowstorm, 155, 260
nonvisualization of aluminum jackets,
    259
of dirt under skeletal remains, 212–213
of skeletal remains, 212–213
old bullets, 260–261
range determination in charred bodies,
    261–262
recovery of lead fragments, 259–260
useful for, 257
usefulness in bullet emboli cases, 216
visualization of shotgun wads, 261

Y

Yaw, 46

Z

Zip guns, 231–232
    converted starter (blank) pistol, 65